T0407557

Microbiology and Aging

Steven L. Percival

Editor

Microbiology and Aging

Clinical Manifestations

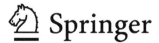 Springer

Steven L. Percival, Ph.D.
ConvaTec, Limited
Global Development Centre
Deeside Industrial Park
Flintshire, UK CH5 2NU
steven.percival@bms.com

ISBN 978-1-58829-640-5   e-ISBN 978-1-59745-327-1
DOI 10.1007/978-1-59745-327-1

Library of Congress Control Number: 2008940880

Printed on acid-free paper.

9 8 7 6 5 4 3 2 1

springer.com

I would like to dedicate this book to Carol, Alex and Tom and my Mum and Dad.
'The cycle of life is a journey of microbiological intrigue'

Preface

The world's population is estimated to reach 8.9 billion by 2050 with 370 million people of 80 years of age or older. Ageing is an incurable disease and defined as the 'deregulation of biochemical processes important for life', but for the purpose of this book, ageing is better defined as the biological process of growing older. Ageing is part of natural human development.

As you will see throughout this book, the microbiological burden on the host is enormous and clinically significant, and will undoubtedly have a role to play in the ageing process. As humans are living longer, there is a greater propensity to infection. This risk is substantially heightened in elderly individuals who are predisposed to infection. While the process of ageing and its effects on the host's microbiology are poorly documented and researched, data obtained from gut studies have shown that microbiological changes take place over time suggesting significance to the host. Do the microbiological changes that occur within and upon the host influence the process of ageing or is it the biological changes of the host that affects the microbiology? Does this therefore affect our propensity to disease? As the host's microbiology changes with ageing, is this significantly beneficial or severely detrimental to the host? Are there ways of enhancing life expectancy by reducing certain bacteria from proliferating or conversely by enhancing the survival of beneficial bacteria?

This book considers the microbiology of the host in different regions of the body and how these vary in the different age groups. Chapter 1 of the book focuses on ageing theories with Chap. 2 considering the human indigenous flora and how this is affected during ageing. Chapter 3 highlights the main infections associated with an elderly population, while Chap. 4 reviews the process of skin ageing and its associated microbiology. Chapter 5 reviews the ageing lung and Chap. 6 reviews influenza in the elderly. Chapter 7 highlights the changes that occur in the oral microflora and host defences with advanced age with Chap. 8 reviewing the influence of the gut microbiota with ageing. Chapter 8 focuses on the gut and its associated immunity. The remaining four chapters of the book consider clostridium and the ageing gut, *Helicobacter pylori* and the hygiene hypothesis and the benefits of probiotics. The microbiology theory of autism in children is reviewed in

Chap. 13. The final chapter of the book examines how the beneficial microbiology of the host leads to human decomposition.

This book encompasses a collection of reviews that highlight the significance of and the crucial role that microorganisms play in the human life cycle.

Flintshire, UK   Steven L. Percival

Contents

Contributors

Joseph F. Albright, PhD
Department of Microbiology, Immunology and Tropical Medicine, The George Washington University School of Medicine, Washington, DC, USA

Julia W. Albright, PhD
Department of Microbiology, Immunology and Tropical Medicine, The George Washington University School of Medicine, Washington, DC, USA

Leslie Baumann, MD
University of Miami Cosmetic Center, Miami Beach, FL, USA

Sarah Connor, MSc
Department of Microbiology, Leeds General Infirmary, Leeds, UK

Caterina Hatzifoti, PhD
University of Sheffield Medical School, Beech Hill Road, Sheffield, UK

Andrew W. Heath, PhD
University of Sheffield Medical School, Beech Hill Road, Sheffield, UK

Robert C. Janaway, PhD
School of Life Sciences, University of Bradford, Bradford, West Yorkshire, UK

Svitlana Kozytska, PhD
Institut für Molekulare Infektionsbiologie, Röntgenring 11, 97070 Würzburg, Germany

Udo Lorenz, PhD
Institut für Molekulare Infektionsbiologie, Röntgenring 11, 97070 Würzburg, Germany

Sameer K. Mathur, MD, PhD
Section of Allergy, Pulmonary and Critical Care Medicine, Department of Medicine, University of Wisconsin School of Medicine and Public Health, 600 Highland Ave., K4/910 CSC, Madison, WI 53792, USA

Keith C. Meyer, MD, MS
Section of Allergy, Pulmonary and Critical Care Medicine, Department of Medicine, University of Wisconsin School of Medicine and Public Health, 600 Highland Ave., K4/910 CSC, Madison, WI 53792, USA

Caroline Murphy, PhD
Alimentary Pharmabiotic Centre, University College Cork, Cork, Ireland

Eileen Murphy, PhD
Alimentary Pharmabiotic Centre, University College Cork, Cork, Ireland

Knut Ohlsen, PhD
Institut für Molekulare Infektionsbiologie, Röntgenring 11, 97070 Würzburg, Germany

Liam O'Mahony, PhD
Alimentary Pharmabiotic Centre, University College Cork, Cork, Ireland

Rimondia S. Percival, PhD
Department of Oral Biology, Leeds Dental Institute, Clarendon Way, Leeds LS2 9LU, UK

Steven L. Percival, PhD
West Virginia University Schools of Medicine and Dentistry, Robert C. Byrd Health Sciences Center-North, Morgantown, WV, USA

John G. Thomas, PhD
Robert C. Byrd Health Sciences Center-North, West Virginia University Schools of Medicine and Dentistry, Morgantown, WV, USA

Edmund Weisberg, MD
Department of Dermatology, University of Texas Southwestern Medical Center, Dallas, TX, USA

Andrew S. Wilson, PhD
School of Life Sciences, University of Bradford, Bradford, West Yorkshire BD7 1DP, UK

Chapter 1
Ageing Theories, Diseases and Microorganisms

Steven L. Percival

Biology of Ageing

Ageing is a 'progressive decline or a gradual deterioration of physiological function including a decrease in fecundity or irreversible process of loss of viability and increase in vulnerability'.[1,2] It is often referred to as the deregulation of biochemical processes important for life.[1,3,4] However, for the purpose of this book and chapter, ageing is best described as the biological process of growing older. The ageing process is associated with physiological changes, an increased susceptibility to certain diseases, an increase in mortality, a decrease in metabolic rate, a reduction in height and reaction times, a fluctuation in weight, menopause in woman, reduction in olfaction and vision, and, in particular, a decrease in the immune response.[5–7]

Factors known to cause and influence ageing in humans remain diverse, and scientifically problems reside in distinguishing causes from effects.[8] However, there are strong evolutionary and genetic influences known to effect the ageing process and life expectancy.[9–11] The physiological changes that do occur during human ageing increase an individual's susceptibility to various diseases and therefore increase the likelihood of death.

Mechanistic Theories on Ageing

Many ageing theories have been proposed, and scientifically scrutinized. To date, the reasons why humans age are still extensively being researched, but still no overall general consensus regarding the cause of the ageing exists. Nevertheless, what can be agreed upon is the fact that ageing is an 'inescapable biological reality'.[12] However, many scientists hypothesize that ageing is 'a disease that can be cured, or at least postponed'.[13]

S.L. Percival
West Virginia University Schools of Medicine and Dentistry Robert C, Byrd Health Sciences Center-North, Morgantown, WV, USA

S.L. Percival (ed.), *Microbiology and Aging.*
DOI: 10.1007/978-1-59745-327-1_1, © Springer Science + Business Media, LLC 2009

The first ageing theory, founded on genetic principles, can be traced back to the work of Weismann at the end of the nineteenth century.[14] Weismann postulated that evolution introduced ageing to avoid parents, and their more adapted offspring, competing for the same resources. This theory of 'programmed death' was severely criticized, as it seemed very unlikely that such a programme could ever be implemented in natural conditions where practically no individual dies of old age. An alternative theory of ageing, proposed by Peter Medawar, stated that ageing resulted from an accumulation of mutations. Such mutations, known to be detrimental to the host, were considered free to accumulate resulting in death. More recently, in 1957, George Williams proposed a complementary ageing theory known as the 'antagonistic pleiotropy theory'. Agonistic pleiotropy means that a single gene may have an effect on several traits (pleiotropy), and that these effects may affect fitness in opposite ways (antagonistic). This theory states that evolution favours mutations that improve fitness at an earlier age, even at the expense of a reduced fitness later on in life. According to this ageing theory, senescence is a by-product of good adaptation early in life. Even today, this remains a well-respected ageing theory. Evolutionary ageing theories are constantly being challenged by the generation of new findings as a result of long-lived mutant animal models. Data obtained from these studies have resulted in suggestions that Weismann's programmed death theory[15] should be reconsidered specifically, as all evolutionary theories still need experimental confirmation and should not be considered mutually exclusive.[16]

Within the animal kingdom clear differences in the rates of ageing are evident. Many theories exist to suggest reasons for this.[17–20] Such theories, however, lie outside the nature of this book. While many theories have been proposed to help explain human ageing, there still remains a lack of adequate 'ageing' models. Consequently, this makes hypothesis-testing difficult. Testing the many ageing theories is difficult, expensive and time consuming, and discriminating between causes and effects is presently impossible.

To date, the two most respected human ageing theories include the 'programmed theories of ageing' and the 'damage-based theories of ageing'. Programmed ageing theories suggest that ageing is not a random process but driven by genetically regulated processes, as opposed to the damage-based ageing theories which suggest that ageing is a result of damage accumulation products produced by the normal cellular processes of the body as a result of poor repair systems in the body. The damage-based theories imply that ageing is predominately a result of interactions with the environment,[21] as opposed to the programmed theories which are predetermined. However, there does seem to be a large amount of overlap between these theories. Each of the two theories will be considered in turn.

Programmed Theories of Ageing

The programmed theories of ageing defend the idea that ageing is genetically determined: i.e. a programmed and predetermined process. This suggests that the process of ageing is 'genetically regulated'. The significance of this is apparent when we consider certain hormones,[22] such as growth hormone, which are known to decline with age and whose target is the insulin-like growth factor 1 (IGF-1).[22] However, it has been found that by restoring or altering hormonal levels in the younger generation, ageing has not been deterred. In fact, hormone replacement has been shown to prematurely accelerate ageing. Nevertheless, there have been numerous research findings that have shown that the endocrine system is able to influence the ageing process.

Only one single gene has been shown to have a possible direct effect on human longevity. This gene is the apoE gene. The apoE gene codes for a protein in the body that is involved in fat transport. Centenarians have been found to have a high prevalence of the apoE e2 variant (or allele) compared to the e4 variant.[23] The e4 variant is known to cause susceptibility to elevated blood cholesterol, coronary artery disease, and Alzheimer disease (the function of this protein in the brain is not yet known).[24]

In animal studies, several genes have been isolated that have been shown to influence ageing and life span. For example, in the nematode worm, *Caenorhabditis elegans*, the inactivation or loss of a few genes increases its life span fivefold, generally (but not always) at the expense of a reduced fertility.[4,24] Life extension in worms has been linked with the worms' ability to enter a phase called Dauer larva, during which the animal seals its mouth and does not feed. Some mutant worms (with non-functional or missing DAF-2 gene) show an extended life span, and enter this phase whatever the environmental conditions.[25] Similar life extension by genetic means has been observed in other animal models. Examples include the fruit fly, *Drosophila melanogaster*, and the mouse, where longevity is often connected with dwarfism.[26]

The pattern of genes involved in longevity suggests that a common biochemical pathway may be involved in the regulation of ageing of some organisms. It appears that in humans some genes associated with ageing are involved in molecular pathways homologous to that responding to insulin and (IGF-I) in mammals, a pathway regulating glucose intake and its conversion into fat. It is no surprise then that life span is considered to be affected by dietary restriction. It is possible that genes regulating food consumption, and food intake itself, may affect life span.

Most recently, De Magalhaes[8] has suggested a number of genes thought to directly influence mammalian ageing and known to alter the rate of both ageing and age-related debilitation. These genes have been grouped into three broad pathways: namely, the genes involved with DNA metabolism (CKN1, lamin A, WRN, XPD, Terc, PASG, ATM, and p53), and the genes involved with energy metabolism and the growth hormone/IGF-1 axis and oxidative stress (p66shc, MSRA, and Thdx1).[8] The significance of all these genes having a role in human ageing is currently being investigated further.

Damage-Based Theories

The damage-based theories of ageing suggest that aging results from a continuous process of damage accumulation, originating from by-products produced by normal metabolic processes of the body. The damage-based theories are predominantly a result of interactions with the environment,[21] whereas programmed ageing, as mentioned previously, seems to be predetermined and occurs on a fixed schedule. Despite this, ageing could be a result of extrinsic or intrinsic factors that cause an accumulation of damage[27] or a result of changes in gene expression that are either programmed or derived from DNA structural changes.[28]

Ageing in animals has been quoted to be multi-factorial, with the changes of ageing considered to be under the guidance of biological clocks.[29] As humans exhibit a gradual ageing process compared to animals, this suggests that the mechanisms of ageing, in particular the existence of biological clocks, may be different in humans when compared to animals.

Energy Consumption Hypothesis

In 1908 Max Rubner[30] suggested a relationship between body size, metabolic rate, and longevity/ageing. Essentially, this theory suggested that bigger animals live longer than smaller animals because they spent fewer calories per gram of body mass. The energy consumption theory suggested that animals are born with a limited amount of potential energy and the faster they use this stored energy the quicker they die. However, the rate of living theory evolved as a continuation of the energy consumption hypothesis, which essentially hypothesized that the faster the metabolic rate, the faster the biochemical activity and, therefore, the faster an animal would age.

In 1935 McCay[31] first recognized that dietary restriction extended longevity. The theory suggested that a decrease in calories possibly has an effect on the metabolic rate. This theory was investigated and shown to extend the life of rodents. In addition, dietary restrictions have been shown to result in a significant retardation and decline in immunological competence and decline in tumour development in rodents. Irrespective of these and other findings, the dietary restriction theory is at present flawed with many unanswered questions still remaining.

Free Radical Theory

In 1954 Rebeca Gerschman and collegues[32] first proposed the concept that free radicals were toxic. Such free radicals are referred to as reactive oxygen species (ROS), which originate from exogenous sources such as ionizing and ultraviolet radiation, and from endogenous processes caused by cellular activity, i.e. waste products of metabolism. In 1956 Harman proposed the 'free radicals theory' which described that ROS were the source of damage which accumulates in cells.[33] This theory simply argues that ageing results from the damage generated by ROS. Because there are numerous enzymes to restrict the damage inflicted by the ROS, this suggests a strong reason why these ROS must be of some biological significance.[34] However, much of the evidence for this theory has come from research in transgenic fruit flies and not humans.

ROS encompass many chemical species, mostly superoxide anions, hydroxyl radicals, and hydrogen peroxide (H_2O_2). These small molecules (compared to proteins and nucleic acids) are chemically very active, and can therefore cause a great deal of damage and disruption to cells.[35] Reactive radicals of nitrogen (nitric oxide and derivatives) and of oxygen (superoxide anion, hydrogen peroxide, hydroxyl radical) can inflict considerable damage on macromolecules (protein, nucleic acids, complex lipids), which give rise to carcinogens (e.g. nitrosamines) and trigger (or sometimes prevent) apoptoic death of cells, i.e. macrophages and vascular epithelial cells. Unless mechanisms for scavenging these reactive species are effective, the damage inflicted by free radicals is known to substantially increase cell death.

ROS are by-products produced in the mitochondria (the main source of ROS). The efficiency of the mitochondrial electron transport and energy-generating processes deteriorate with age, resulting in increased levels of oxidizing free radicals and ultimately leading to cell death or deterioration. The control of ROS levels and production is fundamentally important in the human body, but it is interesting to note that ROS may not just be causing random damage but may also be used as signalling molecules in various cellular processes of the body.[35] The significance of this warrants further investigation. To further complicate the picture, it has been shown that the pathways that control ROS levels are ageing themselves.[35] These pathways have been found to be less efficient at an older age. In addition to this, Weindruch[36] has found that some animals are known to age more slowly because they produce less ROS.

The human body has evolved mechanisms to control the detrimental effects of harmful chemicals and ROS. One mechanism involves the use of superoxide dismutase (SOD), which has no function other than disposing of superoxide anions. Another enzyme known to be very beneficial in suppressing the effects caused by ROS is methionine sulphoxide reductase A (MSRA). This enzyme is able to catalyse the repair of protein-bound methionine residues known to be oxidized by ROS. Presence of this enzyme suggests that ROS are biologically significant. Interestingly, overexpression of MSRA in Drosophila has been shown to increase longevity.[37]

It is universally accepted that ROS have a role to play in pathologies of the body but the exact influence ROS have on mammalian ageing is as yet undetermined and inconclusive.

DNA-Damage Theory

The DNA-damage theory was first proposed by Leo Szilard in 1959,[38] and suggests that damage to DNA causes ageing. However, it is doubtful whether DNA damage accumulation alone is able to drive the ageing process. Nevertheless, as with a number of the ageing theories proposed, any changes that do occur in DNA may have a role to play in ageing. To date, the essence of these changes and the mechanisms that are involved are as yet undetermined.

Interestingly, accelerated ageing has been noted in humans because of certain genetic mutations. Two rare diseases, namely, Werner's syndrome (WS) and Hutchinson–Gilford's syndrome, produce conditions which are similar to an accelerated ageing process due to DNA damage.[39] In addition to this, ROS have also been shown to damage DNA.[40]

Microorganisms and Ageing

Ageing/senescence has been documented in a number of microorganisms. For example, by measuring ageing by reproductive output, ageing has been shown to exist in *Caulobacter crescentus*.[41] In addition to this, ageing has been reported in *Escherichia coli* cells, following nutrient depletion. In this example, *E. coli* has been shown to lose its ability to reproduce and recover from injury. Furthermore, it has been shown that when *E. coli* divides, one of the newly formed colonies inherits the oldest end, or pole, of the 'mother'. This newly formed cell has been shown to have a diminished growth rate, decreased offspring production, and an increased incidence of death,[42] which are all characteristics of ageing.

Ageing and Disease/Infection

The world's population by the year 2050 is estimated to become 8.9 billion (as published by the Department of Economic and Social Affairs). With this increase comes an increase in the number of ageing and aged individuals. For example, in 1998, 66 million people in the world were 80 years of age or older. This figure is projected to become 370 million by the year 2050.

By the year 2030, in the US alone, it is estimated that one in five people will be expected to be 65 years and older.[43,44] Changes within the immune functions are known to occur during the ageing process which pre-disposes the elderly population, when compared to the younger population, to many types of infectious agents.[44–47] As well as a change in the types of microorganisms associated with infections comes a greater diversity of pathogens associated with an elderly population compared to that of a younger one.[44–47] This will have effects on recovery and clinical outcome.

A number of pathologies associated with human ageing are highlighted in Fig. 1.1,[48] and the leading causes of death in humans can been seen in Table 1.1. Specific conditions highlighted in the table include diabetes, heart disease, cancer, arthritis, and kidney disease, with heart disease the number one cause of death in people aged 85 (Fig. 1.2[48]) followed then by cancer, cerebrovascular diseases,

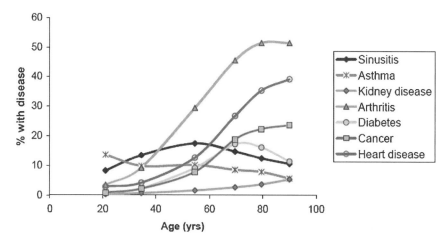

Fig. 1.1 Prevalence of selected chronic conditions, expressed in percentages, as a function of age for the US population (2002–2003 dataset). (Source: National Center for Health Statistics Data Warehouse on Trends in Health and Aging. Courtesy and permission from Dr João Pedro de Magalhães. http://www.senescence.info/definitions.html)[48] (See Color Plates)

Table 1.1 Death by underlying or multiple causes, expressed in rates per 100,000 people or in percentage of the total deaths, for the 2001 US population in two age groups: 45–54 years and 85 years of age and older. (Source: National Center for Health Statistics Data Warehouse on Trends in Health and Aging. Courtesy and permission from Dr João Pedro de Magalhães. http://www. senescence.info/definitions.html)[48]

Cause of death	45–54 years		Over 85 years	
	Incidence	% of deaths	Incidence	% of deaths
Diseases of the heart	92.8	21.66	5,607.5	37.48
Malignant neoplasm	126.3	29.48	1,747	11.68
Cerebrovascular diseases	15.1	3.52	1,485.2	9.93
Parkinson's disease	0.1	0.02	1,312.8	8.77
Alzheimer's disease	0.2	0.05	703.2	4.70
Pneumonia	4.6	1.07	676.5	4.52
Chronic lower respiratory diseases	8.5	1.98	638.2	4.27
Diabetes melittus	13.6	3.17	318.6	2.13
Certain infectious and parasitic diseases	22.9	5.35	243.8	1.63
Atherosclerosis	0.5	0.12	177.3	1.19
Others	143.8	33.57	2,050.9	13.71

Parkinson's and Alzheimer's diseases, pneumonia, and chronic lower respiratory diseases. Infections in the elderly population are commonly due to pyogenic bacteria. Conditions that are highly prevalent in this age group include pneumonia, urinary tract infections, endocarditis, bacteraemia, and skin and soft tissue infections.[44] Certain conditions such as meningitis are rare in the very old but are more significant in a younger population. In addition to this, viral infections in the older population, when compared to the younger population, are infrequent occurrences.

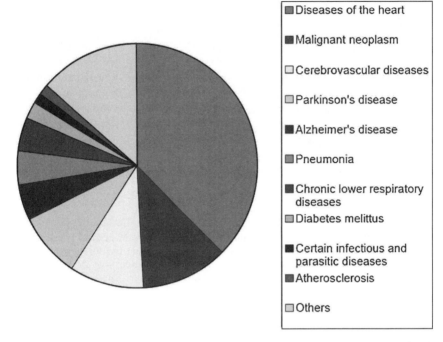

Fig. 1.2 Death by underlying or multiple cause, expressed in rates per 100,000 people, as a function of age for the 2001 US population aged 85 and older (Source: http://www.cdc.gov/nchs/nhcs.htm. National Center for Health Statistics Data Warehouse on Trends in Health and Aging. Courtesy and permission from Dr João Pedro de Magalhães. http://www.senescence.info/definitions.html)[48] (See Color Plates)

Exceptions to this, however, include herpes zoster reactivation (shingles),[49] influenza,[50] and gastroenteritis.[51]

If we work from present figures, within the next 50 years there will be 20 million elderly persons hospitalized with pneumonia, septicaemia, and urinary tract infections. Also, because of the increased usage of prosthetic devices by the ageing population, infections associated with these devices are increasing exponentially.[52] The statistics quoted for diseases and infections in the US are approximately the same within most developed countries. In developing countries, statistics are significantly different, with most infections and deaths attributed to tuberculosis, leishmamiasis, malaria, and the effects of enteric bacteria. In addition to this, the prevalence of nosocomial infections has been shown to increase substantially with age because of the increased risk of infection per day of hospitalization.[53] Most infections in the elderly have a poorer outcome when compared to younger adults.[54] This is due to a number of factors including late diagnosis of therapy, increased frequency of co-morbidities, and poor tolerance to drugs, to name but a few. To help improve this situation, vaccinations are necessary, i.e. an annual influenza vaccination and a pneumococcal vaccination.[55] However, vaccinations are much less effective in the sick and also institutionalized elderly people.

Increased Sensitivity of Infection in the Elderly

The elderly population is much more sensitive to infection when compared to the younger population for a number of reasons. One reason is due to immunosenescence, another is due to malnutrition, and others are a result of anatomic and also physiological changes. As mentioned previously, the immune system becomes less effective in the elderly, which enhances an individual's susceptibility to infection. Malnutrition in the elderly is known to be major cause in decreasing immune function.[56,57]

Both anatomical and physiological changes in humans are characteristics of the ageing process. For example, the body has many non-immune host defensive mechanisms that prevent infections. As we age, these defence mechanisms, e.g. mucociliary clearance or rapid urine flow, are affected, which leads to efficient removal of bacteria from the human body. Within the lungs, for example, frequent infections, particularly in the elderly, are highly prevalent when compared to the younger population. Colitis and gastroenteritis are also common conditions of the elderly. This is principally due to the fact that ageing is associated with a decrease in gastric acidity and changes in the intestinal flora and intestinal mucus,[58] together with increase in the usage of antibiotics, which in turn increase problems associated with *Clostridium difficle*.

Does Infection Contribute to Ageing?

Ageing, as mentioned previously, is a risk factor for infection but it would seem, on the basis of the evidence to date, that infection, due to exogenous or indigenous microorganisms, may contribute to the ageing phenomenon. This hypothesis is considered conceivable, as pathogens are known to cause tissue and cellular destruction. In addition, the immune response of the body clearly has an effect on invading pathogens but at the same time does cause damage to the host itself.[59] Furthermore, latent or chronic infections contribute to the ageing process. For example, latent infections may periodically be reactivated, and those microorganisms known to avoid the immune system may contribute to the ageing process.

Inflammation, due to bacteria, is documented in many diseases and associated with the ageing process. *Chlamydia pneumoniae*, *Helicobacter pylori*, cytomegalovirus, herpes simplex virus, and also those responsible for periodontitis[60–64] are considered significant to atherosclerosis, but it is probable that viruses and bacteria have an aggravating influence on an individual with a genetic susceptibility to disease.[65]

Conclusion

Ageing is part of natural human development. This suggests that both ageing and human development are regulated by the same genetic processes.[66–68] In many animal species it has been suggested that ageing is a product of evolution and that ageing may be an unintended result of evolution. This theory does seem unlikely in humans, however. Evolution does not favour the concept of a long life but favours and optimizes reproductive mechanisms. Many ageing theories do overlap, and how the microbiology of the host affects the ageing process has not been reported. As you will see throughout this book, the microbiological burden on the host is enormous and clinically significant and undoubtedly will have a role to play in the ageing process.

As humans are living longer, there is a greater propensity to infection. This risk is substantially higher in elderly individuals who are predisposed to infection. While the process of ageing and the effects ageing has on the hosts' microbiology, and vice versa, are poorly documented and researched, data obtained from gut studies suggest that microbiological changes take place in the human host over time suggesting significance to the host. Do the microbiological changes that occur within and upon the host influence the process of ageing, or are they the biological changes of the host that affect the microbiology? Does this therefore affect our propensity to disease? As the host's microbiology changes with ageing, is this significantly beneficial or severely detrimental to the host? Are there ways of enhancing life expectancy by reducing certain bacteria from proliferating or, conversely, by enhancing the survival and proliferation of beneficial bacteria delay ageing? As you will see throughout this book, the whole area of ageing is complex and to date ageing remains an incurable disease.

The role microorganisms may play in influencing ageing is unquestionably significant to human life, longevity, and disease. Microbiological changes that do occur, specifically in the gut during ageing, may provide some useful research findings that may shed some light on the effects microorganisms have on human development and ageing.

Acknowledgement I would like to thank Dr João Pedro de Magalhães for his help with this chapter by providing information contained in his Web site http://www.senescence.info/definitions.html.

References

1. Comfort A. Ageing: The Biology of Senescence. Routledge and Kegan Paul, London. 1964.
2. Partridge L, Gems D. Mechanisms of ageing: public or private? Nat Rev Genet 2002;3:165–175.
3. Williams GC. Pleiotropy, natural selection, and the evolution of senescence. Evolution 1957;11:398–411.
4. Finch CE. Longevity, Senescence, and the Genome. The University of Chicago Press, Chicago and London. 1990.
5. Craik FIM, Salthouse TA. Handbook of Aging and Cognition. Erlbaum, Hillsdale. 1992.
6. Hayflick L. How and Why We Age. Ballantine Books, New York. 1994.
7. Spence AP. Biology of Human Aging. Prentice Hall, Englewood Cliffs, NJ. 1995.

8. De Magalhaes JP. Open minded. Ageing Rev 2005;4:1–22.
9. Holliday R. Understanding Ageing. Cambridge University Press, Cambridge. 1995.
10. Finch CE, Tanzi RE. Genetics of aging. Science 1997;278:407–411.
11. Finch CE. Variations in senescence and longevity include the possibility of negligible senescence. J Gerontol Biol Sci 1998;53A:B235–B239.
12. Olshansky SJ, Hayflick L, Carnes BA. No truth to the fountain of youth. Sci Am 2002;286:92–95.
13. Guarente L, Kenyon C. Genetic pathways that regulate ageing in model organisms. Nature 2000;408(6809):255–262.
14. Weismann A. On Heredity. Clarendon Press, Oxford. 1891.
15. Hamilton G. Clock of ages. New Sci 2003;2392:26–29.
16. Promistlow DE, Pletcher SD. Advice to an aging scientist. Mech Ageing Dev 2002;123:841–850.
17. Austad SN. Why We Age: What Science Is Discovering About the Body's Journey Through Life. Wiley, New York. 1997.
18. Austad SN. Diverse aging rates in metazoans: targets for functional genomics. Mech Ageing Dev 2005;126(1):43–49.
19. Warner H, Miller RA, Carrington J. Meeting report – National Institute on Aging Workshop on the Comparative Biology of Aging. Sci Aging Knowledge Environ 2002;17:5.
20. De Magalhaes JP. Is mammalian aging genetically controlled? Biogerontology 2003; 4:119–120.
21. Holliday R. The multiple and irreversible causes of ageing. J Gerontol A Biol Sci Med Sci 2004;59(6):B568–B572.
22. Hammerman MR. Insulin-like growth factors and aging. Endocrinol Metab Clin North Am 1987;16(4):995–1011.
23. Perls T, Kunkel L, Puca A. The genetics of aging. Curr Opin Genet Dev 2002;12:362–369.
24. Finch CE, Ruvkun G. The genetics of aging. Annu Rev Genomics Hum Genet 2001;2:435–462.
25. Tatar M, Bartke A, Antebi A. The endocrine regulation of aging by insulin-like signals. Science 2003;299(5611):1346–1351.
26. Holzenberger M, Dupont J, Ducos B, Leneuve P, Geloen A, Even PC, Cervera P, Le Bouc Y. Igf-1 receptor regulates lifespan and resistance to oxidative stress in mice. Nature 2003;421 (6919):182–187.
27. Cutler RG. Evolution of human longevity: a critical overview. Mech Ageing Dev 1979;9 (3–4):337–354.
28. Campisi J. Aging, chromatin, and food restriction – connecting the dots. Science 2000;289 (5487):2062–2063.
29. Olson CB. A review of why and how we age: a defense of multifactorial aging. Mech Ageing Dev 1987;41(1–2):1–28.
30. Rubner M. Das Problem der Lebensdauer und seine Beziehungen zu Wachstum und Ernäh-rung. München; Berlin: Verlag von R. Oldenburg. 1908;208S.
31. McCay CM, Crowell MF, Maynard LA. The effect of retarded growth upon length of the life span and upon the ultimate body size. J Nutr 1935;10(1):63–75.
32. Gerschman R, Gilbert DL, Nye SW, Dwyer P, Fenn WO. Oxygen poisoning and x-irradiation: a mechanism in common. Science 1954;119(3097):623–626.
33. Harman D. Aging: a theory based on free radical and radiation chemistry. J Gerontol 1956;11 (3):298–300.
34. Beckman KB, Ames BN. The free radical theory of aging matures. Physiol Rev 1998;78 (2):547–581.
35. Finkel T, Holbrook NJ. Oxidants, oxidative stress and the biology of ageing. Nature 2000;408 (6809):239–247.
36. Weindruch R. The retardation of aging by caloric restriction: studies in rodents and primates. Toxicol Pathol 1996;24(6):742–745.

37. Ruan H, Tang XD, Chen ML, Joiner ML, Sun G, Brot N, Weissbach H, Heinemann SH, Iverson L, Wu CF, Hoshi T. High-quality life extension by the enzyme peptide methionine sulfoxide reductase. Proc Natl Acad Sci USA 2002; 99(5):2748–2753.
38. Szilard L. On the nature of the aging process. Proc Natl Acad Sci USA 1959;45(1):30–45.
39. Martin GM, Oshima J. Lessons from human progeroid syndromes. Nature 2000;408 (6809):263–266.
40. Hamilton ML, Van Remmen H, Drake JA, Yang H, Guo ZM, Kewitt K, Walter CA, Richardson A. Does oxidative damage to DNA increase with age? Proc Natl Acad Sci USA 2001;98(18):10469–10474.
41. Ackermann M, Stearns SC, Jenal U. Senescence in a bacterium with asymmetric division. Science 2003;300(5627):1920.
42. Stewart EJ, Madden R, Paul G, Taddei F. Aging and death in an organism that reproduces by morphologically symmetric division. PloS Biol 2005;3(2):e45.
43. Anon. US Bureau of the census. An aging world: 2001. Available at http://www.census.gov/prod/2001pubs/p95–1.pdf.
44. Yoshikawa TT. Epidemiology and unique aspects of aging and infectious diseases. Clin Infect Dis 2000;30:931–933.
45. Marrie TJ. Community-acquired pneumonia in the elderly. Clin Infect Dis 2000; 31:1066–1078.
46. Nicolle LE. Urinary tract infection in geriatric and institutionalized patients. Curr Opin Urol 2002;12:51–55.
47. Leibovici L, Pitlik SD, Konisberger H, Drucker M. Bloodstream infections in patients older than eighty years. Age Ageing 1993;22:431–442.
48. De Magalhaes JP. http://www.senescence.info/definitions.html.
49. Schmader K. Herpes zoster in the elderly: issues related to geriatrics. Clin Infect Dis 1999;28:736–739.
50. Simonsen L. The global impact on influenza on morbidity and mortality. Vaccine 1999;17: S3–S10.
51. Garibaldi RA. Residential care and the elderly: the burden of infection. J Hosp Infect 1999; 43:S9–S18.
52. Stocks G, Janseen HF. Infection in patients after implantation of an orthopaedic device. ASAIO J 2000;46:S41–S46.
53. Emori TG, Banerjee SN, Culver DH et al. Nosocomial infections in elderly patients in the United States, 1986–1990. National Nosocomial Infections Surveillance System. Am J Med 1991;91:289S–293S.
54. Choi C. Bacterial meningitis in the aging adults. Clin Infect Dis 2001;33:1380–1385.
55. Ortqvist A. Pneumococcal vaccinations: current and future issues. Eur Respir J 2001; 18:184–195.
56. Chandra RK. Nutrition, immunity and infection: from basic knowledge of dietary manipulation of immune responses to practical application of immune responses to practical application of ameliorating suffering and improving survival. Proc Natl Acad Sci USA 1996;93:14304–14307.
57. Krabbe KS, Bruunsgaard H, Hansen CM, Møller K, Fonsmark L, Qvist J, Madsen PL, Kronborg G, Andersen HO, Skinhøj P, Pedersen BK. Ageing is associated with a prolonged fever response in human endotoxemia. Clin Diagn Lab Immunol 2001;8:333–338.
58. Klontz KC, Alder WH, Potter M. Age-dependent resistance factors in the pathogenesis of foodborne infectious disease. Aging (Milano) 1997;9:320–326.
59. Franceschi C, Bonafe M, Valensin S et al. Inflamm-aging. An evolutionary perspective on immunosenescence. Ann NY Acad Sci 2000;908:244–254.
60. Shay K. Infectious complications of dental and periodontal diseases in the elderly population. Clin Infect Dis 2002;34:1215–1223.
61. Ngeh J, Anand V, Gupta S. Chlamydia pneumoniae and atheroscerosis – what we know and what we don't. Clin Microbiol Infect 2002;8:2–13.

62. Epstein SE. The multiple mechanisms by which infection may contribute to atheroscerosis development and course. Circ Res 2002;90:2–4.
63. Danesh, J, Collins R, Peto R. Chronic heart disease: is there a link? Lancet 1997;350:430–436.
64. Sorlie PD, Nieto FJ, Adams E, Folsom AR, Shahar E, Massing M. A prospective study of cytomegalovirus, herpes simplex virus 1, and coronary heart disease: the atherosclerosis risk in the communities (ARIC) study. Arch Intern Med 2000;160:2027–2032.
65. Itzhaki RF, Lin WR, Shang D, Wlcock GK, Fargher B, Jamieson GA. Herpes simplex virus type 1 in brain and risk of Alzheimer's disease. Lancet 1997;349:241–244.
66. Medvedev ZA. An attempt at a rational classification of theories of ageing. Biol Rev Camb Philos Soc 1990;65(3):375–398.
67. Zwaan BJ. Linking development and aging. Sci Aging Knowledge Environ 2003;2003 (47):32.
68. De Magalhaes JP, Church GM. Genomes optimize reproduction: aging as a consequence of the development program. Physiology (Bethesda) 2005;20:252–259.

Chapter 2
Indigenous Microbiota and Association with the Host

John G. Thomas and Steven L. Percival

Human Development, Microorganisms, and 'Normal Flora'

The association between man and microorganism started during the early stages of human evolution. It is therefore of no surprise that the concept of bacteria influencing human development is of significance. In spite of this, evidence that bacteria may influence a specific host's development has largely been derived from research findings obtained from invertebrate models. Nevertheless, the initial findings generated from these invertebrate models may have some relevance to both animal and human development. For example, research has shown that bacteria, such as *Vibrio fischeri*, are capable of affecting morphological changes in the marine squid *Euprymna scolopes*. The 'commensal' relationship between *V. fischeri* and *E. scolopes* occurs when the squid hatches from its eggs. As the eggs hatch, within a few hours, *V. fischeri*, located in the sea water, colonize the newly formed squid. *V. fischeri* are then thought to induce morphological changes in the developing light organ of the squid, brought about by diffusible communication signals released by the bacteria. Although the communication between bacteria and the mammalian cells was first studied in the 'vibrio–squid model', the theory and science behind this is thought to have direct relevance to infections and diseases in humans. This would therefore indicate some degree of organization and co-ordination at the molecular level which may be applicable to human development. As bacteria do play a role in human development, it is probable that bacteria contribute significantly to human ageing. In fact, evidence for this has been documented in germ-free mice, wherein the mice had been infected with *Bacteroides thetaiotaomicron*. *Bacteroides* were found to affect the expression of various host genes known to have an influence on things such as nutrient uptake, metabolism, angiogenesis, mucosal barrier function,

J.G. Thomas and S.L. Percival
West Virginia University Schools of Medicine and Dentistry Robert C, Byrd Health Sciences Center-North, Morgantown, WV, USA

S.L. Percival (ed.), *Microbiology and Aging*.
DOI: 10.1007/978-1-59745-327-1_2, © Springer Science + Business Media, LLC 2009

and the development of the enteric nervous system.[1] In addition to this study, it has been found that the commensal bacteria associated with the host may be able to influence the normal development and function of the mucosal and gut immune system.[2–8] Consequently, on the basis of these and other similar studies, it is plausible to hypothesize that bacteria–host interactions have a role to play in the morphogenesis of mammals and therefore a link to the ageing phenomena.

Indigenous Microbiota (Normal Flora)

During early development (in the mother's womb), 'man' is generally not exposed to microbes. It is not until entry into the outside world that microorganisms become significant. These significant microorganisms, which are able to colonize the host, often become companions for life. Such 'companion' micoorganisms have been referred to as the 'normal' microflora which are considered to exist in a symbiotic relationship with 'man'. However, when we consider any form of symbiotic relation-ship, the microorganisms found on and within the body are in a mutualistic relation-ship with the host. This mutualistic relationship occurs when both human and bacteria benefit. However, in some instances this mutualistic relationship becomes one of paratism, when the microbe or human suffers at the expense of the other, or commensalism, where either the human or microbe benefits and the other remains unaffected. Historically the human–microbe relationship is considered to be one of commensalism. Nevertheless, it would appear that the microflora and animal/human relationship is not one of commensalism. This is because each partner has the ability to influence the other. Therefore, the commensal flora of the body is often better described as the 'indigenous microbiota', as suggested by Dubos.[9]

The healthy human contains approximately 10 times more bacteria than normal human cells.[10] The bacterial load on or within the host constitutes more than 2,000 different phylotypes. Despite this number, only 8 of 55 main divisions of bacteria have been shown to be present on or in the human host, suggesting some degree of host selection. The selected group of microbes associated with the host has been referred to as the 'microbiome'.[11] These 'selected microbes' are considered to use the human host merely as 'an advanced fermentor to maximise the productivity of the microbiome'.[12] The capacity of the indigenous microbiota to cause harm and disease to the host is severely limited by the host's immune system which helps to maintain a microbe–host homeostasis, which in turn helps to prevent the generation of significant microbial disturbances. However, if disturbances to the indigenous microbiota do occur, such as after surgical procedures or with chronic wounds, a person's host defences are often compromised, predisposing them to changes in their microflora and initiation of infections and diseases.

A number of indigenous bacteria are considered to be pathogenic, particularly those which have inherent multi-drug resistance. Such indigenous bacteria reside in the gut, the skin, and oropharynx but generally do not cause disease.

In the human mouth, some 500–700 different microbial taxa, considered to be part of the indigenous microbiota, have been identified compared to 500–1,000 in the colon. Despite these numbers, it is very difficult to define the true community of microbes in different regions of the body. This is principally due to the complexities of the communities in the human body and the variations in the indigenous microbiota that exist between age, sex, and hygiene. In addition, the different sampling methods that are often used in studies, combined with the changes that take place with microbial nomenclature, affect the correct interpretation of the findings.[13]

Microbiota Differences in Children and Adults

The indigenous microbiota of children and adults at different anatomical sites is considered significant. Initially this is due to the fact that young children have immature immune systems, no teeth, and different diets and are not exposed to the same environmental microbes as adults. For example, the initial microbiota colonising the gut of small children are predominately *Bifidobacterium* spp. compared to adults guts which are predominantly colonized by *Bacteroides*. In the elderly population, a decline in the effectiveness of the immune system in conjunction with poor health, diet, and hygiene leads to changes in the 'normal' microbiota. Specific microbiological changes that have been observed in the elderly population include[13] a decrease in *Veillonella* and *Bifidobacteria* species in the gut; increased levels of Clostridia, enterobacteria, and lactobacilli; an increase in urinary tract infections (UTI); an increase colonization in the oropharynx by *Candida albicans* and *Klebsiella*; increased levels of enetrobacteria and streptococci on the skin; and increased levels of Gram-negative bacteria in the eye and oral cavity.

The Development of the Indigenous Microbiota

The development of the indigenous microbiota begins soon after birth. Upon and within the neonate, colonization of pioneering bacteria occurs within 24 h. In many regions of the body, the microbes generally begin to proliferate in a heterogeneous manner. Autogenic and allogenic factors then prevail, leading to the adhesion and removal of certain microbial populations. Such changes are referred to as microbial succession, and are known to occur in areas where microbial communities exist.[14] Over time, the microbiology diversity and density in certain regions of the body become more stable (see Table 2.1) and less dynamic, eventually culminating in the formation of 'climax communities'. Consequently, regions of the body begin to develop a defined microflora. Such a defined microflora will be found on the skin or cutaneous regions of the body, the upper respiratory tract, oral cavity, gastrointestinal tract, and genital tract. This microflora, however, is subject to change specifically when modifications in the diet and the host immune system occur. The lack of

Table 2.1 Numbers of bacteria documented to inhabit locations of the adult body

Location	Population size
Skin	10^1–10^6 cm^{-1}
Saliva	10^8 ml^{-1}
Dental plaque	10^{12} g^{-1}
Ileal contents	10^8 ml^{-1}
Colon (faeces)	10^{10} g^{-1}
Vagina	10^8 ml^{-1}

research into the microbiological changes that occur with advancing age prevents us from gaining a better understanding of the benefits of the microflora and therefore the therapeutic procedures that could be implemented. In fact, there is mounting evidence that probiotics (discussed further in the book), and their significance to human health, is growing in acceptance for human well-being.

To date, the microbiology of the human microbiota is as yet incomplete despite more than a century of culture-based investigations. Many species of microbes have yet to be recovered from the host, and molecular techniques have been used only occasionally in a number of these environments.

Each anatomical site known to have its own microbiota will be considered in turn.

Skin

In the mother's uterus the unborn baby's skin is sterile. Following birth, colonization of the baby's skin occurs. As the skin is a barrier to many pathogenic bacteria, it restricts microorganisms attaching. While the skin is a highly effective organ in preventing the growth and invasion of pathogens, it is well documented that skin infections do occur – a frequent occurrence during the later years of life.

The outermost layer of the epidermis of the skin provides a very good barrier to the effects of environmental pressures. In fact, the keratinocytes, which are dead in the outermost layer of the skin, are continually being sloughed off and as such this prevents exogenous bacteria from colonizing. As the moisture content of the skin is very low, the bacterial growth on the skin is limited. The acidic pH of the skin also helps to suppress bacterial growth.

Indigenous bacteria that are known to colonize the skin are able to produce antimicrobials such as bacteriocin and toxins that inhibit pathogens from attaching. For example, bacteria such as *Staphylococcus epidermidis* are able to bind to keratinocyte receptors on the skin and once attached are known to prevent *S. aureus* from attaching.

The microbes that make up the largest proportion of normal skin flora include the Gram-positive bacteria such as Staphylococcus, Coryneform bacteria, and Micrococci (see Table 2.2). Gram-negative bacteria occur rarely as part of the normal skin flora. However, *Acinetobacter* spp. have been found routinely on the perineum and

Table 2.2 Commonly isolated microorganisms identified on a normal healthy skin

Genus	Species
Staphylococcus	S. aureus, S. capitis, S. capitis, S. auricularis, S. cohnii, S. epidermidis, S. haemolyticus, S. hominis, S. saccharolyticus, S. saprophyticus, S. simulans, S. warneri, S. xylosus
Acinebacter	A. johnsonii, A. baumannii
Malassazia	M. furfur
Micrococcus	M. luteus, M. lylae, M. kristinae, M. sedentarius, M. roseus, M. varian
Corynebacterium	C. jeikeium, C. urealyticum, C. minutissimum
Propionibacterium	P. acnes, P. avidum, P. granulosum

axilla. Staphylococci found on the skin are generally coagulase-negative and have included *S. epidermidis*, *S. haemolyticus*, and *S. hominis*. In the main, these coagulase negative staphylococcus (CNS) constitute a non-pathogenic group of bacteria that colonize the skin. However, CNS have been known to cause nosocomial infections, particularly in patients with intravascular catheters.

Micrococci, predominately *Micrococcus luteus*, are found in abundance on the skin surface. Most species of micrococcus are non-pathogenic; however, *M. sedentarius* has been known to cause pitted keratolysis. Coryneformes are also found on the skin.

The number of bacteria detected on the skin surface is about 10^{12}, which is equivalent to 10^4 cm^{-2}, which equates to about one bacterium per 100 μm^2. This indicates therefore that the bacteria are not evenly distributed but exist in microcolonies on the skin surface often growing as biofilms.

Mouth

In 1683, Antonie van Leeuwenhoek first observed the presence of microorganisms in the mouth, but it was not until 1890 that oral bacteria were considered to have a role to play in disease.[15] Today we know that the oral microbiota is beneficial to the host, as indicated by their ability to suppress the effects of exogenous microorganisms. However, imbalances and certain bacteria associated with the normal microbiota in the mouth can lead to oral diseases and cause soft-tissue infections and abscesses. Microorganisms in the mouth and throat are present in high numbers, with levels present in saliva at 10^8 or 10^9 ml^{-1}.

Colonization of the human mouth by bacteria occurs within the first 6–10 h after birth.[16] After 8–10 h, the bacteria, often only transient, that have been identified in a baby's mouth have included staphylococcus, streptococcus, coliforms, and enterococci, to name but a few. From 0 to 2 months, the most common bacteria isolated from the oral microbiota of the infant have included mainly the viridans streptococci such as *Streptococcus salivarius*, *S. oralis*, *S. mitis* biovar 1 together with *Neisseria* spp., *Staphylococcus* spp., and *Prevotella* spp. As the infant gets older (6–12 months), other microorganisms begin to appear in the mouth. These have included the ones mentioned above and *S. sanguis*, *Actinomyces* spp., *Fusobacterium* spp. (specifically *F. nucleatum*), and *Capnocytophaga*. At 12 months, in addition to the microbes mentioned above, other microbes such as *S. mutans*, *Clostridium* spp., *Peptostreptococcus* spp., *Prevotella intermedia* and *pallens* together with *Porphyromonas gingivalis* begin to colonize the oral microbiota of the infant's mouth. Many transient microorgansims appear in the newborn's mouth, which eventually become part of the resident microbiota or go on to colonize other regions of the body. It is during the teething and the weaning processes that newborns become more significantly exposed to bacteria.

   S. salivarius has been isolated frequently on the first day of a baby's life,[17] whereas during the teething process *S. sanguis* is documented to be the first colonizer of teeth.[18] *S. mutans* are also early colonizers of the teeth but these bacteria have been shown to take a longer time to colonize the teeth surface.[18,19] Over time, as biofilms (plaque) begin to form on the tooth surface, the microbiota becomes more complex and heterogeneous. The microbiota found in plaque isolated from children (4–7 years old) seems to be similar to that of adults.[20–22] Major microbiota changes in the mouth occur up to age of 19 as a result of the ageing process, possibly brought about by changes in hormones.[21,22] *Bacteroides* and *Spirochaetes* have been documented in the mouth of children. Levels have been shown to increase around puberty. Contrary to this, levels of *Capnocytophaga* spp. and *A. naeslundii* have been shown to decrease with advancing age. At adolescence, black pigmented anaerobes and *Spirochaetes* begin to increase in numbers in the mouth and form a significant component of the oral microbiota.

   Over 45 years ago, the number of bacteria that had been identified to be present in the adult mouth was as low as 30. Today, because of the advancement in microbial identification procedures, this number is documented to be much higher, with some 700 different species of bacteria now having been recognized.[23] In Table 2.3 the commonly encountered and cultured bacteria can be seen, but this is no definitive and complete list of oral bacterial genera, as this table constitutes only a select list of frequently isolated microbes. While the microbiota in the mouth is very heterogenous, principally due to the fact that the oral microbiota is under a constant flux from the shedding of epithelial cells, saliva flow, diet, and the effects of the innate immune response, the dental plaque does show a very high degree of homeostasis.

   A large number of microorganisms have been detected in the adult mouth that do not reside there for long periods. These are transient oral microbiota bacteria derived from food or from the other regions of the body. These bacteria are considered insignificant but are capable of causing opportunistic infections in debilitated individuals. The bacteria known to cause diseases such as dental caries and peridonotal diseases are caused by the resident microflora found colonizing the teeth. Oral pathogens such as *S. mutans* have been linked to caries,[24] as have *Actinobacillus actinomycetemcomitans*. Treponema has been linked with periodontal disease. These bacteria, however, are considered to constitute part of the indigenous microbiota of the mouth.

Table 2.3 Commonly occurring cultured bacteria isolated from the oral cavity

Microorganism	Species
Actinomyces	*A. israelli, A. viscosus, A. naeslundii*
Prevotella	*P. melaninigenica, P. intermedia, P. loescheii, P. denticola*
Porphyromonas	*P. gingivalis, P. assacharolytica, P. endodontalis*
Lactobacillus	*L. casei, L. brevis, L. plantarum, L. salivarius*
Fusobacterium	*F. nucleatum, F. naviforme, F. russii, F. peridonticum, F. alocis, F. sulci*
Bifidiobacterium	*B. dentium*
Streptococcus	*S. anginosus, S. gordonii, S. mitis, S. mutans, S. oralis, S. rattus,*
	S. salivarius, S. sanguis
Campylobacter	*C. rectus, C. sputorum, C. curvus*
Rothia	*R. dentocariosa*
Capnocytophaga	*C. ochracea, C. sputagena, C. gingivalis*
Propionibacterium	*P. acnes*
Eubacterium	*E. alactolyticum, E. brachy, E. nodarum*
Veillonella	*V. parvula, V. atypical, V. dispar*
Peptostreptococcus	*P. anaerobius, P. micros*
Neisseria	*N. flavescens, N. mucosa, N. sicca, N. subflava*
Haemophilus	*H. parainfluenzae*
Selenomonas	*S. sputigena, S. flueggei*
	Corynebacterium matruchotii
Actinobacillus	*Actinobacillus*
Capnocytophaga	*Capnocytophaga*
Bacteroides	*B. buccae, B. buccalis, B. denticola, B. oralis*
Wolinella	*W. curva, W. recta*

On the palate, lips, cheeks, and floor of the mouth, the microbiota is considered sparse.

The tongue generally harbours a polymicrobial microbiota. A study conducted in 1966[25] has shown that the predominant bacteria found on the human tongue are Streptococci (35%), Gram-positive rods (16%), *Veillonella* (16%), Gram-negative rods (6%), non-pigmenting *Bacteroides* (5%), and *Peptostreptococcus* spp. (4%), and the rest were Gram-positive cocci. Recent studies using 16s rRNA have shown that the tongue contains a very diverse microbiota and these may act as a reservoir for bacteria associated with periodontal diseases.

Upper Gastrointestinal Tract

The dominant population of bacteria residing in the upper gastrointestinal (GI) tract of a healthy adult human has included *Pseudomonas* spp., *Micrococcus* spp., *Bacillus* spp. as well as lactobacilli, bifidiobacteria, and streptococci.[26] However, the microbial composition of the indigenous microbiota of the GI tract is affected by sex, age, and diet, which significantly alter the microflora. However, depending on the individual, it is generally appreciated that a well-balanced, healthy gut has a microbiota which generally remains stable throughout adulthood. The host and bacterial association is a mutually beneficial relationship important for providing nutritional benefits, angiogenesis, and immunity.

Oseophagus

The normal microbiota of the oesophagus is an area that has been poorly researched. As it is the route by which food is passed from the mouth to the stomach, it is likely to be composed of its own microflora. From a 16S rRNA study of the oesophagus, 95 species of bacteria have been identified.[27]

Stomach

The acidity of the stomach kills many ingested microbes[28] and as such is considered to be sterile. The resting pH of the stomach is about 2, but as the gastric mucosa ages it becomes less efficient in secreting acid. At this point the stomach is not a great bacteriocidal agent, allowing for the development of a stomach microflora. The development of a stomach microflora is acknowledged to occur in 10% of the population at the age of 50 and 50% at the age of 70. However, this does vary in regions of the world particularly where poor diets are common. In individuals who have a resting gastric pH of below 5, the microbiota is dominated by *Streptococcus, Lactobacillus, Veillonella,* and *Micrococci.* Above a pH of 5, more acid-tolerant bacteria reside; e.g. *Bacteroides* spp. *Helicobacter pylori* has been isolated from the gastric mucosa of a high percentage of individuals and as such is considered to be part of the 'normal' microbiota of the adult stomach. *Helicobacter pylori* will be discussed further in the book. Common bacteria that have been cultured from a healthy adult's stomach can be seen in Table 2.4.

Table 2.4 Common bacteria (genera) isolated from the stomach in healthy individuals

Bacteria
Streptococcus, Lactobacillus, Staphylococcus, Micrococcus, Neisseria, Pseudomonas, Haemophilus, Veillonella, Bacteroides, Enterobacteria, Bifidiobacterium

Table 2.5 Common bacteria (genera) isolated from the upper small intestine (adapted from[29,30]) (ND - Not detected)

Bacteria	Frequency of isolation range of numbers
Streptococcus	6/10, ND-10^4
Lactobacillus	3/10, ND-10^4
Staphylococcus	1/10, ND-10^2
Micrococcus	1/10, ND-10^2
Veillonella	1/10, ND-10^2
Fungi/yeasts	2/10, ND-10^4
Bacteroides	6/10, ND-10^4
Enterobacteria	4/10, ND-10^4
Bifidiobacterium	1/10, ND-10^3

Small Intestine

From the stomach to the colon the bacterial population increases from 10^4 to 10^7 ml^{-1}. Within the small intestine the bacteria that predominate are mainly Gram-positive strains. These constitute about 10^5–10^7 cfu ml^{-1} of fluid. Such bacteria found here include the lactobacilli and enterococci. At the lower end of the small intestine, the flora begins to change and anaerobic bacteria and coliforms begin to dominate the microbiota. The major organisms that are found in the upper regions of the small intestine are mainly Gram-positive bacteria. However, low numbers of *E. coli* and *Bacteroides* have been isolated. The upper small intestine is considered to be sterile, as bacteria are exposed to proteolytic enzymes, bile salts, and the innate immune response together with a rapid flow through of fluid that restricts bacterial colonization and proliferation.

The lower small intestine, which is composed of the distal and terminal ileum, is a region where peristalsis is slower and bile salts are present. This favours the formation of a resident microbial flora. Commonly isolated bacteria that have been cultured from the upper intestine can be found in Table 2.5.

Colon

The microbiological development of the human gut can be divided into a number of stages:[31]

Stage 1: The microflora of the infant. This is the first stage of bacterial attachment and the development of a 'sub-climax' microflora.
Stage 2: Transitional flora. It is here that growth and inactivation of the microflora begins. The diet and environmental conditions are important factors affecting this community. The role the transient flora has in determining the climax community in the gut is presently unknown.

Stage 3: Adult climax community: Decline in microbiota. This is the stage that is associated with ageing possibly leading to the decline in the human host's ability to sustain and control the equilibrium of its microflora.[32]

Microflora of the Infant's Gut

At birth the neonate intestines are sterile but within 24 h become quickly colonized with microbes acquired from both the mother and the external environment.[33] Within the first 17 days of life, a microbiota would have developed in the GI tract of infants. This microbiota has been shown to be significant to disease, particularly atopic infections.[34] The microbiota of the infant gut was studied sometime ago,[35,36] but today only a small number of studies are being undertaken to advance this area further.

Following the birth of a baby, the initial inoculum of bacteria entering the GI tract originates from the region by which it is delivered, i.e. cervical or vaginal microflora. Ultimately, the baby can be colonized only by those microorganism to which it is exposed and by organisms that are capable of forming a permanent community on the gut mucosa. The early colonizers of new born babies have include *E. coli* and streptococci, which are able to utilize the many nutrients in the large intestine. As these bacteria grow, they produce short-chain fatty acids that remove oxygen, making the environment anaerobic. With breast-fed babies, these bacteria will be replaced by Bifidobacterium. Host factors will also have a role to play in controlling the colonization of many strains of bacteria in the developing gut.

Immunoglobulin A is a very important antibody found in mucosal secretions of the gut. Levels in children, up to the age of 2 years, are considered to be very low in comparison to those in an adult.[37] In breast-fed infants, owing to the high levels of immunoglobulin A in breast milk, many bacteria are prevented from gaining access to the mucosal cells. Breast milk is also known to stimulate the growth of bifido-bacterium, which is very important in preventing colonization by pathogenic bacteria. A dominance of Bifidobacteria has been reported in the guts of breast-fed babies.[38–40] Conversely, formula-fed babies have guts that are predominantly colonized with bacteria such as Bacteriodes and contain only low levels of Bifido-bacterium. Bacteria such as the coliforms, micrococci, and streptococci appear very early in the faecal flora of breast-fed babies. As the diet changes, Gram-negative enterobacteria become more prominent, and bacteria such as bacteriodes, entero-cocci, and clostridia begin to increase in numbers in the baby's gut. In comparison, in adults the bacteria found in the faeces are predominately bacteriodes and bifidobacteria. These are obligate anaerobes and outnumber *E. coli* (10^7–10^8 g^{-1}) by 1,000:1 to 10,000:1. The indigenous microbiota of infants does not 'climax' until solid food begins,[26,36] and once weaning begins the gut microbiota soon develops a microbiology similar to that of an adult.[41] During the weaning

Table 2.6 Commonly occurring bacteria isolated from human faeces

Bacteria
Acidaminococcus, Bacteroides, Bifidiobacterium, Clostridium, Coprococcus, Enterobacter, Enterococcus, Escherichia, Eubacterium, Fusobacterium, Klebsiella, Lactobacillus, Megamonas, Megasphaera, Methanobrevibacter, Methanosphaera, Peptostreptococcus, Proteus, Ruminococcus, Veillonella

process, facultative anaerobes such as Streptococci and coliforms start to decline. These bacteria are soon superseded by Bacteriodes, which become established as the dominant bacteria in the intestine. Pioneering bacteria of the GI tract are reported to be enterobacteria, principally *E. coli* and enterococcus, staphylococcus, and streptococci, followed then by obligate anaerobes, bifidobacteria, and Bacteriodes.[42]

Andrieux et al.[43] studied the inter-individual variation and the influence of age on metabolic characteristics of the faecal microflora from persons of three age groups. The results form their study showed significant differences between elderly persons and younger adults and children, but the major metabolic characteristics of the faecal microflora were not found to be greatly altered by the ageing process. Probiotics are considered significant for a healthy gut, but it has been found that probiotics administered in the first months of life did not significantly interfere with long-term composition or quantity of gut microbiota.[44]

Adult Indigenous Microbiota in the Colon

The human GI microbiota, specifically in the adult colon, is composed of a very complex community of microorganisms (see Table 2.6). Viruses, for example, constitute a large component of this ecosystem, and well over 1,200 different viral genotypes have been identified in human faeces isolated from a healthy adult gut equating to 10^9 virions per gram of dry faeces.[45]

The dominant bacterial phyla known to inhabit the adult gut include the Actinobacteria, Bacteroidetes, Firmicutes,[46] and Proteobacteria. While there are numerous studies that have documented the diversity of the microbiota of the GI tract,[47] in terms of species composition, differences in healthy individuals' microbiota have complexed the true composition and 'climax community' of the adult gut. Subsequently, this has been, and still remains, a very challenging area of research.

A large number of authors estimate that the gut contains between 400 and 500 different species of culturable bacteria.[48] However, modern molecular techniques, prior to 2006, have shown that these numbers are much higher, more than 1,000 species,[12,49,50] indicating that a large number of the bacteria living in the GI tract are in fact non-culturable at present.[51]

The defensive mechanisms of the body have a role to play in helping to control the microbial composition of the gut and maintain it as a 'climax community'. Changes in the bacteriology of the colonic microflora occur during the ageing process. This has been shown to be significant for bacteria such as *Bacteroides* and *Bifidiobacteria*, which are thought to provide both beneficial and protective functions to the host. These shifts in dominant species in the adult colon may help us to understand the decreased functionality of the human microbiota during ageing and its significance. To date, this has not been explored in great detail.

It is probable that the gut is a self-regulating system that functions to control, among other things, the gut 'climax community'. As this community is highly resistant to invading bacteria and well adapted to this niche, it is probable that any invading bacteria would require time to adapt to this way of life. But, to date, despite intensive studies in gut microbiology, the exact mechanisms by which the body controls the composition and distribution of certain microflora are largely unknown. Diet has been researched, and there is evidence that this may affect the microbiota in the gut of animals but this remains controversial in humans. Even changing diets to a vegetarian one has produced no real effect on the predominant microflora in the gut.[52]

Age-related changes to the bacterial genera and species have been identified in the adult gut.[28] A number of studies, as mentioned previously, have shown that bacteriodes decline in numbers with advancement of age.[53–55] These bacteria are very important in the gut and are involved in polysaccharide digestion. If metabolic activities therefore change in the gut with advancing age, other bacteria within the ecosystem will be affected. In fact, within elderly populations there is evidence of a rise in proteolytic bacteria. These include clostridium, propionibacteria, and fuso-bacteria.[53,55,56] Increases in levels of clostridium have been observed in healthy individuals when compared to younger adults.[55] The consequence of this could be an increase in bile acid transformations, resulting in the development of harmful metabolites in the colon. Also the cell material released from some bacteria is known to increase in the elderly population. These are thought to contribute to arthritis.[57]

Bifidobacteria occur in excess of 10^{10} g^{-1} dry weight of faeces.[28] During the ageing process, and most notably within an elderly population, there is a marked change in the levels of Bifidobacteria,[55,58,59] indicating a decline in colonic microbial stability. While a wide range of Bifidobacteria exist both in the adult and infant gut, in the elderly population *Bifidobacterium adolescentis*, *B. angulatum*, and *B. longum* seem to be the most dominant species.[53,59,60]

Respiratory Tract

The respiratory system is responsible for transporting air to the lungs where both oxygen and carbon dioxide exchange can take place. Initially air is conducted from the nose, which then passes through the pharynx, larynx, trachea, bronchi, and then through the bronchioles to the alveoli. It is the areas found above the bronchi that are known to be heavily colonized by microorganisms. The distal airways, i.e. bronchi and bronchioles, and the lungs are generally sterile.

During breathing, air, which contains many fine particles including micoorganisms, is inhaled through the nose. The bacteria that are inhaled become trapped in the mucus found on top of the nasal mucosa. The mucociliary escalator then transports the mucus containing the bacteria into the pharynx. Mucus is then swallowed and the microorganisms will then be killed by the acid in the stomach. Within the nasal fluid many different antimicrobials can be found. These include lysozyme, lactoferrin, IgA, and IgG, among others. These agents are important in helping to reduce infection and disease. They are also important in determining the composition of the indigenous microbiota of the respiratory system.

At birth, as with most sites in the human body, the respiratory tract is sterile. However, a number of studies have shown that some neonates do harbour bacteria. These have included *Bacillus subtilis*, *E. coli*, and *Staphylococcus epidermidis*, which are generally acquired from the mother during birth. Following birth, the primary bacteria found colonizing the oropharynx are alpha haemolytic streptococci. However, there are very few studies available that have characterized the microbiology of the respiratory tract of infants, which prevents a comprehensive analysis of the microbiology in this area. The majority of studies that are available for analysis have concentrated on studying the nasopharynx and the effects of specific pathogens colonizing this site. In most of these studies staphylococci have been the most frequently isolated bacteria. Levels of staphylococci in the nasopharynx have been shown to decrease with age. During the first 6 months of life, the main bacteria found colonizing the nasopharyngeal have included *S. aureus*, *S. epidermidis*, *Streptococcus mitis* and *pneumoniae*, *Moraxella catarrhalis*, *Neisseria* sp., Enterobacteriaceae, and *H. influenzae*. After 6 months, the levels of certain bacteria in the nasopharyngeal region begin to decrease. These have included *Staphylococcus aureus*, but other bacteria such as *Streptococcus pneumoniae*, *Moraxella catarrhalis*, and *H. influenzae* have been shown to increase in numbers during the ageing process. Also, bacteria such as *N. meningitides* are generally not isolated from children within the first 2 years of life. However, it is well documented that the carriage of *N. meningitides* increases during the ageing process.

Microorganisms that are considered to be part of the indigenous microbiota of the adult respiratory tract are many. Such ones have included *Streptococcus pyogenes*, *Neisseria* spp., *Haemophilus* spp., *Staphylococcus aureus*, CNS, *Propionibacterium* spp., *Prevotella* spp., *Corynebacterium* spp., *Moraxella* spp., and *Streptococcus pneumoniae*, to name but a few. In the nasal cavity of adults a vast array of bacteria have been found, which include, in order of proportions, *Corynebacterium* spp., *Staphylococcus* spp., *Streptococcus* spp., *Aureobacterium* spp., *Rhodococcus* spp., and *Heamophilus* spp. Within the nasopharynx region, because of high levels of available nutrients, many different bacteria have been isolated. A selection of these bacteria that have been isolated from the respiratory tract of a healthy adult is shown in Table 2.7.

Table 2.7 Common bacteria found in the upper respiratory tract

Region and bacterial numbers	Infants (1–18 months)	Children/adults
Anterior Nares	*Staphylococcus aureus, S. epidermidis, Corynebacterium* sp.	*Staphylococcus aureus, S. saprophyticus, S. epidermidis, S. hominis, haemolyticus, cohnii, Corynebacterium jeikeum, C. minutissimum, C. xerosis, Propionibacterium acnes, P. avidum, Neisseria* sp., *Corynebacterium* sp.
Nasopharynx	*Staphylococcus aureus, S. epidermidis, Stretococcus pneumonia, Streptococcus mitis, Moraxella catarrhalis, Neisseria* spp., *Haemophilus influenzae, Enterobacteriaceae*, alpha haemolytic streptococci	All the above plus: CNS, alpha haemolytic streptococci, *Stretococcus pneumonia, Moraxella catarrhalis, Haemophilus influenzae, H. parainfluenzae, Neisseria meningitides, N. mucosa, N. sicca, N. subflava, Fusobacterium* sp., *Prevotella* spp., *Porphyromonas* spp., *Peptostreptococcus* spp.
Oropharynx	All the above (nasopharynx) plus: *Streptococcus anginosus, S. constellatus, S. intermedius, S. sanguis, S. oralis, S. mitis, S. acidominimus, S. morbillorum, S. salivarius, S. uberis, S. gordonii, S. mutans, S. cricetus, S. rattus, S. sobrinus, S. crista, S. pneumoniae, S. pyogenes, Haemophilus parainfluenzae, Mycoplasma salivarius, M. orale*	All the above (nasopharynx) plus: *Streptococcus anginosus, S. constellatus, S. intermedius, S. sanguis, S. oralis, S. mitis, S. acidominimus, S. morbillorum, S. salivarius, S. uberis, S. gordonii, S. mutans, S. cricetus, S. rattus, S. sobrinus, S. crista, S. pneumoniae, S. pyogenes, Haemophilus parainfluenzae, Mycoplasma salivarius, M. orale*

In general, age has an effect on the carriage of certain indigenous bacteria. Age has been shown to affect the prevalence of *Streptococcus pneumoniae, H. influenzae*, and *M. catarrhalis*.

In the respiratory tract an infection occurs when the immune system is compromised, a pathogen is virulent, and a high inoculum is available. It is probable that oral microbes infect the respiratory tract. This suggests a significant role the oral flora plays in respiratory tract infections.

N. meningitidis, Streptococcus pneumoniae, and *H. influenzae* are the main causative agents of meningitis.[61] *N. meningitidis* is the main cause of meningitis, and worldwide it is responsible for over 500,000 cases – its attack and fatality ratio is higher in children (highest incidence is in children 6–24 months) than adults.

Pneumonia is a major cause of both morbidity and mortality worldwide. Many bacteria including anaerobic Gram-negative rod-shaped bacteria are considered significant to pneumonia. *Streptococcus pneumoniae* is a major cause of lobar pneumonia, which is known to affect infants less than 2 years old and the elderly.[61] It is estimated that over a million children are affected and die from this disease. Sinusitis is another indigenous related infection that affects infants more than adults. The major organism responsible for acute sinusitis is *Streptococcus pneumoniae* together with *Haemophilus influenzae*, and *Moraxella catarrhalis*. *Porphyromonas* spp. and *Fusobacterium* spp. are responsible for chronic sinusitis.

Children, particularly, below the age of 15 years, are also affected by bacteria that cause otitis media. The bacteria responsible for this include *S. pneumoniae*, *Haemophilus influenzae*, and *Moraxella catarrhalis*.

Other infections caused by the indigenous microbiota include epiglottitis and bronchitis.

UTI (Including Vagina)

The urinary system is composed of the kidneys (generally two), two ureters, a bladder, and a urethra. Anatomically, the systems in males and females do differ significantly. The microorganisms that are found first in the urethra are determined by age. In general though, the more predominant bacteria found colonizing the urethra include *Lactobacillus* sp., *Streptococcus* sp., *Fusobacterium* sp., *Staphylococcus* sp., *Corynebacterium* sp., CNS, *Bacteroides* sp., and an array of Gram-positive anaerobic bacteria. There are very few studies that have focussed on the indigenous flora of the urethra in both females and males. The main bacteria found colonizing the urethra of males are very similar to those in females and are generally members of the cutaneous microbiota.

The main microorganisms found colonizing the reproductive system of females include *Lactobacillus* spp., *Staphylococcus* spp., *Corynebacterium* spp., *Enterococcus* spp., *Fusobacterium* spp., *Bacteroides* spp., *Porphyromonas* spp., *Clostridium* spp., *Candida albicans*, and *Propionibacterium* spp. The genital tract, specifically of woman, can be a potential reservoir of infection. Early studies have shown that a 'healthy' vagina is colonized only with Lactobacilli. During puberty, production of oestrogen occurs, the vaginal wall thickens, and glycogen is deposited. Lactobacilli are then able to metabolize the glycogen in the vagina and produce large amounts of lactic acid. This results in the development of an acid pH that reduces the probability of other pathogenic bacteria attaching. Today we know that a homogenous population, of just Lactobacillus, is not evident in the normal vagina. In fact, the vagina can be colonized with a vast array of aerobic and anaerobic bacteria in the presence or absence of lactobacillus. Interestingly, the flora of the vagina does not overlap with the indigenous flora found in the GI tract, despite its close proximity. However, the dominant bacteria found in the healthy vagina includes lactobacillus and diphtheroids,[62,63] with the prevalence of lactobacillus reported to be between 45 and 96%.

Within premenopausal women, anaerobic Gram-positive cocci have been reported to occur in abundance together with *Bacteroides*.

Oestrogen seems to have a major effect on the microflora of the vagina, and during the menstrual cycle bacterial adherence and colonization seem to be affected. However, to date, research that has looked into this area remains inconsistent. For example, the microbiology of the vagina between pre- and post-menopausal women has shown no relationship with changes in hormonal levels. There are only relatively few reports that have studied the microflora of women at the post-menopausal stage of life, but reports in the 1930s have shown that lactobacilli is substantially reduced.[64] During the post-menopausal stage, the flora remains the same but there is a greater incidence of Gram-negative bacilli reported when compared to pre-menopausal women.

In addition, there have been no significant differences documented in the microflora of the vagina between pregnant and non-pregnant women. However, there are reports that in pregnant women Lactobacillus levels may be significantly higher than in non-pregnant women.

Overall, to date, research seems to suggest that within the vagina, soon after birth, lactobacilli infect. During the child-bearing years, lactobacilli, *S. epidermidis*, and corynebacteria predominate. Other bacteria that have been documented to occur here include viridans streptococci, enterococci, Group B streptococci, non-pathogenic neisseriae and enteric bacilli, *Acinetobacter* spp., *Haemophilus vaginalis*, and Mycoplasma.

Eyes

It is still debatable whether microorganisms that can be detected in the eye constitute a transient flora or a resident microflora. Most studies that have been undertaken have shown that in healthy adults most do not yield any bacteria that can be cultured. Any bacteria that have been identified have been common bacteria that constitute the normal microbiota of the skin.[65,66] Principally, most studies completed to date have been conducted using culturable and not molecular techniques.

The microbiota of the ocular in infants is often determined by the birth route. For example, with a normal vaginal delivery, the conjunctiva of the eye is colonized by the vaginal microbiota of the mother. Fewer bacteria have been isolated from babies that have been delivered by caesarean section, and bacteria commonly found are those which constitute part of the normal skin microbiota. The common bacteria identified on the conjunctivae of vaginally delivered babies include lactobacillus and bifidobacteria compared to propionibacteria and corynebacterium which are found on the conjunctivae of caesarean-delivered babies. After 5 days following birth, the microbiota of the conjunctivae is dominated by coagulase-negative staphylococci, coryneforms, streptococci, and propionibacteria. As the baby grows, the microbiota remains the same for a long time but levels of *Streptococcus pneumoniae* have been shown to decrease.

In healthy adults, the conjunctivae have some bacteria evident.[67,68] However, this population is considered small. The usual bacteria isolated have included *S. epidermidis* and *Propionibacterium acnes* (anaerobic diptheroids); however, non-haemolytic streptococci, *S. pneumoniae*, *S. aureus*, anaerobic streptococci, lactobacilli, corynebacteria, and enteric bacteria have also been documented to occur but less frequently.

The eye does seems to select for the survival only certain species of bacteria, as certain bacteria are found consistently in samples that are taken from the conjunctivae. Studies that have been done on the eye have shown that the right- and left-eye microbiota are very similar.

Central Nervous System

Many pathogens including bacteria, virus and fungi, and, now, prion proteins are known to cause inflammatory processes and neuronal degeneration specifically of the central nervous system (CNSys). The CNSys is considered sterile but very vulnerable to infectious agents. This is because during ageing the blood–brain barrier and also the immune responses become compromised. As we start to age, infectious agents are able to avoid the normal responses of the body.[69] Viruses such as herpes can be transferred trans-cellularly into the CNSys from infected nerves. Also, with an increase in oxidative stress located at or within neurons, this makes them more vulnerable to many viruses and prions infection. In addition to this, a decline in the immune function during ageing makes neurons more vulnerable so that both the brain and the spinal cord become 'hot spots' for infections. This has been shown to be the case with diseases such as tuberculosis[70] and other agents such as the West Nile virus and Lyme disease.

Prions have been shown to be transmittable between humans, and there is a high probability of transmission from animals and animal products to humans. Prions are known to affect the CNSys, and disorders such as scrapie in sheep, bovine spongiform encephalopathy in cattle, Kuru, Creutzfeldt–Jakob disease, Gerstmann–Straussler–Scheinker disease, and fatal familial insomnia in humans are a result of a prion disease. These diseases are caused by the accumulation of insoluble aggregates of prion protein, and abnormal (scrapie) forms (PrPsc) of a normal protein called the cellular prion protein (PrPc). Prion diseases are well known to have a long incubation period, and it is well documented that these prion diseases are more common in the elderly. Prions cause death of neurons by inducing oxidative stress, triggering apoptosis, and disrupting calcium homeostasis.[71] Inflammatory processes may also contribute to the pathogenesis of prion disorders.[72] Therefore, changes of brain cells and neurons during normal ageing make neurons more susceptible to the toxicity of prions.

It has been hypothesized that infections that occur during childhood could increase the risk of age-related neurodegenerative disorders, but evidence for this remains controversial at present.[73]

A number of viruses are known to infect cells in the nervous system and are able to remain in the neurons for a very long time, often a lifetime. Such viruses include herpes simplex-1, Sindbis virus, rabies, and also measles.[74–77] Transient infections are thought to trigger neurodegenerative cascades when infections occur in aged individuals, which increase the risk of certain diseases.

Certain viruses are also known to damage and also kill myelinating cells of the central and peripheral nervous system. The most common demyelinating disorder found in humans is multiple sclerosis. There is growing evidence that infectious agents may have a role to play in multiple sclerosis. In fact, a review by Steiner et al.[78] has shown associations with canine distemper, human hepes virus-6, parainfluenza virus, measles virus, and *C. pneumoniae*. Synapses have also been shown to be vulnerable to infectious agents.[79]

Adverse Effects of the 'Normal' Microbiota of the Host

The 'normal' microbiota of the host does not always have a beneficial role to play.[80] This essentially is due to the fact that closely related organisms can be both commensal and pathogenic. The indigenous microbiota is capable of causing disease but their pathogenicity is limited principally by the actions of the immune response and competition from other bacteria that occupy the same niche. Within the host, commensals greatly outnumber disease-producing bacteria so that pathogenicity is a rare occurrence. In some instances, however, the indigenous microbiota of the host may become pathogenic. Such examples include *S. mitis* and *S. salivarius*, known to inhabit the oropharynx but which are known to be associated with bacteraemia following dental extraction. Ultimately, the microbiota of the host may be trying to obtain a stable climax community within all the human-specific niche environments. Changes in this community will therefore have possible detrimental effects on the host. Mechanisms used to control these changes to the 'normal' microbiota need to be effectively applied by the host. For that reason, the need for a state of microbiological homeostasis or balance in each microbiological niche of the host is warranted.

As the human body is composed of a wide variety of microorganisms present within a stable ('quasi' steady state) community, changes such as ageing and the physiological and metabolic changes that are associated with it would significantly alter this 'homeostasis'.

Many conditions are known to affect the human host and lower the resistance of the host either generally or at specific sites in the body. Such factors can include malnutrition, debilitation from other diseases, radiation damage, shock, sub-clinical or asymptomatic infections, and also disturbances with the bacterial antagonism resulting from things such as the use of antimicrobial therapy and localized obstructions to the excretory organs, to name but a few.

With endogenous disease, their origins have no definable incubation period, they are not communicable, and they do not result in clinically recognizable immunity and tend to occur and recur slowly over years and involve bacterial agents that are found as part of the indigenous microbiota. These agents have low intrinsic pathogenicity and cause disease when they appear either in unusual body sites or in enormously increased concentrations in or near their usual sites.

Conclusion

Microbes have inhabited this planet approximately 4 billion years before the existence of man, which suggests a significant role for them in human life. However, despite decades of microbiological research, very little is known as to how many microbes affect the health of humans and how the microbiology of the human host changes as humans age.

It is appreciated that the occurrence of specific bacteria at specific niche sites in the body may be a predetermined phenomena rather than a random association. The first encounter between microbes and the human host occurs at birth, and the pioneering bacteria, as well as age of acquisition, is thought to have effects on human development, ageing, and disease. This has been shown to be the case in pre-term babies. A recent publication has shown that colonization of the gut by bifidobacteria and lactobacillus is delayed in pre-term infants[81] and that colonization with potentially pathogenic bacteria (especially *E. coli*) is significantly increased. This delayed colonization by beneficial bacteria does seem to have significant effects on infection rates and disease. In addition to this, the route by which a baby enters the world may well influence the initial pioneering bacteria of the human host. In the United States alone, one-quarter of all babies are born by caesarean. These newborn babies will not inherit microbes from the maternal vagina but acquire bacteria from the external environment. Does this have significant long-term implications to the host? This question is at present being investigated with no clear-cut answers. Pockets of research have shown that with a vaginal birth the microorganisms that are passed from mother to baby are dominated by Gram-positive cocci. This principally will depend on whether the baby is breast fed or formula fed. Contrary to this, it is now being documented, specifically in oral cavity studies, that the host may actually select the microorganisms that colonize and then become indigenous to them. With this in mind, the route by which a baby is delivered will have little effect on which microorganisms will eventually become the microbiota. If it is true that the body may select certain bacteria, it would be logical to suggest that the indigenous microbiota will have positive effects on human development and therefore this would have an effect on human ageing.[82,83]

References

1. Xu J, Gordon JI. Inaugural Article: Honor thy symbionts. Proc Natl Acad Sci USA 2003;100:10452–10459.
2. Mazmanian SK, Liu CH, Tzianabos AO, Kasper DL. An immunomodulatory molecule of symbiotic bacteria directs maturation of the host immune system. Cell 2005;122:107–118.
3. Rakoff-Nahoum S, Paglino J, Eslami-Varzaneh F, Edberg S, Medzhitov R. Recognition of commensal microflora by Toll-like receptors is required for intestinal homeostasis. Cell 2004;118:229–241.

4. Weinstein PD, Cebra JJ. The preference for switching to IgA expression by Peyer's patch germinal center B cells is likely due to the intrinsic influence of their microenvironment. J Immunol 1991;147:4126–4135.
5. Cebra JJ. Influences of microbiota on intestinal immune system development. Am J Clin Nutr 1999;69:1046S–1051S.
6. Shanahan F. The host-microbe interface within the gut. Best Pract Res Clin Gastroenterol 2002;16:915–931.
7. Backhed F, Ding H, Wang T, Hooper LV, Koh GY, Nagy A, Semenkovich CF, Gordon JI. The gut microbiota as an environmental factor that regulates fat storage. Proc Natl Acad Sci USA 2004;101:15718–15723.
8. Ley RE, Backhed F, Turnbaugh P, Lozupone CA, Knight RD, Gordon JI. Obesity alters gut microbial ecology. Proc Natl Acad Sci USA 2005;102:11070–11075.
9. Dubos R, Schaedler RW, Costello R, Hoet P. Indigenous, normal, and autochthonous flora of the gastrointestinal tract. J Exp Med 1965;1(122):67–76.
10. Tlaskalová-Hogenová H, Stepánková R, Hudcovic T, Tuckov L, Cukrowska B, Lodinová-Zádníková R, Kozáková H, Rossmann P, Sokol D, Funda DP, Borovská D, Reháková Z, Sinkora J, Hofman J, Drastich P, Kokesová A. Commensal bacteria (normal microflora), mucosal immunity and chronic inflammatory and autoimmune diseases. Immunol Lett 2004;93(2/3):97–108.
11. Blaser MJ. Host-Pathogen Interactions: Defining the Concepts of Pathogenicity, Virulence, Colonization, Commensalisms, and Symbiosis, Ending the War Metaphor: The Changing Agenda for Unravelling the Host-Microbe Relationship, Institute of Medicine, Forum on Microbial Threats, The National Academy Press, Washington, DC. 2005, pp. 115–130.
12. Nicholson JK, Holmes E, Wilson ID. Gut microorgaism, mammalian metablolism and personalized health care. Nat Rev Microbiol 2005;3:1–8.
13. Wilson M. Microbial Inhabitants of Humans: Their Ecology and Role in Health and Disease. Cambridge University Press, UK. 2004.
14. Tannock GW. Normal Flora: An Introduction to Microbes Inhabiting the Human Body. Chapman & Hall, London. 1995.
15. Miller WD. The Micro-organisms of the Human Mouth. S.S. White Dental MFGC., Philadelphia. 1980.
16. Socransky SS, Manganiello SD. The oral microbiota of man from birth to senility. J Periodontol 1971;42:485–496.
17. Tagg JR, Pybus V, Phillips LV. Application of inhibitor typing in a study of transmission and retention in the human mouth of the bacterium *Stretococcus salivarius*. Arch Oral Biol 1983;28:911–915.
18. Carlsson J, Grahnén H, Jonsson G. Lactobacilli and streptococci in the mouth of children. Caries Res 1975;9(5):333–339.
19. Ikeda T, Sandham HJ. Prevalence of *Streptococcus mutans* on various tooth surfaces in Negro children. Arch Oral Biol 1971;16:1237–1240.
20. Frisken KW, Tagg JR, Laws AJ, Orr MB. Suspected periodontopathic microorganisms and their oral habitat in young children. Oral Microbiol Immunol 1987;2:60–64.
21. Delaney JE, Ratzan SK, Kornman KS. Subgingival microbiota associated with puberty: studies of pre-, circum- and postpubertal human females. Pediatr Dent 1986;8:268275.
22. Wojcicki CJ, Harper DS, Robinson PJ. Differences in periodontal disease-associated microorganisms of subgingival plaque in prepubertal, pubertal and postpubertal children. J Periodontol 1987;58:219–223.
23. Fujimoto C, Maeda H, Kokeguchi S, Takashiba S, Nishimura F, Arai H, Fukui K, Murayama Y. Application of denaturing gradient gel electrophoresis (DGGE) to the analysis of microbial communities of subgingival plaque. J Periodontal Res 2003;38:440–445.
24. Emilson CG, Krasse B. Support for and implications of the specific plaque hypothesis. Scan J Dent Res 1985;93:96–104.

25. Theilade E, Wright WH, Jensen S, Loe H. Experimental gingivitis in man. II. A longitudinal clinical and bacteriological investigation. J Periodontal Res 1966;1:1–13.
26. Roberts AK, Van-Bierevliet J-P, Harzer G. Factors of human milk influencing the bacterial flora of infant faeces. In Composition and Physiological Properties of Human Milk (Schraub J, ed.), Elsevier, Amsterdam. 1985, p. 259.
27. Pei Z, Bini EJ, Yang L, Zhou M, Francois F, Blaser MJ. Bacterial biota in the human distal oesophagus. Proc Natl Acad Sci USA 2004;101:4250–4255.
28. Finegold SM. Normal indigenous intestinal flora. In Human Intestinal Microflora in Health and Disease (Hentges DJ, ed.), Academic Press, New York. 1983, pp. 3–31.
29. Borriello SP. Microbial flora of the gastrointestinal tract. In Microbial Metabolism in the Digestive Tract (Hill MJ, ed.), CRC Press, Boca Raton, FL. 1986.
30. Drasar BS, Shiner M, McLeod G. Studies on the intestinal flora. I. The bacterial flora of the gastrointestinal tract in healthy and achlorhydric persons. Gastroenterology 1969;56:71–79.
31. Drasar BS, Roberts AK. Control of the large bowel microflora. In Human Microbial Ecology (Hill MJ and Marsh PD, eds), CRC Press, Boca Raton, FL. 1990, pp. 89–110.
32. Hebuterne X. Gut changes attributed to aging: effects on intestinal microflora. Curr Opin Clin Nutr Metab Care 2003;6:49–54.
33. Bourlioux P, Koletzko B, Guarner F, Braesco V. The intestine and its microflora are partners for the protection of the host: report on the Danone Symposium "The Intelligent Intestine", held in Paris, June 14, 2002. Am J Clin Nutr 2003;78:675–683.
34. Penders J, Thijs C, van den Brandt PA, Kummeling I, Snijders B, Stelma F, Adams H, van Ree R, Stobberingh EE. Gut microbiota composition and development of atopic manifestations in infancy: the KOALA Birth Cohort Study. Gut 2007;56(5):661–667.
35. Cooperstock MS, Zedd AA. Intestinal flora of infants. In Human Intestinal Microflora in Health and Disease (Hentges DJ, ed.), Academic Press, New York. 1983, p. 79.
36. Roberts AK. The development of the infant faecal flora, Ph.D. Thesis, CNAA. 1988.
37. Jatsyk GV, Kuvaeva IB, Gribakin SG. Immunological protection of the neonatal gastrointestinal tract: the importance of breast feeding. Acta Paediatr Scand 1985;74:246–249.
38. Bullen CL, Tearle PV, Willis AT. Bifidiobacteria in the intestinal tract of infants: an *in vivo* study. J Med Microbiol 1976;9:325–333.
39. Stark PL, Lee A. The microbial ecology of the large bowel of breast-fed and formula-fed infants during the first year of life. J Med Microbiol 1982;15:189–203.
40. Harmsen HJ, Wildeboer-Veloo AC, Raangs GC, Wagendorp AA, Klijn N, Bindels JG, Welling GW. Analysis of intestinal flora development in breast-fed and formula-fed infants using molecular identification and detection methods. J Pediatr Gastroenterol Nutr 2000;30:61–67.
41. Mackie RI, Sghir A, Gaskins HR. Developmental microbial ecology of the neonatal gastrointestinal tract. Am J Clin Nutr 1999;69:1035–1045.
42. Rotimi VO, Duerden BI. The development of the bacterial flora in normal neonates. J Med Microbiol 1981;14:51–62.
43. Andrieux C, Membré JM, Cayuela C, Antoine JM. Metabolic characteristics of the faecal microflora in humans from three age groups. Scand J Gastroenterol 2002;37(7):792–798.
44. Rinne M, Kalliomäki M, Salminen S, Isolauri E. Probiotic intervention in the first months of life: short-term effects on gastrointestinal symptoms and long-term effects on gut microbiota. J Pediatr Gastroenterol Nutr 2006;43(2):200–205.
45. Zhang T, Breitbart M, Lee WH, Run JQ, Wei CL, Soh SWL, Hibberd ML, Liu ET, Rohwer F, Ruan YJ. RNA viral community in human feces: prevalence of plant pathogenic viruses. PLoS Biol 2006;4:108–118.
46. Backhed F, Levy RE, Sonnenburg JL, Peterson DA, Gordon JI. Host-bacterial mutualism in the human intestine. Science 2005;307:1915–1920.
47. Blaut M, Collins MD, Welling GW, Dore J, van Loo J, de Vos W. Molecular biological methods for studying the gut microbiota: The EU human gut flora project. Br J Nutr 2002;87(2):S203–S211.

48. Rajilic-Stojanovic M. Diversity of the human gastrointestinal microbiota: novel perspectives from high throughput analyses, Ph.D. Thesis, Wageningen University, Wageningen, the Netherlands. 2007.
49. Noverr MC, Huffnagle GB. Does the microbiota regulate immune responses outside the gut? Trends Microbiol 2004;12:562–568.
50. Philips ML. Interdomain interactions: dissecting animal-bacterial symbioses. Bioscience 2006;56:376–381.
51. Suau A, Bonnet R, Sutren M, Godon JJ, Gibson GR, Collins MD, Dore J. Direct analysis of genes encoding 16S rDNA from complex communities reveals many novel molecular species within the human gut. Appl Environ Microbiol 1999;65:4799–4807.
52. Moore WEC, Cato EP, Holdeman LV. Anaerobic bacteria of the gastrointestinal flora and their occurrence in clinical infections. J Infect Dis 1969;119:641–649.
53. Hopkins MJ, MacFarlane GT. Changes in predominant bacterial populations in human faeces with age and with *Clostridium difficile* infection. J Med Microbiol 2002;51:448–454.
54. Bartosch S, Fite A, Macfarlane GT, McMurdo ME. Characterization of bacterial communities in feces from healthy elderly volunteers and hospitalized elderly patients by using real-time PCR and effects of antibiotic treatment on the fecal microbiota. Appl Environ Microbiol 2004;70(6):3575–3581.
55. Woodmansey EJ, McMurdo ME, Macfarlane GT, Macfarlane S. Comparison of compositions and metabolic activities of fecal microbiotas in young adults and in antibiotic-treated and non-antibiotic-treated elderly subjects. Appl Environ Microbiol 2004;70(10):6113–6122.
56. Hopkins MJ, Sharp R, Macfarlane GT. Variation in human intestinal microbiota with age. Dig Liver Dis 2002;34:S12–S18.
57. Severijnen AJ, van Kleef R, Hazenberg MP, van de Merwe JP. Cell wall fragments from major residents of the human intestinal flora induce chronic arthritis in rats. J Rheumatol 1989;16 (8):1061–1068.
58. Mitsuoka T, Hayakawa K, Kimura N. The faecal flora of man. II. The composition of bifidobacterium flora of different age groups (author's transl). Zentralbl Bakteriol Orig A 1974;226(4):469–478.
59. He F, Ouwehand AC, Isolauri E, Hashimoto H, Benno Y, Salminen S. Comparison of mucosal adhesion and species identification of bifidobacteria isolated from healthy and allergic infants. FEMS Immunol Med Microbiol 2001;30(1):43–47.
60. He F, Ouwehand AC, Isolauri E, Hosoda M, Benno Y, Salminen S. Differences in composition and mucosal adhesion of bifidobacteria isolated from healthy adults and healthy seniors. Curr Microbiol 2001;43(5):351–354.
61. Long SS. Capsules, clones and curious events: pneumococcus under fire from polysaccharide conjugate vaccine. Clin Infect Dis 2005;41(1):30–34.
62. Hunter CA Jr, Long KR. A study of the microbiological flora of the vagina. Am J Obstet Gynecol 1958;75(4):865–871.
63. Levison ME, Corman LC, Carrington ER, Kaye D. Quantitative microflora of the vagina. Am J Obstet Gynecol 1977;127:80–85.
64. Cruickshank R, Sharman A. The biology of the vagina in the human subject. II. The bacterial flora and secretion of the vagina at various age periods and their relation to glycogen in the vaginal epithelium. J Obstet Gynaecol Br Emp 1936;32:208–212.
65. Armstrong RA. The microbiology of the eye. Ophthalmic Physiol Opt 2000;20:29–41.
66. Wilcox M, Stapleton F. Occular bacteriology. Med Microbiol Rev 1996;7:123–131.
67. Ramachandran L, Sharma S, Sankaridurg PR, Vajdic CM, Chuck JA, Holden BA, Sweeney DF, Rao GN. Examination of the conjunctival microbiota after 8 hours of eye closure. CLAO J 1995;21:195–199.
68. Kirkwood BJ. Normal flora of the external eye. Insight 2007;32(1):12–13.
69. Carter JA, Neville BG, Newton CR. Neurocognitive impairment following acquired central nervous system infections in childhood; a systematic review. Brain Res Brain Res Rev 2003;43:57–69.

70. Hosoglu S, Geyik MF, Balik I, Aygen B, Erol S, Aygencel TG, Mert A, Saltoglu N, Dokmetas I, Felek S, Sunbul M, Irmak H, Aydin K, Kokoglu OF, Ucmak H, Altindis M, Loeb M. Predictors of outcome in patients with tuberculous meningitis. Int J Tuberc Lung Dis 2002;6 (1):64–70.
71. Haughey NJ, Mattson MP. Calcium dysregulation and neuronal apoptosis by the HIV-1 proteins Tat and gp120. J Acquir Immune Defic Syndr 2002;31(2):S55–S61.
72. Eikelenboom P, Bate C, Van Gool WA, Hoozemans JJ, Rozemuller JM, Veerhuis R, Williams A. Neuroinflammation in Alzheimer's disease and prion disease. Glia 2002;40(2):232–239.
73. Martyn CN. Infection in childhood and neurological diseases in adult life. Br Med Bull 1997; 53:24–39.
74. Kristensson K, Dastur DK, Manghani DK, Tsiang H, Bentivoglio M. Rabies: interactions between neurons and viruses. A review of the history of Negri inclusion bodies. Neuropathol Appl Neurobiol 1996;22:179–187.
75. Griffin DE. A review of alphavirus replication in neurons. Neurosci Biobehav Rev 1998; 22:721–723.
76. Schneider-Schaulies J, ter Meulen V, Schneider-Schaulies S. Measles virus interactions with cellular receptors: consequences for viral pathogenesis. J Neurovirol 2001;7:391–399.
77. Mettenleiter TC. Pathogenesis of neurotropic herpesviruses: role of viral glycoproteins in neuroinvasion and transneuronal spread. Virus Res 2003;92:197–206.
78. Steiner I, Nisipianu P, Wirguin I. Infection and etiology and pathogenesis of multiple sclerosis. Curr Neurol Neurosci Rep 2001;1:271–276.
79. Labetoulle M, Kucera P, Ugolini G, Lafay F, Frau E, Offret H, Flamand A. Neuronal pathways for the propagation of herpes simplex virus type 1 from one retina to the other in a murine model. J Gen Virol 2000;81:1201–1210.
80. McFarland LV. Normal flora: diversity and functions. Microb Ecol Health Dis 2000;12:193–207.
81. Westerbeek EA, van den Berg A, Lafeber HN, Knol J, Fetter WP, van Elburg RM. The intestinal bacterial colonisation in preterm infants: a review of the literature. Clin Nutr 2006;25(3):361–368.
82. Stappenbeck TS, Hooper LV, Gordon JI. Developmental regulation of intestinal angiogenesis by indigenous microbes via Paneth cells. Proc Natl Acad Sci U S A 2002;99:15451–15455.
83. Alekshun MN, Levy SB. Commensals upon us. Biochem Pharmacol 2006;71:893–900.

Chapter 3
Infections in the Elderly

Knut Ohlsen, Svitlana Kozytska, and Udo Lorenz

Introduction

Infections continue to be a major cause of morbidity and mortality in elderly patients. According to a recent study, hospitalizations for infectious diseases represent the second highest proportion of all discharges among older adults.[1] The problem is of increasing importance because of the demographic changes anticipated for the future decades. These changes will lead to a substantial increase in the number of older persons in the world. While in the industrialized countries the average life expectancy will rise moderately by 6–8 years in the next five decades, the increase in the developing world will be 20 years, resulting in an average life expectancy in these regions of 70 years. It is expected that the percentage of people aged 65 and older will increase in the more developed regions, rising from 15.3% in the year 2005 to 25.9% in 2050 (http://www.un.org/esa/population/publications/WPP2004/WPP2004_Vol3_Final/Chapter2.pdfUN-report and http://www.un.org/esa/population/publications/WPP2004/WPP2004_Vol3_Final/Chapter2.pdfUN-report).

In 2050, almost every second person in the industrialized world will be older than 55 years, and especially very old persons will have a substantial impact on the population structure. Likewise, population dynamics in the rapidly developing countries such as China, India, and Brazil shows similar characteristics. These dramatic changes in age structure of the population have major implications for all national health care systems. In the United States, elderly people aged 65 and older constituted 12% of the population in 2005, but they comprised 34% of the hospitalizations (http://www.hcup-us.ahrq.gov/reports/factsandfigures/HAR_2005.pdf). It is well known that the rates of hospitalization and length of hospital stays increase with

K.Ohlsen, and S. Kozytska,
University of Würzburg, Institute for Molecular Infection Biology, Röntgenring 11, 97070 Würzburg, Germany

U. Lorenz
University of Würzburg, Centre for Operative Medicine, Department of Surgery, Oberdürrbacher Str. 6, 97080 Würzburg, Germany

S.L. Percival (ed.), *Microbiology and Aging.*
DOI: 10.1007/978-1-59745-327-1_3, © Springer Science + Business Media, LLC 2009

age. There are several reasons why especially older persons are jeopardized by pathogenic agents. Older adults more often have chronic diseases such as diabetes mellitus, atherosclerosis, rheumatism, and vascular diseases and therefore are more susceptible to common infections. In addition to multiple, chronic, comorbid diseases, an impaired immune system, a decreased protection by vaccines, prolonged stay in hospitals, permanent catheterization, invasive procedures, malabsorption, or polypharmacy are further reasons why older patients have a higher risk to contract an infection. On the other hand, infections in the elderly pose specific problems due to the lack of signs and symptoms that are common in younger adults, such as fever and leukocytosis.

In this review the most important types of infections in the elderly are introduced.

Urinary Tract Infections

Urinary tract infections (UTIs) are the second most common infections in the elderly (Fig. 3.1). Many of these infections occur in the setting of urethral catheterization and neurogenic bladders with increased residual urine.[2] In addition, gender-specific factors contribute to an increased risk for developing UTI, such as prostatic hypertrophy in man, an increase in vaginal pH, vaginal atrophy due to postmenopausal estrogen depletion, and incomplete emptying of the bladder in women. These factors favor the colonization of the urinary tract by bacteria.

UTIs due to catheterization are especially common in nursing homes. The diagnosis of asymptomatic bacteriuria or chronic UTIs is often problematic because classical clinical manifestations such as dysuria, fever, and urinary frequency may be absent or masked in older patients. Usually the intestinal flora serves as source of infection. Several pathogens have been recognized to be responsible for causing UTIs including *Escherichia coli*, *Klebsiella* sp., *Proteus* sp., *Pseudomonas aeruginosa*, enterococci, coagulase-negative staphylococci and *Candida* sp. Mostly, UTI start as bladder infections and often evolve to encompass the kidneys. Importantly, up to 25% of patients requiring a urinary catheter for >7 days develop catheter-associated UTI, which account for 40% of all nosocomial infections.[3] However, short-term catheterization also presents a considerable risk factor. The main indications for catheterization are incontinence, obstruction, and perioperative monitoring. The number of patients developing UTIs due to catheterization could be lowered by an improved catheter management. In a European study, the indication for bladder catheterization was inadequate or unnecessary in up to 31% of the cases.[4] Importantly, catheter-associated UTIs are often asymptomatic, and therefore are unrecognized by healthcare workers. In many cases, these infections become chronic owing to a high rate of recurrence. Secondary bloodstream infections are uncommon, and in those cases where sepsis developed, in only 3% of all patients the microorganism recovered from the urine was also isolated by blood culture. *Escherichia coli* is the cause of the majority (>35–70%) of UTIs in all ages. The group of *E. coli* bacteria that causes UTI is specifically called uropathogenic *E. coli* (UPEC).[5] It is currently not known whether the virulence potential of a

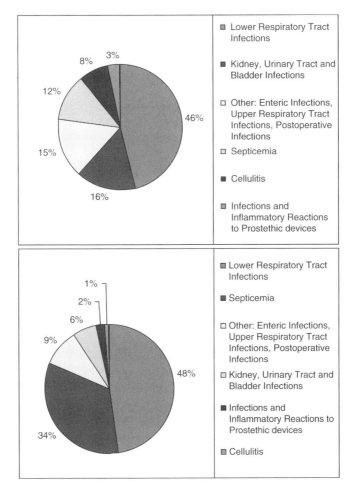

Fig. 3.1 Proportion of infectious disease hospitalizations (**a**) and infectious disease-related deaths (**b**) according to infectious disease group among patients 65 years or older in the United States from 2000 through 2002 (adapted from Ref. 1) (See Color Plates)

pathogen causing UTIs differs between young and older patients. Many virulence properties of UPEC enable the pathogen to colonize the urinary tract such as adhesins, e.g., type 1 and P fimbriae, Ag43 and toxins, e.g., hemolysin. Adherence to the urinary tract epithelium is often the first step in establishment of UTI, as adherent bacteria are able to resist the hydrodynamic forces of urine flow. In addition, the bacteria interact with functions of the host including cell signaling pathways. Among the adhesins, P fimbriae show the strongest disease association in clinical studies. P fimbriae contribute to the establishment of bacteriuria by binding to the α-D-galactopyranosyl-(1-4)-β-D-galactopyranoside receptor epitope in the globoseries of glycolipids[6,7] and activate innate immune responses in animal models and in the human urinary tract.[7] Type 1 fimbriae also enhance colonization and induce immune responses in the mouse UTI model.[8,9] Type 1 fimbriae confer binding to D-mannosylated proteins, such as uroplakins, which are abundant in the bladder.[10]

Symptomatic UTIs should be treated with antimicrobials. Although resistance rates are increasing, fluoroquinolones and trimethoprim/sulfamethoxazole have remained the antibiotic treatments of choice for therapy of uncomplicated UTIs. Fluoroquinolones such as ciprofloxacin have been recommended in acute pyelonephritis in older patients because of increased bacterial eradication, tolerability, and fewer adverse side effects.[11] In every case, treatment should be directed to the microorganism identified in the urine considering resistance profiles. Importantly, polymicrobial infections occur in about 30% of patients, especially, if the UTI is related to catheterization. These patients should be treated with broad spectrum antibiotics targeting also Gram-positive bacteria such as enterococci and staphylococci.

Pneumonia

Pneumonia is a leading cause of death in the elderly and a complex relationship exists between age and the incidence and mortality of pneumonia[12] (Fig. 3.1). For example, the incidence rate was increased by age groups from 2 of 1,000 hospital discharges in individuals younger than 60 years to 17 of 1,000 hospital discharges in patients older than 70 years.[13] Hospital mortality doubled with age from 7.8% in those aged 65–69 years to 15.4% in those aged 90 years and older.[14] Hospitalization rates for pneumonia have increased among U.S. adults aged 64–74 years and aged 75–84 years during the past 15 years. Among those aged 85 years or older, at least 1 in 20 patients was hospitalized each year because of pneumonia. Concomitantly, the proportion of comorbid chronic diseases has increased.

The development of pneumonia in elderly patients differs from that in younger individuals because of a complex array of factors. First, the major risk factor for developing pneumonia in the elderly is the presence of other serious illnesses (e.g., cardiopulmonary disease, renal insufficiency, diabetes mellitus, neurologic disorders, endocrine disease, and, especially, neoplastic disease) and those affect also the outcome of pneumonia. Pneumonia is often the terminal event after prolonged serious illness. The mortality rate from pneumonia in patients older than 65 years ranged from 9 per 100,000 in the absence of health-risk conditions, to 979 per 100,000 when two or more health-risk conditions exist.[15] In this regard, depression of the immune system in elderly appears to be less important than the presence of concomitant diseases, since defense mechanisms (e.g., humoral and complement systems, macrophage, and neutrophil function) are relatively intact in elderly patients. Second, the presenting symptoms of pneumonia in the elderly can be subtle with confusion or tachypnea rather than classic symptoms such as fever, chills, and rigors. Patients aged 65–74 years and 75 years had mean numbers 2.9 and 3.3 fewer symptoms, respectively, than those aged 18–44 years.[16] Another presentation is that of an acute decompensation of a more obvious underlying disease (e.g., congestive heart failure, chronic obstructive pulmonary disease, or diabetes mellitus).[17] Third, colonization and adherence of the respiratory tract with potentially pathogenic Gram-negative and Gram-positive bacteria occur more often in the elderly than in younger persons, owing in part to such factors as repeated antibiotic therapy, endotracheal intubation and other mechanical devices, smoking, malnutrition, surgery, and pharmacologic alterations of the oral and/or gastric pH. Other predisposing factors for developing pneumonia are aerosolization of pathogens with inhalation of microparticles (e.g., *Mycobacterium tuberculosis*, *Legionella* spp., influenza virus, and the invasive, multidrug-resistant *Streptococcus pneumoniae*) and silent aspiration of gastric contents with Gram-negative bacilli, sometimes in association with anaerobes or anaerobic bacteria that normally reside in the gingival crevices (e.g., peptostreptococci, fusobacteria, black-pigmented anaerobes). Notable, gastric and jejunostomy feeding tubes do not necessarily prevent aspiration.[18] Furthermore, the aging lung impairs the elasticity and mucociliary clearance within the lung.[19] Elderly patients also may have a less effective cough due to underlying illness, weakness, and coexisting pulmonary disease. As already stated, the characteristic clinical features of fever, cough, and sputum production are often subtle and incompletely expressed in elderly patients. The classical constellation of pneumonia in the elderly of cough, fever, and dyspnea might be absent in 56% of patients.[20] Instead, elderly patients with pneumonia commonly present with acute confusion or delirium and deterioration of the baseline function. Tachypnea and tachycardia may be presenting signs.

Chest X-ray is usually diagnostic, and multilobe involvement is seen more often in elderly patients. The diagnosis should not be exclusively made on the basis of expectorated sputum, because expectorated sputum does not distinguish colonization from true pulmonary infection. Transtracheal aspiration, transthoracic aspiration, and bronchoscopy using a protected brush may produce reliable results but are rarely used in elderly patients for routine diagnostic evaluation. Treatment of pneumonia includes antimicrobial drug therapy, respiratory supportive care, and, if needed, drainage of empyemas or significant pleural effusions. Recommendations for antimicrobial drug use depend on the specific organism. In the case of negative cultures, the therapy should be empiric and it is therefore important to anticipate the types of pathogens that might be expected in different settings (Table 3.1). In community-acquired pneumonia (nonhospitalized elderly persons), a limited number of pathogens is responsible for disease. *S. pneumoniae* infections are diagnosed most often, and are believed to cause most of the infections that lack a definitive diagnosis. An increasing incidence of drug-resistant pneumococci up to 25% is recognized.[21] Other causes include *Haemophilus influenzae*, influenza virus and other viruses, mixed bacterial or mixed viral and bacterial infections, Gram-negative bacilli, *Staphylococcus aureus*, and atypical pneumonia organisms (e.g., *Mycoplasma* species, *Legionella* species, *Coxiella* species, or *Chlamydia* (*C. pneumoniae* or *C. psittaci*). In nursing home-acquired pneumonia (institutionalized elderly persons), bacterial pneumonia is due to *H. influenzae*, Gram-negative rods (including *Klebsiella* and *Pseudomonas*), streptococci other than the pneumococcus, and *S. aureus*. In hospital-acquired pneumonia (hospitalized elderly persons),

Table 3.1 Major etiologies of pneumonia in elderly persons (%)

Organism	Community	Nursing home	Hospital
Streptococcus pneumoniae	30–60	12–24	6–15
Staphylococcus aureus	5	5–26	3–15
Haemophilus influenzae	7–15	5–20	–
Gram-negative bacilli (including *Klebsiella, Pseudomonas, Acinetobacter, Enterobacter*)	5–15	12–35	40–75
Gram-negative cocci (*Moraxella catarrhalis*)	5–10	a	–
Viral infection	a	a	–
Mycobacterium tuberculosis	a	a	–
Polymicrobial	20–25	40–50	30–40
"Atypical" organisms (*Mycoplasma pneumoniae, Legionella* species, *Chlamydia pneumoniae, Coxiella burnetii*)	5	5	–

[a]Recognized as important etiology, but frequency in elderly is unclear

Gram-negative bacilli including *P. aeruginosa, Klebsiella, Acinetobacter* spp., and *Enterobacter* spp. as well as Gram-positive cocci such as *S. aureus* are the major causes.[22]

Currently, vaccination is available only for prevention of influenza as well as pneumococcal pneumonia and *Haemophilus influenzae* type b (HiBb). Vaccination against influenza and *Streptococcus pneumoniae* is recommended for all persons older than 65 years or for persons with significant underlying immunodeficiency, renal disease, diabetes, or malignancy. There is some controversy regarding the use of pneumococcal vaccines. In a recent meta-analysis examining the effectiveness of pneumococcal vaccination, no evidence was found that the vaccine was less efficacious for the elderly, institutionalized people, or those with chronic disease.[23]

With increasing rates of institutionalization and hospitalization of the elderly, they are necessarily exposed to more virulent pathogens and increasing antimicrobial resistance. Although the understanding of its pathogenesis is constantly improving, an accurate diagnosis of pneumonia remains a difficult clinical problem. The subtle nature of clinical signs, symptoms, and X-ray findings can present a misleading picture. Thus, the vigilance for recognizing pneumonia and initiating treatment in elderly patients should be higher than in younger adults. By recognizing pathogens associated with the clinical setting in which pneumonia develop (community, nursing home, or hospital) and appreciating the risk factors associated with these settings, a rational basis for initial therapy can be derived. Many effective antibiotics are available, and considering the high risks of pneumonia, treating elderly patients requires increased efforts in disease prevention.

Sepsis and Bacteremia

The incidence of sepsis is disproportionately increased in older patients, and age is an independent predictor of mortality.[24] Sepsis and septic shock are associated commonly with bacterial infection, but bacteremia may not be present. Bacteremia is the presence of viable bacteria within the liquid component of blood. Bacteremia may be transient, as is seen commonly after injury to a mucosal surface, primary (without an identifiable focus of infection), or more commonly secondary to an intravascular or extravascular focus of infection. Because of comorbidities, immunosupression, use of foreign body devices, and increased use of invasive methods, elderly persons are at high risk for sepsis. There is a trend that the average age of patients with sepsis increases consistently over time.[25] The relative frequency of specific causative organisms has shifted over time, as indicated by the emergence of fungal pathogens and the recent pre-eminence of Gram-positive organisms.[25,26] The most important pathogens causing sepsis are the Gram-positive species *Staphylococcus aureus*, *S. epidermidis*, *Enterococcus faecalis* and *E. faecium*, and Gram-negatives such as *E. coli*, *Klebsiella* spp., *Proteus mirabilis*, *Pseudomonas aeruginiosa*, *Acinetobacter* spp. as well as fungi such as *Candida albicans* and *Aspergillus* spp.[27] The dramatic augmentation that has been noted in the bacteremic cases due to Gram-positive cocci and fungi is attributable to several reasons including increasing occurrence of antimicrobial resistance, widespread use of invasive procedures and immunosuppressive drugs, chemotherapy, and transplantation. Many of these pathogens are normal inhabitants of the human body colonizing the skin (*S. epidermidis*) or gastro-intestinal tract (enterococci, *E. coli*) and have been historically regarded as apathogenic or with low pathopotency. However, these pathogens are now being recognized to infect especially immunocompromised persons in intensive care units, carrier of foreign bodies, and older patients. Importantly, all these opportunistic pathogens have the capacity to acquire multiple antibiotic resistance traits.[28]

For example, *Staphylococcus epidermidis* is primarily a normal inhabitant of the healthy human skin and mucosal microflora. In recent decades, however, the bacterium emerges as a common cause of nosocomial infections.[29] Mostly, these infections occur in association with the use of medical devices and they preferentially affect immunocompromised and critically ill patients causing acute bacteremia and septicemia. The ability of *S. epidermidis* to form biofilms on medical devices is regarded as a major virulence mechanism (Fig. 3.2). It is interesting to note that some *S. epidermidis* clones are especially successful in establishing nosocomial infections. Molecular analysis has revealed that these clones are biofilm positive, express multiple resistance traits, and often harbor a specific insertion element IS256. Moreover, multilocus sequence typing (MLST) identified ST27 (now reclassified as ST2) as the predominant clonal type.[30] Obviously, there is a strong selection towards specific virulence properties in hospitals that enable *S. epidermidis* bacteria to survive and to cause infections under these conditions. Interestingly, the capacity to form thick multilayered biofilms on polymer and metal surfaces[31] is associated mostly with the synthesis of an extracellular polysaccharide, the so-called polysaccharide intercellular adhesin (PIA). The enzymes involved in PIA production are encoded by the *icaADBC* operon.[32] Numerous studies have shown that the *icaADBC* genes are more prevalent in *S. epidermidis*

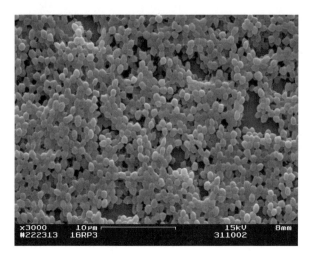

Fig. 3.2 Scanning electron microscopic image of *S. epidermidis* RP 62A biofilm

strains from device-associated infections than in commensal isolates.[33,34] There-fore, this genetic information has been regarded as a discriminating factor between pathogenic and nonpathogenic *S. epidermidis* strains. Biofilm-positive bacteria are less susceptible to the action of antibiotics and are shielded from the host immune system through the slimy polysaccharide matrix.

Symptoms of sepsis are usually nonspecific and include fever, chills, and constitutional symptoms of fatigue, malaise, anxiety, or confusion. These symptoms are not pathognomonic for infection and may be seen in a wide variety of noninfectious inflammatory conditions.[35] They may be absent in serious infections, especially in elderly individuals. The therapy of sepsis and bacteremia has some priorities. The blood must be cleared rapidly of bacteria by adequate antibiotic therapy. Certain antimicrobial agents may cause the patients to get worse. It is believed that certain antimicrobials trigger more LPS to be released, causing more problems for the patient. Antimicrobials that do NOT cause the patient to get worse are carbapenems, ceftriaxone, cefepime, glycopeptides, aminoglycosides, and qui-nolones. Prompt institution of empiric treatment with antimicrobials is essential (see Annane et al. for review[35]). The early institution of antimicrobials has been shown to decrease the development of shock and to lower the mortality rate. After the appropriate samples are obtained from the patient, a regimen of antimicrobials with a broad spectrum of activity is needed. This is because antimicrobial therapy is almost always instituted before the organisms causing the sepsis are identified. Furthermore, the original focus of infection must be treated by removal of foreign bodies, drainage of purulent exudate, particularly for anaerobic infections, and removal of infected organs: debride or amputate gangrenous tissues. Despite aggressive treatment, mortality ranges from 15% in patients with bacteremia and sepsis to 40–60% in patients with septic shock.[36–38]

Skin and Soft-Tissue Infections

Skin and soft-tissue infections (SSTIs) are a common cause of morbidity in older patients primarily due to *Streptococcus* and *Staphylococcus* species. Dry, atrophied, pruritic skin with a reduced capacity for immunologic defense and mechanical repair predisposes the elderly patient to a variety of skin infections. Risk factors such as diabetes and conditions that worsen the skin circulation, such as heart failure, trauma, chronic skin conditions (e.g., eczema) and obesity, facilitate the entry of pathogens into the skin.

Cellulitis

Cellulitis is an infection of the dermis and subcutaneous tissue. Symptoms include local erythema, edema, pain, and tenderness. More complicated infections are marked by systemic symptoms, such as fever and leukocytosis, and can develop into a life-threatening emergency. Erysipelas is a form of cellulitis that affects only the top layers of the skin and is characterized by particularly sharp demarcations and lymphatic inflammation. Superficial cutaneous edema surrounding hair follicles anchored to the dermis sometimes produces a classic dimpled appearance of the skin resembling an orange peel ("peau d'orange").[39] Bullous erysipelas occurs in more or less 5% of the patients and is prevalent in elderly persons and in patients with diabetes mellitus.[40] Potential complications of cellulitis and erysipelas include spread of the infection with septicemia, thrombophlebitis, septic arthritis, osteomyelitis, and endocarditis. Erysipelas is preferentially found on the extremities and within the face. *S. pyogenes* (beta-hemolytic streptococci belonging to Lancefield group A), and *S. aureus* are the most common causes of cellulitis and erysipelas, but erysipelas and bacteremia with a non-haemolytic, streptolysin S-deficient *S. pyogenes* have also been reported.[41,42] With the sequencing of several *S. pyogenes* genomes have come major advances in understanding the pathogenesis of group A *Streptococcus*-associated diseases. Group A *Streptococcus* shows enormous and evolving molecular diversity driven by horizontal transmission between group A *Streptococcus* strains and other streptococci. Acquisition of prophages accounts for much of the diversity, conferring both virulence through phage-associated virulence factors and increased bacterial survival against host defenses.[43,44] One of the key bacteriophage-encoded virulence factors is a putative "hyaluronidase", HylP1, a phage tail-fiber protein responsible for the digestion of the *S. pyogenes* hyaluronan capsule during phage infection.[45] Among the many factors involved in the virulence of the pathogen, the M protein and a group of exotoxins known as *streptococcal superantigens* (SAgs) have received considerable attention. The M protein is exposed from the group A *Streptococcus* (GAS) cell surface as a helical coiled-coil molecule that is antiphagocytic, thereby promoting bacterial survival. Soluble M1 protein likely contributes to the excessive T-cell activation and hyperinflammatory response seen in severe invasive streptococcal infections and is a potent inducer of T-cell proliferation and release of Th1-type cytokines.[46] Sequence analysis of the *emm* gene (encoding the M protein) has become an important surveillance tool for investigating the dynamics of GAS infection, and more than 150 *emm* gene sequence types and several *emm* subtypes have been documented.[47]

Cellulitis and erysipelas require antibiotic treatment. In most cases, they should be treated with intravenous antibiotics if the infection is complicated or of significant extent, or present with a coincident disease. The most common antibiotics used to treat cellulitis and erysipelas are penicillins and cephalosporins. For patients allergic to penicillin or suspected of being infected with an antibiotic-resistant organism, vancomycin or clindamycin is recommended.[48,49]

Necrotizing Fasciitis

Necrotizing SSTIs are infrequent but rapidly progressing and life threatening involving the superficial fascial layers of the extremities, abdomen, or perineum. They require immediate medical attention and emergency surgery to prevent morbidity and death. Early diagnosis and prompt treatment are of prior importance in the treatment of this infection. Necrotizing fasciitis occur frequently as a consequence of trauma or surgery but also after innocuous events such as an insect bite. Only one-third of cases are correctly diagnosed as necrotizing fasciitis and more than two-thirds admitted for instances as "cellulitis".[50,51] The three important forms of necrotizing fasciitis are type I, or polymicrobial (e.g., aerobic Gram-negative bacteria (*Escherichia coli*, *Enterobacter* spp., *Klebsiella* spp., *Proteus mirabilis*); anaerobic Gram-negative bacteria (*Bacteroides* spp., *Fusobacterium* spp.); anaerobic Gram-positive bacteria (*Peptoccocus* spp., *Clostridium* spp.), type II, or group A streptococcal (may be in combination with *Staphylococcus aureus*), and type III gas gangrene, or clostridial myonecrosis. In rare cases, *Aspergillus* species, unencapsulated *Haemophilus influenzae* infection may cause necrotizing fasciitis.[52,53] Differentiating necrotizing infections from common soft-tissue infections is critically important. The laboratory risk indicator for necrotizing fasciitis score can be helpful in distinguishing between cases of cellulitis that should respond to medical management alone and necrotizing soft tissue infections that require operative debridement in addition to antimicrobial therapy.[54] Minor skin infections such as furuncles were found to be present in about 20% of patients before developing necrotizing fasciitis. Treatment for necrotizing fasciitis necessitates therapy involving several antibiotics such as gentamicin and clindamycin. Consideration should be given to cover both aerobes and anaerobes.[55]

One of the problems of nursing home and long-term-care facilities (LTCFs) is infections complicated by antimicrobial-resistant pathogens. The residents in LTCFs have a high frequency of colonization with antimicrobial-resistant organisms, including methicillin-resistant *Staphylococcus aureus* (MRSA), vancomycin-resistant enterococci (VRE), penicillin-resistant pneumococci, extended spectrum β-lactamase-producing and fluoroquinolone-resistant Gram-negative organisms.[56]

Importantly, MRSA has emerged as the major nosocomial pathogen during the past two decades, and is now deeply entrenched in both healthcare facilities and the community at large.[57] All MRSA strains have acquired the so-called *mecA* gene that encodes an additional penicillin-binding protein, PBP2a, which confers cross-resistance to all beta-lactams, including penicillins, carbapenems, and cephalosporins. The pathogen is increasingly recognized in infections among persons in the community and also nursing homes without established risk factors for MRSA, and there is ongoing rise in the incidence of community-acquired MRSA in patients with SSTIs.[58,59] MRSA strains associated with furunculosis, cutaneous abscess, cellulitis, and necrotizing fasciitis usually possess genes for Panton–Valentine leukocidin (PVL)[60,61] and sometimes other virulence genes such as those for toxic shock syndrome or exfoliative toxins.[62]

The antibiotic therapy used in SSTIs in the elderly should include MRSA coverage as indicated. In addition, new treatment options for invasive MRSA infections have been developed for anti-MRSA therapy such as linezolid, daptomycin, tigecycline, and quinupristin/dalfopristin. Moreover, a number of new anti-staphylococcal compounds are in development, including novel glycopeptides (dalbavancin, telavancin, and oritavancin), ceftobiprole, and iclaprim.[63]

Onychomycosis

Onychomycosis or tinea unguium is a skin disease of the elderly, most commonly caused by the dermatophyte *Trichophyton rubrum* but can also be caused by Candida and nondermatophyte molds. The prevalence of onychomycosis is nearly 20% in patients aged >60 years and more often in males than females. Elderly patients have specific risk factors for poor response to therapy for onychomycosis, including frequent nail dystrophy, slow growth of nails, and increased prevalence of peripheral vascular disease and diabetes mellitus. There are four types of onychomycosis: distal subungual onychomycosis, proximal subungual onychomycosis, white superficial onychomycosis, and candidal onychomycosis. Distal subungual onychomycosis, which manifests as thickened and friable nails with associated discoloration and subungual hyperkeratosis, is the most prevalent type and accounts for 75–85% of cases. Onychomycosis can provide a portal of entry for other pathogens and can be related to secondary bacterial infections in diabetic patients leading to foot ulcers and gangrene, recurrent cellulitis, and erysipelas.[64,65] The treatment options for the management of onychomycosis are oral therapies, topical nail lacquer, mechanical or chemical treatments, or a combination of one or more of these modalities.[66] Terbinafine is the drug of choice for dermatophyte onychomycosis, with greater mycological cure rates, less serious and fewer drug interactions, and a lower cost than continuous itraconazole therapy. Adjunct debridement may improve the clinical and complete cure rates compared with terbinafine alone. Unlike other oral antifungal agents, its action against dermatophytes is fungicidal as opposed to fungistatic but it is only effective against dermatophytes while other agents are also effective against nondermatophytes.[67]

Herpes Zoster

Herpes zoster, known as shingles, is caused by reactivation from previous varicella zoster virus (VZV) infection and affects millions of people worldwide. It primarily affects older adults and those with immune system dysfunction, most likely as a result of reduced or lost VZV-specific cell-mediated immunity. Varicella zoster virus infection is the pathogenic etiology of chickenpox, also referred to as *varicella*, an infection that usually happens in prepubescent children. After a chickenpox infection, VZV remains latent in an individual's dorsal root and cranial nerve ganglia even for decades. Herpes zoster is a transient disease characterized by a dermatomal rash that is usually associated with significant pain. Post-herpetic neuralgia (PHN) is the term used for the condition that exists if the pain persists after the rash has resolved.[68] Postherpetic neuralgia is particularly frequent and severe in the elderly, occurring in 25–40% of patients over the age 60 with herpes zoster. The overall incidence of herpes zoster in Europe is approximately 3 per 1,000 people per year and more than 10 per 1,000 people per year in those aged >80 years.[69] A patient with zoster usually first notices unilateral dysesthesia and pain on one side of the body almost in line (dermatomal) before any rash occurs. Within 1–3 days after the initial pain, clusters of grouped vesicles on an erythematous base or urticarial-like plaques develop.

The optimal treatment of herpes zoster and post-herpetic neuralgia requires early antiviral therapy and pain management. Acyclovir, valacyclovir, and famcyclovir can be used to treat zoster and are used for 7 days. Both the vaccine against VZV (Varivax) and the newly released vaccine against herpes zoster (Zostavax) may lead to substantial reductions in morbidity from herpes zoster and PHN in people over 60 years of age. Durability of vaccine response and possible booster vaccination will still need to be determined. In addition, current evidence suggests that multiple medications are effective in reducing the pain associated with PHN. These include tricyclic antidepressants, antiepileptics, opioids, NMDA receptor antagonists as well as topical lidocaine (lignocaine) and capsaicin.[70]

What is the Consequence of an Older Society for Infectious Disease Research?

The management of infections in the elderly as well as research on the impact of microbes on health of elderly persons is very important in the future. Importantly, the demographic transition to an "older society" requires new concepts to manage infections of the elderly in its whole including the investigation of virulence properties of microbes, epidemiology, ecology, immunology, vaccines, and treatment. However, the education of physicians and healthcare workers also needs to be improved. The investigation of such complex areas demands the close collaboration between basic research scientists and physicians and all other professionals involved in geriatric medicine. The major aim of the combined efforts should be to decrease morbidity and mortality of infections in the elderly. This could be achieved by improvement of medical care and implementation of new therapies based on novel research findings. For example, a significant proportion of UTIs could be prevented if catheterization procedures could be optimized. Moreover, a better understanding of the complex interplay of viral and bacterial pathogens of the upper respiratory tract and their impact on the outcome of an infection would improve the therapy of pneumonia. Importantly, effective vaccines against the most prevalent pathogens of respiratory diseases especially against *S. pneumoniae* could substantially lower the number of deaths due to pneumonia. Likewise, the number of nosocomial infections caused by antibiotic-resistant bacteria such as multiresistant staphylococci and enterococci, *E. coli*, *Klebsiella* spp., and *Pseudomonas aeruginosa* could be decreased by improvement of hygiene standards, optimization of antibiotic treatment, and novel therapies such as immunotherapy. As it is well recognized that the success of opportunistic pathogens depends on the status of the immune system, it should be discovered how an impaired immune reactivity impact the occurrence, incidence, course, and prognosis of an infection. These issues are of special importance since the success of preventative measures directly depend on immunological properties of older patients. Finally, it is essential to investigate how the colonization of humans by microbes is changing during the course of life. New molecular typing methods allow specifically the characterization of individual colonization patterns. Another important topic of future research is the exploration of the impact of infections and chronic diseases. It is tempting to speculate that bacterial and viral pathogens may be involved in several chronic diseases in addition to the well-characterized role of *Helicobacter pylori* in stomach cancer and lymphoma or the proposed role of chlamydia in coronary heart disease.

Concluding Remarks

The shift of the population structure towards older age groups will impact all segments of a society. This trend will pose new challenges for geriatric medicine, and, especially, infectious disease research has to meet these challenges to explore the specific role of pathogenic agents and infectious diseases in the elderly. There is a strong need to develop new concepts for prevention, diagnosis, and therapy of infections in the largest group of the future population.

References

1. Curns AT, Holman RC, Sejvar JJ, Owings MF, Schonberger LB. Infectious disease hospitalizations among older adults in the United States from 1990 through 2002. Arch Intern Med 2005;165:2514–2520.
2. Bagshaw SM, Laupland KB. Epidemiology of intensive care unit-acquired urinary tract infections. Curr Opin Infect Dis 2006;19:67–71.
3. Warren JW. Catheter-associated urinary tract infections. Int J Antimicrob Agents 2001; 17:299–303.
4. Bouza E, San Juan R, Munoz P, Voss A, Kluytmans J. A European perspective on nosocomial urinary tract infections II. Report on incidence clinical characteristics and outcome (ESGNI-004 study). European Study Group on Nosocomial Infection. Clin Microbiol Infect 2001;7:532–542.
5. Klemm P, Hancock V, Schembri MA. Mellowing out: adaptation to commensalism by Escherichia coli asymptomatic bacteriuria strain 83972. Infect Immun 2007;75:3688–3695.
6. Oelschlaeger TA, Dobrindt U, Hacker J. Virulence factors of uropathogens. Curr Opin Urol 2002;12:33–38.
7. Roberts JA, Marklund BI, Ilver D, Haslam D, Kaack MB, Baskin G, Louis M, Mollby R, Winberg J, Normark S. The Gal(alpha 1–4)Gal-specific tip adhesin of Escherichia coli P-fimbriae is needed for pyelonephritis to occur in the normal urinary tract. Proc Natl Acad Sci USA 1994;91:11889–11893.
8. Anderson GG, Palermo JJ, Schilling JD, Roth R, Heuser J, Hultgren SJ. Intracellular bacterial biofilm-like pods in urinary tract infections. Science 2003;301:105–107.
9. Snyder JA, Haugen BJ, Buckles EL, Lockatell CV, Johnson DE, Donnenberg MS, Welch RA, Mobley HL. Transcriptome of uropathogenic Escherichia coli during urinary tract infection. Infect Immun 2004;72:6373–6381.
10. Bouckaert J, Mackenzie J, de Paz JL, Chipwaza B, Choudhury D, Zavialov A, Mannerstedt K, Anderson J, Pierard D, Wyns L, Seeberger PH, Oscarson S, De Greve H, Knight SD. The affinity of the FimH fimbrial adhesin is receptor-driven and quasi-independent of Escherichia coli pathotypes. Mol Microbiol 2006;61:1556–1568.
11. Talan DA, Stamm WE, Hooton TM, Moran GJ, Burke T, Iravani A, Reuning-Scherer J, Church DA. Comparison of ciprofloxacin (7 days) and trimethoprim-sulfamethoxazole (14 days) for acute uncomplicated pyelonephritis in women: a randomized trial. JAMA 2000;283:1583–1590.
12. Kochanek KD, Murphy SL, Anderson RN, Scott C. Deaths: final data for 2002. Natl Vital Stat Rep 2004;53:1–115.
13. Gross PA, Rapuano C, Adrignolo A, Shaw B. Nosocomial infections: decade-specific risk. Infect Control 1983;4:145–147.
14. Kaplan V, Angus DC, Griffin MF, Clermont G, Scott Watson R, Linde-Zwirble WT. Hospitalized community-acquired pneumonia in the elderly: age- and sex-related patterns of care and outcome in the United States. Am J Respir Crit Care Med 2002;165:766–772.
15. Schneider EL. Infectious diseases in the elderly. Ann Intern Med 1983;98:395–400.
16. Metlay JP, Schulz R, Li YH, Singer DE, Marrie TJ, Coley CM, Hough LJ, Obrosky DS, Kapoor WN, Fine MJ. Influence of age on symptoms at presentation in patients with community-acquired pneumonia. Arch Intern Med 1997;157:1453–1459.
17. Musgrave T, Verghese A. Clinical features of pneumonia in the elderly. Semin Respir Infect 1990;5:269–275.
18. DiSario JA, Foutch PG, Sanowski RA. Poor results with percutaneous endoscopic jejunostomy. Gastrointest Endosc 1990;36:257–260.
19. Huchon G. Lung diseases in the elderly. Respiration 1998;65:343–344.
20. Granton JT, Grossman RF. Community-acquired pneumonia in the elderly patient. Clinical features epidemiology and treatment. Clin Chest Med 1993;14:537–553.

21. Hofmann J, Cetron MS, Farley MM, Baughman WS, Facklam RR, Elliott JA, Deaver KA, Breiman RF. The prevalence of drug-resistant *Streptococcus pneumoniae* in Atlanta. N Engl J Med 1995;333:481–486.
22. Anon. Hospital-acquired pneumonia in adults: diagnosis assessment of severity initial antimicrobial therapy and preventive strategies. A consensus statement American Thoracic Society November 1995. Am J Respir Crit Care Med 1996;153:1711–1725.
23. Hutchison BG, Oxman AD, Shannon HS, Lloyd S, Altmayer CA, Thomas K. Clinical effectiveness of pneumococcal vaccine. Meta-analysis. Can Fam Physician 1999;45: 2381–2393.
24. Martin GS, Mannino DM, Moss M. The effect of age on the development and outcome of adult sepsis. Crit Care Med 2006;34:15–21.
25. Martin GS, Mannino DM, Eaton S, Moss M. The epidemiology of sepsis in the United States from 1979 through 2000. N Engl J Med 2003;348:1546–1554.
26. Wisplinghoff H, Bischoff T, Tallent SM, Seifert H, Wenzel RP, Edmond MB. Nosocomial bloodstream infections in US hospitals: analysis of 24179 cases from a prospective nationwide surveillance study. Clin Infect Dis 2004;39:309–317.
27. Bearman GM, Wenzel RP. Bacteremias: a leading cause of death. Arch Med Res 2005; 36:646–659.
28. Livermore DM. Bacterial resistance: origins epidemiology and impact. Clin Infect Dis 2003;36:S11–S23.
29. von Eiff C, Peters G, Heilmann C. Pathogenesis of infections due to coagulase-negative staphylococci. Lancet Infect Dis 2002;2:677–685.
30. Kozitskaya S, Olson ME, Fey PD, Witte W, Ohlsen K, Ziebuhr W. Clonal analysis of *Staphylococcus epidermidis* isolates carrying or lacking biofilm-mediating genes by multilocus sequence typing. J Clin Microbiol 2005;43:4751–4757.
31. Gotz F. *Staphylococcus* and biofilms. Mol Microbiol 2002;43:1367–1378.
32. Heilmann C, Schweitzer O, Gerke C, Vanittanakom N, Mack D, Gotz F. Molecular basis of intercellular adhesion in the biofilm-forming *Staphylococcus epidermidis*. Mol Microbiol 1996;20:1083–1091.
33. Cho SH, Naber K, Hacker J, Ziebuhr W. Detection of the icaADBC gene cluster and biofilm formation in *Staphylococcus epidermidis* isolates from catheter-related urinary tract infections. Int J Antimicrob Agents 2002;19:570–575.
34. Galdbart JO, Allignet J, Tung HS, Ryden C, El Solh N. Screening for *Staphylococcus epidermidis* markers discriminating between skin-flora strains and those responsible for infections of joint prostheses. J Infect Dis 2000;182:351–355.
35. Annane D, Bellissant E, Cavaillon JM. Septic shock. Lancet 2005;365:63–78.
36. Rangel-Frausto MS, Pittet D, Hwang T, Woolson RF, Wenzel RP. The dynamics of disease progression in sepsis: Markov modeling describing the natural history and the likely impact of effective antisepsis agents. Clin Infect Dis 1998;27:185–190.
37. Annane D, Aegerter P, Jars-Guincestre MC, Guidet B. Current epidemiology of septic shock: the CUB-Rea Network. Am J Respir Crit Care Med 2003;168:165–172.
38. Alberti C, Brun-Buisson C, Burchardi H, Martin C, Goodman S, Artigas A, Sicignano A, Palazzo M, Moreno R, Boulme R, Lepage E, Le Gall R. Epidemiology of sepsis and infection in ICU patients from an international multicentre cohort study. Intensive Care Med 2002;28:108–121.
39. Liang SY, Mackowiak PA. Infections in the elderly. Clin Geriatr Med 2007;23:441–456.
40. Musette P, Benichou J, Noblesse I, Hellot MF, Carvalho P, Young P, Levesque H, Courtois H, Caron F, Lauret P, Joly P. Determinants of severity for superficial cellutitis (erysipelas) of the leg: a retrospective study. Eur J Intern Med 2004;15:446–450.
41. Denis O, Simonart T. Involvement of *Staphylococcus aureus* in Erysipelas. Dermatology 2006;212:1–3.
42. Sonksen UW, Ekelund K, and Bruun BG. Case of bacteraemic cellulitis by a non-haemolytic strain of *Streptococcus pyogenes*. Scand J Infect Dis 2007;39:262–264.

43. Currie BJ. Group A streptococcal infections of the skin: molecular advances but limited therapeutic progress. Curr Opin Infect Dis 2006;19:132–138.
44. Ohlsen K, Hacker J. Infections in the elderly. Int J Med Microbiol 2005;294:471–472.
45. Smith NL, Taylor EJ, Lindsay AM, Charnock SJ, Turkenburg JP, Dodson EJ, Davies GJ, Black GW. Structure of a group A streptococcal phage-encoded virulence factor reveals a catalytically active triple-stranded beta-helix. Proc Natl Acad Sci USA 2005;102: 17652–17657.
46. Påhlman LI, Olin AI, Darenberg J, Mörgelin M, Kotb M, Herwald H, Norrby-Teglund A. Soluble M1 protein of *Streptococcus pyogenes* triggers potent T cell activation. Cell Microbiol 2008;10(2):404–414
47. Li Z, Sakota V, Jackson D, Franklin AR, Beall B. Array of M protein gene subtypes in 1064 recent invasive group A *Streptococcus* isolates recovered from the active bacterial core surveillance. J Infect Dis 2003;188:1587–1592.
48. Stevens DL, Bisno AL, Chambers HF, Everett ED, Dellinger P, Goldstein EJ, Gorbach SL, Hirschmann JV, Kaplan EL, Montoya JG, Wade JC. Practice guidelines for the diagnosis and management of skin and soft-tissue infections. Clin Infect Dis 2005;41:1373–1406.
49. Werlinger KD, Moore AY. Therapy of other bacterial infections. Dermatol Ther 2004; 17:505–512.
50. Kwan MK, Saw A, Chee EK, Lee CS, Lim CH, Zulkifle NA, Saarey NH, Mohamad Hussien MN. Necrotizing fasciitis of the lower limb: an outcome study of surgical treatment. Med J Malaysia 2006;61:17–20.
51. Wong CH, Chang HC, Pasupathy S, Khin LW, Tan JL, Low CO. Necrotizing fasciitis: clinical presentation microbiology and determinants of mortality. J Bone Joint Surg Am 2003; 85-A:1454–1460.
52. Johnson MA, Lyle G, Hanly M, Yeh KA. *Aspergillus*: a rare primary organism in soft-tissue infections. Am Surg 1998;64:122–126.
53. Stumvoll M, Fritsche A. Necrotizing fasciitis caused by unencapsulated *Haemophilus influenzae*. Clin Infect Dis 1997;25:327.
54. Anaya DA, Dellinger EP. Necrotizing soft-tissue infection: diagnosis and management. Clin Infect Dis 2007;44:705–710.
55. Weinberg JM, Scheinfeld NS. Cutaneous infections in the elderly: diagnosis and management. Dermatol Ther 2003;16:195–205.
56. Esposito S, Leone S, Noviello S, Lanniello F, Fiore M. Antibiotic resistance in long-term care facilities. New Microbiol 2007;30:326–331.
57. Foster TJ. The *Staphylococcus aureus* "superbug". J Clin Invest 2004;114: 1693–1696.
58. Moran GJ, Krishnadasan A, Gorwitz RJ, Fosheim GE, McDougal LK, Carey RB, Talan DA. Methicillin-resistant *S. aureus* infections among patients in the emergency department. N Engl J Med 2006;355:666–674.
59. Gillet Y, Issartel B, Vanhems P, Fournet JC, Lina G, Bes M, Vandenesch F, Piemont Y, Brousse N, Floret D, Etienne J. Association between *Staphylococcus aureus* strains carrying gene for Panton-Valentine leukocidin and highly lethal necrotising pneumonia in young immunocompetent patients. Lancet 2002;359:753–759.
60. Lorenz U, Abele-Horn M, Bussen D, Thiede A. Severe pyomyositis caused by Panton-Valentine leucocidin-positive methicillin-sensitive *Staphylococcus aureus* complicating a pilonidal cyst. Langenbecks Arch Surg 2007;392:761–765.
61. Tristan A, Bes M, Meugnier H, Lina G, Bozdogan B, Courvalin P, Reverdy ME, Enright MC, Vandenesch F, Etienne J. Global distribution of Panton–Valentine leukocidin positive methicillin-resistant *Staphylococcus aureus* 2006. Emerg Infect Dis 2007;13:594–600.
62. Mertz PM, Cardenas TC, Snyder RV, Kinney MA, Davis SC, Plano LR. *Staphylococcus aureus* virulence factors associated with infected skin lesions: influence on the local immune response. Arch Dermatol 2007;143:1259–1263.
63. Micek ST. Alternatives to vancomycin for the treatment of methicillin-resistant *Staphylococcus aureus* infections. Clin Infect Dis 2007;45(3):S184–S190.

64. Scheinfeld N. Infections in the elderly. Dermatol Online J 2005;11:8.
65. Scher RK, Tavakkol A, Sigurgeirsson B, Hay RJ, Joseph WS, Tosti A, Fleckman P, Ghannoum M, Armstrong DG, Markinson BC, Elewski BE. Onychomycosis: diagnosis and definition of cure. J Am Acad Dermatol 2007;56:939–944.
66. Gupta AK, Tu LQ. Therapies for onychomycosis: a review. Dermatol Clin 2006;24:375–379.
67. Loo DS. Onychomycosis in the elderly: drug treatment options. Drugs Aging 2007;24: 293–302.
68. Christo PJ, Hobelmann G, Maine DN. Post-herpetic neuralgia in older adults: evidence-based approaches to clinical management. Drugs Aging 2007;24:1–19.
69. Volpi A, Gross G, Hercogova J, Johnson RW. Current management of herpes zoster: the European view. Am J Clin Dermatol 2005;6:317–325.
70. Schmader K. Herpes zoster and postherpetic neuralgia in older adults. Clin Geriatr Med 2007;23:615–632.

Chapter 4
Skin Aging and Microbiology

Leslie Baumann, Edmund Weisberg, and Steven L. Percival

Introduction

There are two primary skin aging processes, intrinsic and extrinsic. Intrinsic aging refers to the natural course of genetically programmed cellular aging. Extrinsic aging, or premature cutaneous aging, occurs as the result of exogenous forces, including smoking, excessive alcohol consumption, poor nutrition, pollution, and particularly solar exposure, and is, by definition, preventable. The effects of solar exposure, most notably wrinkling and undesired pigmentation, are so prevalent that a subcategory of extrinsic aging, called *photoaging*, is studied quite extensively. While the sun is the primary exogenous causative agent in skin aging, it is not the only etiologic factor. This chapter will focus on the microbiology of skin aging, on various internal and environmental elements involved in the aging process, on extrinsic cutaneous aging due to the influence of the sun, and on the role of the sun in potentially altering the normal course of intrinsic, or natural, aging.

Factors and Theories Pertaining to Cutaneous Aging

Intrinsically aging skin is smooth and unblemished, and manifests normal geometric patterns, with some exaggerated expression lines. Such skin is characterized histologically by epidermal and dermal atrophy, evening or flattening of the epidermal rete ridges, as well as decreased numbers of fibroblasts and mast cells.[1,2] Further, increases occur in the number of collagen fibrils and in the ratio of collagen III to collagen I.[3] Nevertheless, the etiologic pathways of intrinsic skin aging are less understood and have been studied far less than the mechanisms of extrinsic skin aging. Chronological aging is understood, though, to be a dynamic, multifactorial cascade of events mediated by genetic, hormonal, and metabolic processes.

L. Baumann, E. Weisberg, and S.L. Percival
University of Miami Cosmetic Center, Miami Beach, FL, USA

S.L. Percival (ed.), *Microbiology and Aging.*
DOI: 10.1007/978-1-59745-327-1_4, © Springer Science + Business Media, LLC 2009

Exposure to the sun is easily considered the most significant factor in the exogenous aging of the skin. In fact, chronic sun exposure is cited as the primary cause of 80% of facial aging.[4] The extrinsic aging of the skin, seen most often in consistently exposed areas including the face, chest, and extensor surfaces of the arms, results from the cumulative effects of lifelong ultraviolet radiation (UVR) exposure. The clinical presentation is characterized by rhytides, pigmented lesions (e.g., ephelides, lentigines, and patchy hyperpigmentation), and depigmented lesions (e.g., guttate hypomelanosis). In addition, skin tone and elasticity is diminished in photoaged skin. Such skin is increasingly fragile and manifests areas of purpura due to blood vessel weakness, and benign lesions (e.g., acrochordons, keratoses, and telangiectases). On the Glogau scale, which measures the level of clinical photodamage, patients with a significant history of sun exposure typically score higher than expected for their age, while patients with a history of minimal sun exposure usually score lower than expected for their age.

The sine qua non elastosis renders an easy histopathologic identification of photoaged skin. Other important alterations are notable, however. Epidermal atrophy and discrete changes in collagen and elastic fibers help distinguish photoaged skin. Specifically, fragmented, thickened, and more soluble collagen fibers are exhibited in severely photoaged skin.[5] Elastic fibers also become fragmented and undergo progressive cross-linkage and calcification.[6] Continued UVR exposure has been shown to exacerbate these distinct signs of deterioration in collagen and elastic fibers already induced by prior photoaging. In general, aging skin is characterized by increased inelasticity, fragmentation, and collagen bundle fragility.[2]

Chemistry of Intrinsic Aging: Telomeres

At a cellular level, telomeres, the specialized structures at the ends of eukaryotic chromosomes, are thought to play an integral role in the intrinsic aging process. Intact telomeres are essential for the extension of a cell's life span.[7] Interestingly, telomere length shortens with age. This process of erosion of telomeres is now thought of as a veritable internal aging clock, as it serves as one method to measure aging and as the basis for a currently favored theory on aging.[8] One fascinating implication of this theory figuratively places aging and cancer on opposite sides of the same coin. The cellular reverse transcriptase enzyme that stabilizes or lengthens telomeres, known as telomerase, is expressed in approximately 85–90% of all human tumors; however, it is absent in many somatic tissues.[9,10] Consequently, most cancer cells, as opposed to healthy cells, are not programmed for apoptosis, or cell death. In other words, telomerase presence is correlated with telomere stability and tumorigenesis, whereas the absence of telomerase is associated with telomere shortening, somatic tissue aging, and a limit to cellular replicative capacity. Significantly, the epidermis is one of the few regenerative tissues known to express the ribonucleoprotein telomerase.[11] Further, an investigation of progressive telomere shortening in 52 specimens of normal human epidermis and 48 specimens of lingual epithelium collected at autopsy from subjects who died between 0 and 101 years of age revealed that the telomere shortening associated with aging is characterized by tissue-specific loss rates.[12] A fascinating recent study on nevus counts helps to illustrate this dichotomy. Melanoma risk has been traditionally linked to a high nevus count as well as the proclivity to form nevi. Researchers conducting a 10-year study of 1,897 Caucasian women between 18 and 79 years old examined whether telomere length measurements in white cells are associated with nevi count and size. Interestingly, investigators found, after adjusting for age, that subjects with the highest nevus counts exhibited greater average telomere length and that subjects with more than 100 nevi had a biological age averaging 6–7 years younger than subjects manifesting fewer than 25 nevi. These findings suggest that individuals with several moles may age slower than those with few moles.[13] In other words, on one side of the coin is the greater risk of melanoma among those with numerous nevi; on the other side, these same individuals may have a reduced rate of senescence.

Although there are several prominent theories that contribute to our understanding of aging, the natural, progressive shortening of telomeres may be the primary mechanism of cellular aging in skin.[2] In addition, telomeres and other cellular components are subject to low-grade oxidative damage due to aerobic cellular metabolism, a process that contributes to intrinsic aging.[14] Much remains to be learned about telomeres and telomerase and their relationship to aging, as well as cancer. Current data provide no indication that medical intervention can safely extend the lengths of telomeres. Therefore, no topical skin care products, systemic drugs, or other treatment options are yet available that can target telomerase. It is thought that telomerase-based therapies may eventually be developed to inhibit telomerase with the intention of also imparting anti-proliferative and apoptosis-inducing effects unrelated to the role the enzyme plays in shortening telomeres during mitosis.[10]

Werner Syndrome (WS), an autosomal recessive disorder in which the causative gene, WRN, encodes a member of the RecQ-like subfamily of DNA helicases, appears to have the potential to play a didactic role regarding our understanding of the aging process.[15] The Werner protein (WRN), a multifunctional nuclear protein exhibiting $3'$–$5'$ exonuclease and ATP-dependent helicase activities, is involved in several DNA metabolic pathways, but is available at reduced levels to WS patients.[16] WS is characterized by signs of accelerated aging and the premature onset of various age-related disorders. In particular, WS patients experience a higher incidence of sarcomas and other tumors of mesenchymal origin than the population at large.[17] In a decade-old study, mouse embryo fibroblasts derived from homozygous WS embryos were demonstrated to have premature loss of proliferative capacity.[15] More recently, researchers observed that telomere reserve exhaustion and telomere dysfunction induced several Werner-like symptoms, including hair graying, alopecia, cataracts, osteoporosis, type II diabetes, and premature death in a mouse model.[18] Further, telomere shortening was cited as the main cause in this model of other observations, such as accelerated replicative senescence and chromosomal instability, particularly nonepithelial tumors often linked to WS. Further elucidation of the aging process is expected from the study of WS, given the relationship of WS to telomere shortening and the association of cellular aging with the status of telomeres and activity of telomerase.

Free Radicals

The free radical theory of aging, considered an important element in our understanding of intrinsic and extrinsic aging, was proposed in 1956.[19] It is one of the most widely accepted theories that accounts for the aging phenomenon.[20] Free radicals, also known as reactive oxygen species (ROS), arise when oxygen molecules combine with other molecules resulting in an odd number of electrons. An oxygen molecule with paired electrons is stable; oxygen with an unpaired electron is "reactive" because it scavenges electrons from surrounding molecules, rendering them impaired.[21] According to the theory, ROS engendered by oxidative metabolism cause cellular damage, which accumulates and accounts for overall aging.[22,23] Significantly, ROS are also thought to be involved cutaneously in causing photoaging, carcinogenesis, and inflammation. UV-induced skin damage is known to be, at least in part, mediated by reactive oxygen intermediates.[24]

Estrogens

Estrogens are not etiological factors in aging, per se, but this key group of hormones significantly impacts the skin, particularly in raising collagen and glycosaminoglycans content and contributing to skin thickness and moisturization. In addition, estrogens influence hair growth, water retention, wrinkling, vascularity, and pigmentation.[25] Indeed, it is the reduction of estrogen levels that is associated with cutaneous signs of aging. Skin, which is known to respond to estrogen via particular receptors (estrogen receptors alpha and beta), has been shown to age because of the influence of various internal and external processes. Hormone levels change through time and can also be affected by extrinsic factors, including, of course, hormone replacement therapy. Significant improvement in the fine facial wrinkles of postmenopausal women was observed in a double-blind, placebo-controlled study following topical application of a conjugated estrogen cream.[26] In addition, in a large cohort study, postmenopausal women using estrogen were shown, a decade ago, to be less prone to develop wrinkles.[27] It can be said that hormonal treatment represented one of the few promising avenues of countering or slowing the cutaneous effects of aging. The relatively recent cessation of part of the Women's Health Initiative (WHI), which implied elevated risk of coronary artery disease and breast cancer from using hormone replacement therapy (HRT), has eliminated HRT from the recommended armamentarium of treatments for aging skin, however, at least until a safe minimum concentration of estrogen for topical delivery, conferring local effects but no systemic side effects, can be ascertained.[25]

While other hormonally based skin aging treatments appear on the horizon, e.g., phytoestrogens and selective estrogen receptor modulators (SERMs), more remains to be understood regarding the hormonal role in skin aging. Nevertheless, it is clear that hormonal influences are a factor in the dynamic aging process.

Chemistry of Extrinsic Aging

Extrinsic or exogenous aging, by definition, can be prevented, and is thus subject to the volitional control of the individual. Exogenous behaviors or factors such as smoking, poor nutrition, and solar exposure are the primary causes of extrinsic, premature cutaneous aging. Sun exposure, by far the most significant etiologic factor in cutaneous aging so much so that it warrants its own designation – photoaging, is thought to account for 80% of facial aging.[4] While discrete signs and symptoms have been directly linked to solar exposure, photoaging is not an independent process. That is to say, photoaging is thought of as the superposition of UV irradiation onto the already occurring endogenous aging process,[25,28,29] and therefore an accelerating or exacerbating phenomenon. The readily apparent results of chronic sun exposure can be observed simply through comparing skin not typically exposed to the sun, which obviously varies by culture, climate, and individual, with skin routinely exposed to the sun (which, of course, also varies, but the hands, neck, and face are safe bets). Using a Wood's lamp or an ultraviolet camera system renders an even more discernible depiction of the symptoms of photodamage, particularly the epidermal pigment component.

UVR exposure results in skin damage through various mechanisms, such as the development of sunburn cells, as well as thymine and pyrimidine dimers; the production of collagenase, the enzyme primarily involved in the breakdown of collagen; and the induction of an inflammatory response. Sunburn cells, or UV-induced apoptotic cells, have long been employed as markers for the assessment of photodamage. Levels of the enzyme caspase-3, which mediates UV-induced apoptosis, are believed to be reliable indicators of the presence of cellular apotosis.[30] Similar to caspase-3, caspase-7 is a key component in the activation of apoptosis.[31] The etiologic mechanism of photoaging is also believed to involve mast cells and macrophages, which are found in greater abundance in such skin.[32]

Signaling through the tumor-suppressor protein p53 after telomere disruption is also associated with aging as well as photodamage, more directly from UVB than UVA wavelengths.[14,33] More infiltrating mononuclear cells have been shown through histologic examination to be present in skin chronically exposed to the sun as compared to protected skin.[32] Furthermore, photoaging, photocarcinogenesis, and photo-immunosuppression are well known to be consequences of UV exposure, especially the UVA range (320–400 nm).[34] Gaining currency is the theory that as UVR exposure impairs DNA and accelerates the rate of telomere shortening, this chief causal component of extrinsic aging can be considered to be an etiologic factor in cellular aging. Indeed, recent reports suggest that photoaging and chronological aging exhibit overlapping or intersecting features. Telomeres, however, do not appear to be important in the primary mechanisms of extrinsic aging. In fact, in a recent study measuring telomere lengths in 76 specimens of epidermis from sun-protected sites, 24 epidermal specimens from sun-exposed sites, and 60 dermal specimens, telomere length was found to be shorter in the epidermis. Intrinsic aging was revealed by diminished telomere length in the epidermis and dermis with age. However, reduced telomere length was not linked to photoaging in this study, as telomere length was demonstrated to be similar in sun-exposed and sun-protected sites.[35] Theoretically, the lower the number of sunburn cells present, the less significant the level of photodamage. The only known ways to prevent the formation of sunburn cells are sun avoidance and the consistent use of broad-spectrum sunscreens. Both practices can also protect against the formation of thymine dimers.

Characteristics of Aging Skin

Although there are separate but overlapping etiologic pathways related to the processes of intrinsic and extrinsic skin aging, aged skin manifests certain identifiable characteristics regardless of its causal pathway. As skin ages, alterations emerge throughout the epidermis, dermis, and subcutaneous tissue, presenting distinct and vast changes in cutaneous structure and function.

Epidermis

Although it may seem counterintuitive, age-related changes can be more pronounced beneath the surface. That is, alterations in the dermis are more quantifiable and histologically verifiable than changes in the epidermis. In fact, some studies imply that the epidermis thins with age,[5] some even suggesting a 10–50% thinning between 30 and 80 years of age,[36–38] but others offer no such conclusions.[39] Indeed, a recent study of biopsies from three different body areas of 71 human subjects ranging from 20 to 68 years of age found no correlation between epidermal thickness and age or skin type.[40] There is general agreement, though, that the stratum corneum (SC) does not become thinner through the aging process. Histopathologic examination of 83 biopsies from sun-exposed and protected skin in healthy volunteers (ranging from 6 to 84 years old) demonstrated that epidermal thickness was constant across decades in both intrinsically and extrinsically aged skin, with the thickness found to be greater in sun-exposed skin.[41] A different study showed that the spinous layer of a wrinkle was thinner at the base than at its flanks.[42] According to this study, fewer keratohyaline granules are found in the wrinkle base as compared to its flanks.

While debate continues regarding the extent to which changes occur in the epidermal layer with age, alterations are known to emerge in aged skin at the intersection of the epidermis and dermis, known as the dermal–epidermal junction (DEJ). Aged epidermis is characterized by a flattened DEJ with a correspondingly reduced connecting surface area and loss of dermal papillae.[41] In a study of abdominal skin across generations, DEJ surface area averaged 2.64 mm^2 in subjects 21–40 years old, but only 1.90 mm^2 in subjects aged 61–80 years.[43] Such apparent diminution in DEJ surface area is believed to contribute to the greater skin fragility associated with age; it may also hinder nutrient transfer between the dermal and epidermal layers. It is worth noting that in the study by El-Domyati et al., facial and abdominal skin thickness remained virtually unchanged through the decades in their sample of 83 biopsies from sun-exposed and protected skin culled from 38 healthy volunteers ranging from 6 to 84 years old, with the epidermis of facial skin found to be consistently and significantly thicker than abdominal skin.[41]

Decreased Cell Turnover

Although epidermal thickness may remain more or less static through time, and wrinkles appear thinner at their base, age-related changes occur in the epidermal layer above the DEJ. The epidermal turnover rate slows markedly, from 30 to 50%, between the third and eighth decades of life.[44] SC transit time has been demonstrated to last 20 days in young adults and 30 or more days in older adults.[45] A prolonged SC replacement rate, epidermal atrophy, slower wound healing, and less effective desquamation are all associated with such cell cycle lengthening in aged skin. In fact, it has been shown that double the time to re-epithelialize was required for older patients after dermabrasion resurfacing procedures as compared to younger patients.[46] Decelerated cell turnover and its concomitant cascade of alterations in older skin result in heaps of corneocytes that render the skin surface rough and dull in appearance. Many cosmetic dermatologists use hydroxy acids and retinoids to speed up the cell cycle in such skin with the expectation that an accelerated turnover rate will ameliorate skin appearance and speed wound healing after cosmetic procedures.

The number of Langerhans cells also markedly declines with age. Significantly, many such cells experience a functional decline, which has been suggested as an explanation for the reduced immune function of the skin seen in the elderly.[36,47]

Dermis

Dermal thickness decreases by approximately 20% with age.[46] Histologic examination has revealed that aged dermis is relatively acellular and avascular.[1] Normal aged skin is also characterized by reduced collagen production and the development of fragmented elastic fibers. Photoaged skin, in addition to such properties, also manifests disorganized collagen fibrils and the accumulation of abnormal elastin-containing material.[41,48] Collagen, elastin, and glycosaminoglycans, the three primary structural constituents of the dermis, clearly undergo significant change with age; these dermal components have been the focus of the preponderance of anti-aging research directed at the skin.

Collagen

The most abundant protein present in humans as well as the primary structural component of the dermis, collagen imparts strength and support to human skin. As suggested above, over time the structural proteins and primary constituents of the skin decline, manifesting in visible signs of cutaneous aging. Epidermal and dermal atrophy as well as flattening of the rete ridges characterize endogenously aged skin.[1] Rhytides, or wrinkles, present in the epidermal and dermal layers of the skin. However, little is known about the pathogenesis of wrinkles.[49] Alterations in collagen are known to play an integral role in the cutaneous aging process, of which wrinkles are the primary manifestation (along with changes in elasticity and pigmentation). Consequently, collagen-containing topical products intended for "anti-aging" purposes have achieved great, though unwarranted, popularity. There are no products yet available to permanently replace the collagen lost with aging.

Collagen, which comprises 70% of dry skin mass, is actually a dynamic family of proteins.[50] In older skin, collagen exhibits thickened fibrils organized in rope-like bundles that appear to be in disarray, as compared to the patterns identified in younger skin.[1] Further, aged fibroblasts have been shown, in vivo and in vitro, to synthesize lower levels of collagen. With age, the ratio of collagen types in human skin changes, serving as an important histologic marker of cutaneous aging. Collagen I comprises 80% of young skin, with collagen III composing about 15% of total skin collagen; in older skin, the ratio of type III to type I collagen has been demonstrated to increase as a result of a substantial loss of collagen I.[51] The overall collagen content per unit area of skin surface is also known to diminish approximately 1% per year.[52] Significantly, collagen I levels have been demonstrated to decrease by 59% in irradiated skin,[53] a decline ascribed to the extent of photodamage.[54] Collagen I is the most important and copious form of collagen in human skin, but other collagen types are influenced by the aging process and these alterations also occur in the human dermal layer.

Collagen IV, an integral element of the DEJ, confers structural framework for other molecules and contributes significantly to the maintenance of mechanical stability. There have been no significant differences reported in collagen IV levels in sun-exposed skin compared to unexposed skin, but significantly lower collagen IV levels have been noted at the base of wrinkles as compared to the flanks of the same wrinkles. Consequently, it is thought that the loss of collagen IV may adversely affect the mechanical stability of the DEJ, thereby promoting the formation of wrinkles.[42]

Collagen VII is the dominant component in anchoring fibrils, which attach the basement membrane zone to the underlying papillary dermis. In a decade-old study, a significantly lower number of anchoring fibrils were found in patients with chronically sun-exposed skin as compared to normal controls. The investigators speculated that wrinkles may develop as a result of anchoring fibril degradation weakening the bond between the dermis and epidermis.[55] A different study revealed the loss of collagen VII to be more pronounced in the base of the wrinkle (as observed with collagen IV in the same study).[42]

The loss of collagen, while a natural endogenous process, has been demonstrated to be accelerated as a consequence of chronic sun exposure. The cascade of events begins with UVR exposure significantly upregulating the production of several types of collagen-degrading enzymes known as matrix metalloproteinases (MMPs). Initially, UV exposure induces an increase in the level of the transcription factor c-jun. The other transcription factor involved in this chain, c-fos, is abundantly present prior to UV exposure. The combination of c-jun and c-fos then contributes to the development of activator protein-1 (AP-1), which, in turn, activates the MMP genes that stimulate collagenase (MMP-1), gelatinase (MMP-9), and stromelysin (MMP-3) synthesis. Subsequently, collagen degradation is mediated by AP-1 activation and the inhibitory activity of transforming growth factor (TGF)-beta signaling.[56] Ultimately, then, UV irradiation dynamically interferes with collagen by inducing the degradation of existing collagen and hindering the production of type I and type III procollagen, by downregulating gene expression of types I and III procollagen.[28] This occurs immediately following UV irradiation, but chronic effects are seen in diminished procollagen I production in skin that is severely photodamaged, even without recent UV exposure.[28,54,57] Studies in humans have revealed that MMPs, particularly collagenase and gelatinase, are synthesized within hours of UVB exposure.[58] Sustained production of MMPs results from frequent or multiple UVB exposures.[48] It is thought that protracted and chronic long-term elevations in the levels of collagenase and other MMPs likely yield the disorganized and clumped collagen that typifies photoaged skin. The production and activity of these MMPs may represent the mechanism through which collagen I levels decline as a consequence of UV exposure. By characterizing the broad influences of UV in activating cell surface growth factor and cytokine receptors, investigators have determined that extrinsic and intrinsic skin aging are distinguished by increased AP-1 activity and MMP expression, inhibited TGF-beta signaling, decreased collagen production, and elevated collagen degradation.[56] It is thought that any such collagen changes due to endogenous aging are likely to be exacerbated by chronic sun exposure.

Elastin

"Elastosis," an accumulation of amorphous elastin material, results from chronic exposure to the sun. Therefore, such alterations identified in elastic fibers are considered pathognomonic of photoaged skin. As elastotic substances amass, the surrounding collagen meshwork erodes.[48] These changes induced by UV exposure can also be described as a thickening and coiling of elastic fibers in the papillary, or superficial, dermis. Chronic UV exposure can also engender such alterations in the reticular, or deeper, dermis.[59] Investigators conducting electron microscopy examination of elastic fibers in UV-exposed skin have observed decreased numbers of microfibrils, as well as increases in interfibrillar space, the complexity of the shape and arrangement of the fibers, and the number of electron-dense inclusions.[60] It is also worth noting that elastin extracted from the skin of elderly patients has been found to contain small amounts of sugar and lipids and an abnormally high level of polar amino acids.[1] Much less is known about elastin than collagen, in general. Accordingly, the etiologic pathway(s) of elastin alteration due to aging are not as well understood as age-related changes in collagen. Nevertheless, MMPs are believed to be involved in the process because MMP-2 has been shown to degrade elastin.[61]

Despite the lacunae in knowledge regarding the pathogenesis of age-related elastin degradation, the initial response of elastic fibers to photodamage has been established as hyperplastic, yielding an increase in elastic tissue. The magnitude of the hyperplastic response is dependent upon the level of sun exposure. A secondary response to photodamage occurs in aged elastic fibers, but it is degenerative, with skin elasticity and resiliency diminishing.[62,63] In such skin, alterations are observed in the normal pattern of immature elastic fibers, called *oxytalan*, which are found in the papillary dermis. In young skin, these fibers develop into a network that ascends perpendicularly from the outermost papillary dermis to just below the basement membrane of the skin. With age, this network incrementally dissolves.[53] As a result, skin elasticity gradually diminishes with age.[64] It is likely that sagging skin, which is commonly seen in the elderly, may be due, primarily, to such a loss of elasticity.

Glycosaminoglycans

In addition to collagen and elastin, glycosaminoglycans (GAGs), mucopolysaccharide chains with repeating disaccharide units attached to a core protein, are responsible for imparting viscosity and structural integrity that contribute to the outward appearance of the skin. GAGs are also significant molecules because they possess the capacity to bind water up to 1,000 times their volume. The GAG family of carbohydrates, integral components of connective tissue, is quite large, but the most physiologically significant members include hyaluronic acid (HA), dermatan sulfate (both of which are two of the most prevalent GAGs), chondroitin sulfate, heparin, heparin sulfate, and keratan sulfate. Maintenance of hydration in normal skin is ascribed to these compounds, which are also thought to contribute to the maintenance of salt and water equilibrium. GAG levels, especially HA levels, have been found to be decreased in photoaged skin, according to several studies,[65] although some earlier studies suggested no reduction in the level of GAGs in aged skin.[66] This discrepancy in findings is likely due to the fact that HA is produced in the epidermis as well as the dermis. The total HA level in the dermis remains stable in endogenously aging skin, but epidermal HA almost completely dissolves.[67] Despite the previously mentioned discrepancy in results, there is evidence that reduced levels of HA and elevated levels of chondroitin sulfate proteoglycans have been associated with photoaging.[68] Interestingly, these patterns are also observed in scars.

HA, as one of the most important GAGs, can bind 1,000 times its weight in water, and is thought to play a significant role in retaining and maintaining water in the skin. HA, which is found in all connective tissue, is synthesized primarily by fibroblasts and keratinocytes in the skin.[69] Besides the dermis, HA is extant in the epidermal intercellular spaces, particularly the middle spinous layer, but not in the SC or stratum granulosum.[70] In young skin, HA is present at the periphery of collagen and elastin fibers and at their intersection. In aged skin, these connections with HA have been found to have eroded.[65] Indeed, decreased levels of HA are associated with aged skin, which is less plump than youthful skin. The reduction in HA connections and levels, which contribute to its disassociation with collagen and elastin as well as diminished water binding, may be a factor in the characteristic changes associated with aged skin, including wrinkling, altered elasticity, reduced turgidity, and decreased capacity to support the microvasculature of the skin. The role of HA in skin hydration has not been completely elucidated as yet, though. It is known, however, that HA does not penetrate the skin upon topical application.[71] HA has been successfully used as a temporary dermal filling agent in soft-tissue augmentation procedures; no permanent replacements have been yet devised, nor have there yet been any suitable HA-containing topical products that can replace this important GAG.

Melanocytes

The number of melanocytes, the epidermal cells responsible for producing the pigment melanin, declines from 8 to 20% per decade through the aging process. This reduction is observed clinically in older patients as a decline in the number of melanocytic nevi.[1] Aged skin exhibits a diminished capacity to protect itself from the sun because melanin, which declines in the elderly, absorbs carcinogenic UV radiation. Consequently, older people are more susceptible to the development of UV-induced cancers. Accordingly, sun protection remains important for elderly patients even though the majority of an individual's deleterious sun exposure occurs during the first two decades of life. Healthy elderly people should be advised that it is not "too late" to incorporate a sunscreen into their skin care regimens. Inactive melanocytes, which are present in greater abundance with age, are also especially copious in hair follicles, which accounts for the graying of hair.[72]

Vasculature

Several studies have demonstrated that aged skin is comparatively avascular. In one study, investigators noted a 35% decrease in the venous cross-sectional area in aged skin as opposed to young skin.[73] This kind of a decline in the vascular network is particularly salient in the papillary dermis with the disappearance of the vertical capillary loops. Significantly, reduction in vascularity is also associated with diminished blood flow, depleted nutrient exchange, inhibited thermoregulation, lower skin surface temperature, and skin pallor.

Subcutaneous Tissue

The appearance of aged skin is known to be influenced by site-specific gains and losses that occur in subcutaneous tissues. With aging, subcutaneous fat dwindles in the face, dorsal aspects of the hands, and the shins. In other regions, particularly the waist in women and the abdomen in men, fat accumulates with age.[1]

The Role of Free Radicals in Photoaging

As suggested above, the formation and activity of free radicals, also known as ROS, are thought to contribute to the aging process. ROS are composed of oxygen molecules with an unpaired electron and are created by normal metabolic processes as well as various exogenous factors, including UV exposure, pollution, stress, and smoking. In addition, there is evidence that free radicals provoke changes in gene expression pathways, which in turn influences the degradation of collagen and the accumulation of elastin observed in photoaged skin.[61] Significantly, antioxidants act to neutralize free radicals by providing another electron, supplying an electron pair to an oxygen molecule, thereby stabilizing it.

Changes in Skin Appearance

Dry Skin

Aged skin is often characterized by xerosis. Dry, scaly skin can be at least partially attributed to the degradation or loss of skin barrier function with increasing age. In fact, the recovery of hindered barrier function has been shown to be slower in aged skin, yielding an increased susceptibility to developing xerosis. The emergence of dry skin is actually the result of a multifactorial process that includes lower lipid levels in lamellar bodies[74] and a decrease in epidermal filaggrin.[75] Older skin also manifests elevated transepidermal water loss (TEWL), rendering the SC more susceptible to developing dryness in low-humidity environments. Besides xerosis, aged skin also often exhibits roughness, wrinkling, pallor, hyper- or hypopigmentation, laxity, fragility, and benign neoplasms, and is predisposed to easier bruising.

Benign Neoplasms in Aging Skin

The surface texture and appearance of the skin can change dramatically with age. For instance, acrochordons (skin tags), cherry angiomas, seborrheic keratoses, lentigos (sun spots), and sebaceous hyperplasias, among other lesions and cutaneous alterations, are not atypical developments. Removal of these benign neoplasms is a common request among patients of dermatologists and plastic surgeons. Destructive treatment options are varied and plentiful, including hyfrecation and several laser methods.

Treatment of Photoaged Skin

Several in-office procedures and topical agents, most of which are intended to "resurface" the epidermis, are employed for the treatment of photoaged skin. This amounts to removing the damaged epidermis and, in some cases, dermis, and replacing the tissue with remodeled skin layers. Resurfacing techniques have been demonstrated to stimulate the synthesis of new collagen with a normal staining pattern, as compared with the basophilic elastotic masses of collagen emblematic of photoaged skin.[76] Technological advancement and innovation in the expanding fields of tissue engineering and gene therapy may eventually result in the incorporation of growth factors, cytokines, and telomerase into the treatment armamentarium.[77] Several antioxidants, such as vitamins C and E, coenzyme Q10, ferulic acid, green tea, idebenone, pycnogenol, tea tree oil, resveratrol, licochalcone, and silymarin are included in topical skin care products to combat photoaging.

Despite the availability of several treatment options for aged skin, prevention of exogenous aging remains the best approach and should be encouraged to all patients. Such measures refer to patterns of behavior and avoidance, such as avoiding exposure to the sun when reasonable, using sunscreen when sun avoidance is impossible, avoiding cigarette smoke and pollution, again, when feasible, eating a diet high in fruits and vegetables, and also taking oral antioxidant supplements or topical antioxidant formulations.

Regularly using prescription retinoids can also contribute to the prevention or treatment of rhytides, the most salient and frequent sign of cutaneous aging. At the very least, the topical application of all-*trans* retinoic acid (0.025–0.1%), also known as tretinoin, was shown a decade ago to ameliorate the appearance of photoaged skin.[78,79] Interestingly, all-*trans* retinoic acid had previously been demonstrated in photoaged skin to promote the gene expression of types I and III procollagen.[54] It is also believed that tretinoin can inhibit the cascade of cellular events induced by acute UV irradiation that result in the breakdown of collagen.[28,80]

Prevention

Rhytides emerge as a result of alterations in the lower, dermal layers of the skin. This is noteworthy because few skin care product ingredients have the capacity to penetrate deeply enough into the dermis to affect or ameliorate deep wrinkles, despite the advertising for topical formulations intended to combat aging. Consequently, prevention of wrinkle development is promoted as a fundamental approach to anti-aging skin care.[81] It is now well understood that to prevent the formation of wrinkles, it is necessary to halt the degradation of collagen, elastin, and HA, all of which decline with age. Therefore, the preponderance of anti-aging procedures and products are designed or formulated with the goal of salvaging, or even enhancing, at least one of these primary dermal constituents. However, the technology necessary to adequately deliver these compounds into the skin does not yet exist. Indeed, the topical products that contain collagen, elastin, or HA cannot suitably replace the main elements of the skin that subside through aging. Nevertheless, some products do foster the natural synthesis of these substances. For example, by the use of retinoids,[57] vitamin C[82] and copper peptide have been demonstrated to stimulate the synthesis of collagen. Oral vitamin C intake may also promote collagen production.[83] In addition, retinoids have been demonstrated to increase HA[84] and elastin synthesis in animal studies.[85] Glucosamine supplementation has also been reported to increase HA levels.[86] No products have yet been established or approved for enhancing elastin or increasing its production.

Reducing inflammation is another key aspect of wrinkle prevention since inflammation is known to accelerate the degradation of collagen, elastin, and HA. The myriad antioxidants already on the market or under investigation are the focus here, as all display distinguishing characteristics, activity, and bioavailability in scavenging ROS, thereby protecting the skin via various mechanisms that are only beginning to be elucidated. Skin inflammation results from ROS acting directly on cytokine and growth factor receptors in dermal cells and keratinocytes. Although much remains to be learned about the impact of cytokines and growth factors on skin aging, these compounds are known to function synergistically in a complex cascade of events.[87] This mechanism is believed to be induced by UV exposure, which provokes growth factor and cytokine receptors in keratinocytes and dermal cells, contributing to downstream signal transduction by stimulating mitogen-activated protein (MAP) kinase pathways (specifically, extracellular signal-regulated kinase, c-jun N-terminal protein kinase, and p38), which amass in cell nuclei and form cFos/cJun complexes of transcription factor activator protein 1, triggering the activation of the MMPs collagenase, 92-kDa gelatinase, and stromelysin to breakdown collagen and other connective skin.[80,88]

While the roles of cytokines and growth factors in aging skin remain to be fully ascertained, the direct effects of free radicals on the aging process and cutaneous aging are well understood. For example, the MAP kinase pathways, which have been demonstrated to activate collagenase production and therefore the degradation of collagen, are mobilized by free radicals.[88] In fact, in one study, human skin pretreated with the antioxidants genistein and N-acetyl cysteine were shown by Kang et al. to inhibit the UV induction of the cJun-driven enzyme collagenase. Using antioxidants in this context is thought to inhibit photoaging by preventing collagenase production, thereby preserving collagen. It is worth noting that while genistein and N-acetyl cysteine exhibit antioxidant properties, these compounds exerted no effect on UV-induced erythema in this study. Nevertheless, combining antioxidants is considered a viable approach to enhancing the effects of each ingredient, as several antioxidants have evinced a propensity to work synergistically with others. In a randomized, double-blind, parallel-group, placebo-controlled investigation of the effects of combining oral formulations of vitamins C and E, carotenoids, selenium, and proanthocyanidins, participants who took the antioxidant combination before UVB exposure exhibited a difference in MMP-1 production as compared with the placebo group ($p < 0.05$).[89] Like the study by Kang et al., no significant differences were observed between the oral antioxidant group and the placebo group regarding minimal erythema dose of the skin.

One group of subjects received daily administration of a base cream containing 0.05% ubiquinone (better known as coenzyme Q10), 0.1% vitamin E, and 1% squalene, along with an orally administered cocktail of 50 mg of coenzyme Q10 + 50 mg of d-RRR-alpha-tocopheryl acetate + 50 µgrams of selenium, while the second group was treated with base cream only.[90] The patients receiving topical and oral administration of the combined antioxidants exhibited higher levels of coenzyme Q10 and vitamin E in the SC. Significant increases in the concentration of coenzyme Q10, d-RRR-alpha-tocopherol, and squalene were measured in the sebum, though not in the SC or plasma, of the patients treated only with topical antioxidant cream.

Despite the plethora of research and media attention regarding the prevention of the effects of photoaging, it is not yet known which antioxidants may be the most suitable for use in the treatment realm. Combining topical and oral antioxidants, or using formulations that are themselves combinations of antioxidants, will likely be the recommended approach to these compounds in the near future. It is also suggested that antioxidants be combined with sunscreens and retinoids to enhance the protective effects of each type of compound because not all sunscreens have an antioxidant effect and not all antioxidants have a sunscreen effect. However, a recent study has shown that a formulation combining vitamins C and E along with ferulic acid confers both a sunscreen effect and an antioxidant effect.[91]

Some Notable Antioxidants

In recent years, several natural compounds have been found to exhibit antioxidant activity. In light of the previously discussed free radical theory of aging, these compounds are especially compelling insofar as they represent the potential to, in some ways, counteract or decelerate the pace of aging. While an exhaustive survey of natural antioxidants (which include such highly touted botanicals as green tea, feverfew, rosemary, grape seed extract, vitamins C and E, ferulic acid, resveratrol, caffeine, mushrooms, curcumin, etc.) would far exceed the scope of this chapter, a few antioxidant ingredients that have recently gained favor and attention are briefly discussed here, particularly in relation to cutaneous effects and/or photoaging.

Caffeine, consumed in popular beverages such as coffee and tea, as well as in certain foods, is believed to confer significant anti-carcinogenic and antioxidant activity. In a recent study, caffeine applied topically 5 days a week for 18 weeks inhibited carcinogenesis and promoted apoptosis in sunburn cells of hairless SKH-1 high-risk (UVB-pretreated) mice.[92] In another influential study, SKH-1 hairless, tumor-free mice were pretreated with UVB twice weekly for 20 weeks and then topically treated with caffeine or (−)-epigallocatechin gallate (EGCG), once a day 5 days a week for 18 weeks. Investigators noted a reduction in the number of nonmalignant and malignant skin tumors per mouse of 44 and 72%, respectively, in the caffeine group and 55 and 66%, respectively, in the EGCG group.[93] In addition to its effects on such UV-mediated processes, caffeine applied topically after UV exposure has been demonstrated to reduce skin roughness and transverse rhytides in mice.[94]

Coenzyme Q10, a fat-soluble antioxidant present in all cells as an element in the electron transportation chain responsible for energy production, has been demonstrated to confer antiapoptotic activity.[95] This compound, which also occurs naturally in fish, shellfish, spinach, and nuts, has been shown to diminish with age in animals and humans, like the key constituents of the skin.[96] It is also worth noting that while UV light is known to deplete vitamins C and E, glutathione, and coenzyme Q10 from the epidermis and dermis, coenzyme Q10 is consistently the first antioxidant to be eliminated in the skin.

Ferulic acid (4-hydroxy-3-methoxycinnamic acid) is prevalent in the plant world, and present in the cell walls of numerous plants, including grains, fruits, and vegetables.[97,98] This potent antioxidant, when included in cosmetic lotions, is also known to confer photoprotection to skin.[99] In addition, it is a member of the family of polyphenolic compounds known as *hydroxycinnamic acids*, which deliver cutaneous benefits,[100] particularly in sunscreens. As a strong UV absorber, ferulic acid is also incorporated into such products.[101] In fact, it might be most useful when combined with other antioxidants. Investigators found that the inclusion of ferulic acid into a solution including vitamins C and E led to a twofold increase in the skin-protective capacity of the already protective formulation.[91] It is thought that such a combination of topical antioxidants in a broad-spectrum sunscreen has the potential to impart optimal UV protection to the skin.[102]

Feverfew (*Tanacetum parthenium*), a perennial herb with a long history of use in folk medicine,[103] has been demonstrated to exhibit anti-inflammatory properties.[104] Its major sesquiterpene lactone, parthenolide, is known to inhibit nuclear factor-kappaB (NF-κB) and exhibit antiproliferative activity.[105] Parthenolide has been shown in vitro to consistently evince antitumor activity,[106] especially against skin cancer induced by UV irradiation.[104] The broad activity of parthenolide against UVB-induced damage has led to the consideration of this feverfew ingredient for its potential as an agent to prevent cutaneous photoaging.[107]

Green tea (*Cammelia sinensis*) is a popular beverage consumed worldwide and a popular ingredient in personal care products, such as moisturizers, cleansers, shower gels, toothpastes, depilatories, shampoos, and perfumes. Products that include green tea as main ingredients are designed to harness the reportedly potent antioxidant capacity of the polyphenols that occur naturally in the green tea leaf. These polyphenols are known to affect the biochemical pathways involved in cell proliferation, inflammatory responses, and responses of tumor promoters.[108] The active ingredients in the polyphenols of the leaves, known as *catechins*, include epicatechin, epicatechin-3-gallate, epigallocatechin, and the most prevalent one, epigallocatechin-3-gallate (EGCG), which is the most studied constituent and comprises 30–40% of the dry weight of green tea leaves.[109] Green tea polyphenols, particularly EGCG, are considered especially adept at inhibiting the carcinogenic activity of UV radiation and providing broad protection against UV-mediated responses such as sunburn, immunosuppression, and photoaging, and are therefore believed to exhibit skin-protective potential too when included or combined with traditional sunscreens.[110]

Polypodium leucotomos (PL) extract, which is derived from tropical fern, has been shown to possess potent antioxidant properties. In one study, phototoxicity incidence was reduced after oral PL administration in participants receiving PUVA treatment,[111] as well as in normal healthy subjects.[112] In a different study, substantially enhanced membrane integrity, reduced lipid peroxidation, increased elastin expression, and inhibited MMP-1 expression characterized PL-treated keratinocytes and fibroblasts exposed to UV.[113]

Pycnogenol, a plant extract derived from pine bark, grapes, apples and other botanicals, is laden with procyanidins, or condensed tannins (also called *proanthocyanidins*), a group of potent free-radical scavenging compounds. Procyanidins are also found in other parts of these plants and in various other plants known to impart antioxidant activity, such as bilberry, cranberry, black currant, green tea, black tea, blueberry, blackberry, strawberry, black cherry, red wine, red cabbage, as well as in grape seed and grape skin. In one study, pycnogenol concentrations of 0.05–0.2% were used to pretreat Skh:hr hairless mice, resulting in a dose-dependent reduction of the inflammatory sunburn reaction (edema) after minimally inflammatory daily exposures to solar-simulated UV radiation.[114] In a study with 21 human volunteers, oral supplementation with pycnogenol was deemed responsible for mitigating the cutaneous effects of UV radiation, specifically reducing erythema.[115] During supplementation, the UV radiation level necessary to achieve one minimal erythema dose (MED) was significantly elevated. Pycnogenol is also known to confer anti-inflammatory effects, which are thought to occur, at least partly, due to its inhibition of IFN-γ-induced expression of ICAM-1.[116] Notably, procyanidins, which are also rife in grape seed extract, are believed to be capable of stabilizing collagen and elastin, thereby enhancing the elasticity, flexibility, and appearance of the skin.

Resveratrol, a polyphenolic phytoalexin compound also present in the skin and seeds of grapes, as well as in berries, peanuts, and other foods,[117–119] is thought to exhibit potent antioxidant, anti-inflammatory, and anti-proliferative activity.[120,121] In particular, resveratrol is believed to act as a chemopreventive agent against skin cancer as well as an anti-proliferative agent against oral squamous, breast, colon, and prostate cancer cells,[122] inducing apoptosis in such tumor cells.[123] Resveratrol may also have a role to play in treating the cutaneous signs of aging. A recent report demonstrates that resveratrol protects against UVB-mediated cutaneous damages in SKH-1 hairless mice.[124,125] Data on resveratrol are sufficiently convincing that this antioxidant is considered suitable for incorporating into various skin care products (e.g., emollients, patches, sunscreens) designed to prevent skin cancer and other UV-induced conditions.[125]

Rosemary (*Rosmarinus officinalis*), long used as a food spice and in traditional medicine, has been recently shown to possess potent antioxidant capacity, which is ascribed to its component phenolic diterpenes.[126–128] In addition, rosemary extracts have been demonstrated to exhibit anticarcinogenic properties, including reduction of skin tumorigenicity.[129] Specifically, rosemary has been shown to suppress tumorigenesis in the two-stage skin cancer model in mice,[130,131] and exhibit photoprotective properties.[132] A study of human surface lipids in which skin treated with rosemary extract protected against free radical damage engendered by *t*-butyl hydroperoxide has also supported the growing antioxidant reputation of rosemary.[133,134] Finally, investigators studying the role of oxidative stress and sulfdryl (SH) groups in heat shock protein 70 (HSP70) induction in human skin fibroblasts and the effect of antioxidants concluded that the antioxidant activity of hydrophilic rosemary extract exhibits the potential to reduce ROS-induced skin damage while delivering cosmetic benefits.[135]

Silymarin, a naturally occurring polyphenolic flavonoid or flavonolignans constituent of the seeds of the milk thistle plant *Silybum marianu*, has been demonstrated to exhibit antioxidant, anti-inflammatory, and immunomodulatory activity in several animal models and is thought to have the potential to prevent skin cancer as well as photoaging.[136] Silybin, the primary component of silymarin that is thought to account for its salubrious effects, has been shown following systemic administration to be bioavailable in skin and other tissues.[137] Topical application of silybin prior to or immediately after UV exposure has also been noted for strongly protecting against UV-induced epidermal insult by depleting thymine dimer-positive cells.[138]

Sun Avoidance

Sun avoidance remains the obvious and most effective approach to prevent the numerous deleterious effects of UV radiation, but this can often be challenging to achieve. The use of sunscreen is also considered a primary component in anti-aging and skin-protective regimens, particularly products that protect against UVA as well as UVB radiation. In a study on the utility of sunscreens, children that tend to freckle developed 30–40% fewer freckles when treated daily with an SPF 30 sunscreen as compared to children who were not treated with a sunscreen.[139] This study reinforces the long-standing recommendations of dermatologists for patients to protect against sun exposure in order to prevent the formation of such pigmented lesions that not only render an older appearance, but are associated with an elevated risk of melanoma. While avoidance is often impractical as well as an unpopular suggestion among many patients, it is incumbent upon physicians to assess the receptivity of their patients and recommend as stringent a sun-avoidance regimen as they deem their patients will accept. At a minimum, patients should be encouraged to avoid sun exposure between 10 A.M. and 4 P.M. and to avoid tanning beds at any hour. The use of a Wood's light to demonstrate to patients the skin damage that they have already experienced from sun exposure can be a sobering but persuasive method to get patients to implement any or several sun-protective behaviors, including measures such as the use of sunscreens, antioxidants, and retinoids. Daily application of sunscreen is recommended, even when patients intend to stay inside. Because UVA radiation can penetrate glass, patients should also be advised that they can reduce their risk at home and at work by not lingering near sun-splashed windows and by placing UVA shields on windows. The use of sun-protective clothing, such as a broad-brimmed hat and SPF 45 clothing, also serves as a practical complement to a healthy sun-protective regimen when prolonged exposure is anticipated and unavoidable or as a substitute when sun avoidance is not feasible.

Microbiology of the Skin

Human skin is considered an organ and is composed of different tissue types – namely, epidermal, nervous, muscular, and connective. The total surface area of human skin is 1.75 m^2 and it weighs approximately 5 kg. Certain regions of the body such as the axillae, groin, and areas between the toes are well known to support the growth of relatively high densities of bacterial cells. At other sites of the body the density of bacterial populations are considered, in comparison, much lower. Consequently, both the density and composition of the normal flora of the skin will vary between anatomical locales.

The skin, as mentioned previously, is composed of an outer epidermis and an inner dermis. The outermost epidermal layer is 0.5–3 mm thick and this is the layer that is important in microbial adhesion and proliferation of intact skin. The epidermis consists of approximately 90% dead keratinocytes. Other cells found in the epidermis include melanocytes (important for reducing skin damage as they absorb UV light), Langerhans cells (immune response cells), and Merkel cells (cells that have adapted for sensory signals association). The layer below the epidermis is the dermis. It is here that the skin becomes more complex. Found here are collagen and elastin fibers forming connective tissue, hair follicles, sebaceous glands, sudoriferous glands, adipose tissue, nerves veins, and capillaries.

Essentially, the skin provides the first line of defense to microorganisms that wish to adhere.[140–143] Such defenses include a low moisture content, antimicrobial peptides, a slightly acidic (5.5) pH, a high salt content, the presence of lipids and fatty acids, immunoglobulins, and a continual shedding of squames and lysozymes. In addition, airborne pathogens generally have a reduced ability to settle and adhere on skin because of the airflow that occurs continually across the body surface. If microorganisms do reach the skin surface, they are exposed to dead keratinized cells together with a lipid-rich surface coating composed of esters, sterols, alkanes, ceramides, and phospholipids, among others, found between these cells which reduce irreversible adhesion and proliferation. Owing to the very low availability of nutrients and high levels of keratin, which cannot be biodegraded by most bacteria, microbial proliferation is therefore substantially reduced. Skin has its own lymphoid tissue providing both a humoral and cell-mediated response. However, certain regions of the body have skin with a higher moisture content than normal and a neutral or slightly alkaline pH and as such these areas are more effectively colonized by certain groups of bacteria. It is interesting to note that females generally have a lower skin surface pH than men.[144] The significance of this has not yet been determined.

Microflora of the Skin

Despite the vast array of microorganisms found in nature there are only a few that are found colonizing the human skin.[145,146] Bacteria that colonize the skin are referred to as the *resident microorganisms* or "normal microbiota of the skin." Price in 1938[147] first classified the term *resident flora* as constituting those bacteria that were relatively stable in both composition and numbers on the human skin.

He also proposed the term *transient flora* to represent those microorganisms (exogenous) that "lie free" on the skin surface.[147]

To date, both quantitative and qualitative data obtained from skin microbiology studies, over the past 50 years, have generated only small amounts of comparable data. This is because many studies have used different sampling techniques to both quantify and culture microorganisms that are retrieved from the skin at different anatomical sites. Most of the research embarked upon in skin microbiology was accomplished between 1960 and 1980 and based on culturable techniques only to identify bacteria.[148–151] Consequently, this has resulted in a gross underestimation of the true diversity and richness of skin microbiota in different regions of the body. Also, the different microbial recovery methods applied to the various research studies have yielded different quantities of bacteria from the same regions of the body.[148,152,153]

Both ecological and host factors can influence strongly the normal microflora of the skin. Such factors include age, sex,[153,154] body location, hygiene, climate, soaps, occlusion, race, occupation, as well as status as an in- or outpatient in hospitals,[155] to name but a few. For example, an increase in temperature and humidity will increase the colonization rate of bacteria. In one study it was found that bacteria survived longer on wet skin compared to skin that was dry.[156]

Skin Flora from Birth

The fetus is considered microbiologically sterile until soon after birth. Following birth, the skin of a newborn baby is coated with vernix caseosa, which helps to maintain the pH of the skin at 7.4. Over time, the vernix disappears and the pH of the skin becomes more acidic (pH 3.0–5.9).[157] This change in pH aids in the selective colonization of skin by microorganisms.

The pioneering bacteria of the skin are often determined by the mode of delivery of a newborn. For example, following a caesarean section delivery the newborn is colonized with microorganisms from the external environment, including the baby's mother.[158] However, babies born by vaginal delivery are colonized by microorganisms that are found associated with the birth canal.

Early studies that have looked at the microbiology of skin in infants have involved the use of scrub techniques to recover bacteria from the skin surface.[159] The scrub techniques involve the application of detergents to the groin, forehead, axillae, and antecubital fossae of newborns. One study using this technique involved sampling the skin of 25 newborns 2 h following birth. In addition, newborns were also sampled at days 1, 2, and 5 and 6 weeks after birth. Between 76 and 80% of the sampling sites, 2 h following birth, were colonized with aerobic bacteria at a level of 36–51 cfu cm^2. Within 24 h, the levels of bacteria in the groin, and also around the axilla regions of the newborn, had increased to 10^3 cfu cm^2.

Slightly lower numbers of bacteria were detected on the scalp (5.4×10^2 cfu cm^2). After 48 h, bacterial counts had reduced to 5.3×10^2 cfu cm^2, with level of bacteria in the axilla and groin regions reducing to 1.0×10^2 cfu cm^2. At day 5 the number of bacteria on the scalp had increased to 2.7×10^3 cfu cm^2. After 6 weeks of sampling, the numbers of bacteria counted on the newborn's skin were equivalent to that of an adult, i.e., 9.8×10^4 cfu cm^2 at the axilla and 3.2×10^5 cfu cm^2 at the groin. The most commonly isolated bacteria in all instances, on all skin areas sampled, was *S. epidermidis*. After 6 weeks, Gram-negative bacteria became quite common on the skin of children, which is considered to be an uncommon situation on adult human skin. Additional studies carried out on neonates have shown that within 2.5 h following birth no microbes could be cultured in 6–13% of babies.

The microflora of infants seem to vary widely between children. Infants are not colonized early on with a dense microbiota and consequently become very susceptible to colonization by pathogenic microorganisms. Infants are therefore known to carry many pathogenic and potentially pathogenic bacteria on their skin along with normal skin flora, when a comparison is made between older children and adults. The normal flora of the neonate's skin seems to be very stable, and even bathing of babies has been shown not to have a significant effect on the skin flora.[160]

Microorganisms such as *Propionibacterium* and *Malassezia folliculitis* are found in higher numbers during and following puberty. However, colonization of infants with cutaneous *Malassezia* commensal flora by the age of 3–6 months has been documented.[161] *Malassezia* spp. are significant to neonates as potential pathogens, as they have been found to cause neonatal sepsis in immunologically immature infants.[162]

Most cases of skin infections observed in babies are associated with bacteria such as *Staphylococcus aureus* and less predominant organisms such as *S. epidermidis*, coliforms, *Pseudomonas*, and yeast.[163] Aly et al.[157] studied the adherence of *S. aureus* to the nasal mucosal cells in newborns. It was found that the binding of *S. aureus* is lower during the first 4 days of life but increases after 5 days.

On the skin of the face of babies a characteristic age-related effect has been found for levels of resident aerobic and anaerobic bacteria.[164] A study by Leyden et al. found that the density of anaerobic diphtheroids and surface aerobic micrococci were higher in infancy when compared to early childhood.[164] In addition, they concluded that at puberty the quantity of organisms on the skin of the face increases and that this increase is more significant during late adolescence. The quantities of anaerobic and aerobic bacteria evident in early adulthood are considered to remain constant until old age. However, at old age the number of bacteria decreases. This seems to be related to the production of sebum on the skin surface.[164,165]

The skin of neonates becomes a significant infection problem particularly during hospital stays.[166] Transfer of pathogens from the mother's skin is also a significant source of infection in neonates.[167]

Normal Adult Skin Flora

The microflora of the adult human skin is variable with regard to bacterial strains and species,[168] with quantities of bacteria varying from 6×10^2 to 2×10^6 bacterial cells per square centimeter. These numbers do, however, vary, as they are often dependent on sex, age, and colonization site.[169] The adult skin also provides a very inhospitable environment for microbes to proliferate, which seriously restricts the microbial diversity.

The most frequently isolated and cultured bacteria found on the adult skin surface include *Staphylococcus*, *Micrococcus*, *Corynebacterium*, *Propionibacterium*, *Malassezia*, *Brevibacterium*, *Acinetobacter*, and *Dermabacter*. However, the ecology of the skin has been shown to vary as do the methods that have been employed for microbial identification. For instance, molecular techniques recover a wider diversity of microorganisms from skin than can be recovered by culturable techniques.[170–172]

Coagulase-negative staphylococci (CNS) constitute the majority of bacteria found as part of the skin ecosystem. CNS are located on the epidermis and the upper parts of the hair follicles.[173] Eighteen different species of CNS have been isolated from the skin of adult humans[174] and approximately 50% of the staphylococci found colonizing the skin are *Staphylococcus epidermidis*. *S. saprophyticus* is also regularly cultured from the microbiota of the skin but more specifically from areas such as the vagina and rectum. Other CNS isolated from skin have included *S. hominis*, *S. warneri*, *S. haemolyticus*, and *S. capitis*.

Coagulase-positive staphylococci, i.e., *S. aureus*, have also been isolated frequently from adult skin. *S. aureus* is widespread in nature and found principally on human skin, skin glands, and mucous membranes, but more specifically in the anterior nares of humans.[175,176] *S. aureus* is found predominantly in high concentrations on hands and the perineum.[177] But it is not isolated very regularly in certain regions of the body and is therefore considered a transient bacterium.[178]

Kloos and Musselwhite[179] studied the distribution of *Staphylococcus* and *Micrococcus* species and associated coryneform bacteria, *Acinetobacter*, *Klebsiella*, *Enterobacter*, *Bacillus*, and *Streptomyces* on adult skin. Staphylococci and coryneforms were found to be the most predominant and persistent bacteria isolated from the nares and axillae. On the head, legs, and arms, staphylococci, coryneforms, micrococci, and bacilli were the most predominant bacteria. Gram-negative isolates such as *Acinetobacter* were most frequently isolated during the warmer months of the years. *S. aureus* and *S. epidermidis* were the most predominant and persistent staphylococci isolated from the nares. *S. epidermidis* and *S. hominis* were the most predominant and persistent staphylococci isolated from the axillae, head, legs, and arms. *S. capitis* was often isolated from the head and arms and *S. haemolyticus* was often isolated from the head, legs, and arms. *S. simulans*, *S. xylosus*, *S. cohnii*, *S. saprophyticus*, *S. warneri*, and an unclassified coagulase-positive species were only occasionally isolated from skin. In addition to this study, Nagase et al.[176] in 2002 conducted a survey that studied the distribution of *Staphylococcus* species on the skin of animals and humans. In this study, staphylococci were isolated from 12 (100%) of 12 pigs, 17 (89.5%) of 19 horses, 30 (100%) of 30 cows, 73 (90.1%) of 81 chickens, 10 (40%) of 25 dogs, 23 (76.7%) of 30 laboratory mice, 20 (52.6%) of 38 pigeons, and 80 (88.9%) of 90 human beings. The predominant staphylococci isolated from a variety of animal species were novobiocin-resistant species, *S. xylosus* and *S. sciuri*, regardless of the animal host species. The novobiocin-resistant species including *S. xylosus* and *S. sciuri* were only occasionally isolated from human skin. The predominant staphylococci found on human skin were novobiocin-sensitive species, *S. epidermidis* (63.8%), followed by *S. warneri* (28.8%) and *S. hominis* (13.8%).

Micrococci luteus is the most predominant and persistent micrococcus isolated from skin and is found at high densities in regions of the head, legs, and arms.[180] Other micrococci that have been isolated have included *M. varians*, *M. lylae*, *M. sedentarius*, *M. roseus*, *M. kristinae*, and *M. nishinomiyaensis*. *M. lylae* is frequently isolated during the colder months of the year.[179]

Propionibacteria are common inhabitants of hair follicles and sebaceous glands and are prevalent anaerobes of the normal flora of skin. The most predominant species found on the skin of the back, forehead, and scalp is *P. acnes*, which is particularly relevant at puberty, when densities start to peak.

Gram-negative bacteria are not a common occurrence on normal healthy adult skin and as such are often considered transient organisms. Common Gram-negative bacteria frequently found on healthy adult skin include *Acinetobacter* spp. and *Pseudomonas* spp. *Acinetobacter* spp. are considered to constitute 25% of the adult skin microflora, being found in high numbers in the perineum, toe webs, and axillae.[179,181,182] Also as part of the skin, microbiota fungi and yeasts are found, particularly *Malassezia*. These are known to inhabit the hair follicles.[183,184] Seven different species of *Malassezia* have been isolated from skin and include *Mal. furfur*, *Mal. sympodialis*, *Mal. globosa*, *Mal. slooffiae*, *Mal. restricta*, *Mal. obusta* and *Mal. pachydermatis*. Age has been shown to have an effect on its prevalence on skin.[185,186]

From an anatomical point of view, the skin is divided into three distinctive regions. These regions include the moist areas that provide a great breeding ground for bacteria to proliferate, i.e., the groin, toe web areas, and the armpits. The oily areas include the forehead, and the dry areas the forearm.[187] Work by Leyden et al.[187] has shown that coryneforms and bacteria belonging to the micrococcacea group are evident in the toe webs and axillae. In the perineum there were large proportions of micrococcacea, but much lower than in the axilla area, and, as would be expected, in this area there were a large number of Gram-negative rods, possibly fecal in origin.[187] Where oily areas are present on the human body, such as the forehead, the relative levels of micrococcacea and coryneform bacteria were low while the levels of *Propionibacterium* spp. were significantly higher. On the scalp, *Malassezia* spp. occurred in high concentrations.[188,189]

The microbial communities found on adult skin differ in composition, being dictated by the colonizing site, i.e., anatomical site,[190] and also the host.

The diversity and density of bacteria are also governed by environmental perturbations.[191] A large number of sebaceous glands are located on the scalp, together with hair coverage enhancing the moisture content. The major bacteria located here include the propionibacteria, specifically *P. acnes* and staphylococci, specifically *S. capitis*. The forehead has a high acidic pH, variations in temperature, and a very high density of sebaceous and eccrine glands. The main bacteria dominating the forehead, as with the scalp, include propionibacteria, specifically *P. acnes*, staphylococci (specifically *S. capitis*, *S. hominis*, *S. epidermidis*), Micrococci, *Malassezia*, and coryneforms.[168] The hands are composed of regions with variations in microbial densities and diversity. Also, variations in temperature between different regions of the body have an effect on microbial composition. The region beneath the fingernail is very densely colonized specifically, as this region is occluded and therefore conducive to the proliferation of many anaerobic bacteria, fungi, and Gram-negative bacteria.

Yeasts are recovered in higher numbers from the elderly population. This is possibly due to a decrease in sweat production that occurs in the elderly.[192] Within the dry skin areas of the adult, staphylococci represent over 90% of the total population.[187,193] There have been numerous reports on the significant difference between hospitalized patients and healthy people. In hospitalized patients the skin has been shown to shift from a more Gram-positive to a more Gram-negative microflora.[181,194–196]

Bacterial Interactions, Skin Physiology, and Flora on the Skin

As mentioned previously, the presence of a normal skin flora is important to human health owing to their resistance to colonization from invading pathogens and also by their ability to have effects on reactions derived from the body as well as from xenobiotic agents.[197,198] In adults, the skin microflora is generally considered "relatively stable." However, within this relatively stable ecosystem, interactions between bacteria and skin cells are known to occur. Nevertheless, chemical and physical interactions between bacteria on the skin are, to date, very poorly understood. Initial research has shown that major forms of antagonism between bacteria on the skin surface occur.[199] This is very important as a defensive mechanism on adult skin helping to prevent skin infections.

As well as the resident microflora, the skin is composed of a dead layer of keratinized cells, referred to as the *stratum corneum*, which aids in preventing bacterial attachment. As a food source, keratin can be utilized only by a small number of bacteria and as such does not constitute a good food source for colonizing bacteria. Found between these cells are fatty acids, waxes, sterols, and phospholipids, among others, which in combination with dead cells makes the skin surface very dry and virtually uninhabitable by many bacteria. Combined also with a low pH, bacterial growth is inhibited. However, certain regions of the body have a relatively high moisture content and a neutral pH, aiding bacterial adhesion. Other problems for bacteria reside on the skin, namely, the ever-shedding squames that are disseminated together with any adhering bacteria. There is also skin-associated lymphoid tissue that is involved with humoral and cell-mediated responses of the immune system and sweat production and contains lysozymes that are known to cleave beta 1,4 glycosidic bonds found in many Gram-positive (N-acetylglucosamine and N-acetylmuramic acid) and Gram-negative bacteria (peptidoglycan). Consequently, this armory of defensive mechanisms evident in the human body does help to substantially reduce microbial proliferation of the intact skin.[200,201]

The temperature of the human body is regulated at 37°C, but that of the skin is lower, ranging from approximately 31°C in the big toe region to 36.1°C in the groin. Ultimately, certain regions of the body that are more accessible and represent a more favorable environment will enhance the survival and colonization of certain genera of bacteria.

Skin Flora and Infection

The balance between the skin barrier and innate immunity helps to maintain healthy skin. Disturbances in this balance may predispose the host to a number of infections.[202–205] Skin infections have been shown to be more significant as humans age.[206] The "normal" skin flora is considered a significant source of serious infections.[207] For example, micrococci, specifically the species *M. luteus*, have been associated with cases of pneumonia, septic arthritis, and meningitis. *S. epidermidis* is a major inhabitant of the skin and generally comprises greater than 90% of the aerobic resident flora. They are often classified as contaminants of the skin when isolated during infections, and are therefore thought of as mutual bacteria aiding the human innate immune system. Antimicrobial peptides on the surface of the skin have recently been identified as originating from *S. epidermidis*.[208] However, in certain situations *S. epidermidis* can be the cause of a number of life-threatening infections, e.g., biofilm formation on artificial heart values and intravascular catheters. This is principally due to these bacteria being avid biofilm formers resulting in enhanced virulence and resistant to antimicrobial chemotherapy. A "transient" bacterium associated with skin infections is *S. aureus*. *S. aureus* is considered a normal component of the nasal microflora.[209–211] Nearly 86.9 million people (32.4% of the population) are considered to be colonized with *S. aureus*,[212] 20% of the population are considered to be persistently colonized, 60% of the population intermittently carry the bacteria, and 20% are never colonized. *S. aureus* found on healthy human skin generally acts as a commensal and rarely as a pathogen, but it is known to cause minor and self-limiting skin infections. Skin infections due to *S. aureus* include impetigo, folliculitis, furuncles and subcutaneous abscesses, and the scalded skin syndrome.[213,214]

Many diphtheroids are found on the human skin. *Corynebacterium jeikeium* is the most frequently recovered and medically relevant member of the group, particularly in hospitalized patients.[215] In the last few years, *Corynebacterium* diphtheroids have gained interest because of the increasing number of nosocomial infections with which they are associated.[216,217]

Propionibacteria are prevalent in skin-colonizing bacteria. The most well-known ailment associated with *P. acnes* is acne vulgaris, which affects up to 80% of adolescents in the US.[218] In fact, *P. acnes* is able to initiate and also contribute to inflammation during acne episodes. Reports of *P. acnes* being associated with foreign device infections have also been highlighted. Gram-negative rods such as *Acinetobacter* are known to be a cause of skin infections, particularly in patients with wound infections and burns. *Acinetobacter* has been associated with many infections such as endocarditis and respiratory tract infections, among others. *Pseudomonas aeruginosa* is another Gram-negative bacterium that lives innocuously on human skin. However, they are able to infect practically any tissue with which they come into contact. Infections due to *P. aeruginosa* occur primarily in compromised patients.

Skin bacteria are generally very avid biofilm formers. Evidence of biofilms on skin has been documented, and the actual architecture has been observed in dermatitis and eczema. The first reported incidence of biofilms on skin was by *S. epidermidis*.[219] It has been suggested that the severity of eczema is proportional to colonization resistance.[220]

Conclusion

Aging of the skin is a dynamic, multifactorial process governed by intrinsic genetic factors and mediated by extrinsic influences.[221] Intrinsic or natural aging is determined cellularly as a function of heredity and is therefore inevitable through the passage of time. Extrinsic aging, which, like intrinsic aging, manifests in cutaneous alterations, is caused by exogenous sources and is therefore avoidable insofar as the behaviors or exposures that promote such changes can be reasonably avoided. In particular, prolonged, chronic exposure to the sun is best avoided to significantly reduce one's risk of inducing extrinsic skin aging. Addressing and showing examples of the attendant wrinkling and pigmentary changes associated with photoaging and the potentially more serious consequences of chronic sun exposure can be effective approaches for physicians in an attempt to encourage sun-protective behavior, as this method appeals to an individual's strong concern about appearance. The clinical appearance of photoaging is characterized by rough and xerotic skin, mottled pigmentation, and wrinkling. Such cutaneous manifestations, particularly when extensive or severe, may be precursors to actinic keratoses and skin cancer. It is important for physicians to inform patients that photodamage represents the cutaneous signs of premature aging and that "sun tans," which remain popular, qualify as photodamage. Summarizing the role of telomeres in cellular aging and cancer and/or briefly discussing the differences between intrinsic and extrinsic aging might prove useful in convincing patients to reduce or eliminate behaviors that facilitate extrinsic aging and, ideally, reduce the prevalence and incidence of photodamage, photoaging, and photo-induced skin cancers. Apart from sun avoidance, which includes limiting sun exposure to the hours prior to 10 A.M. or after 4 P.M., the only known defenses against photoaging are using sunscreens to block or reduce the amount of UV reaching the skin, using retinoids to inhibit collagenase synthesis and to promote collagen production, and using antioxidants, particularly in combination, to attack and neutralize free radicals.

The skin microflora is a complex ecosystem but to date the ecological studies that have been undertaken to examine this ecosystem in different regions of both the infant and adult have been solely culture-based methods that underestimate the true numbers and diversity of bacteria inhabiting this ecosystem. It is widely accepted that the resident microbial community on infants and adults alike has a significant role to play in human health, and that it is generally positive. However, when imbalances occur, the microbial flora can have a negative effect on human skin.[222] We require a deeper understanding of skin microbiology and the aging process, together with a better understanding of the host factors that are known to affect the biofilm and its overall community and architecture on skin. The role of personal hygiene becomes significant with an aging population. In conclusion, the skin microbiota play a very important role in preventing many pathogens from colonizing the skin and causing disease, in a manner similar to the "barrier effect" produced by intestinal microbes.

References

1. Fenske NA, Lober CW. Structural and functional changes of normal aging skin. J Am Acad Dermatol 1986;15:571–585.
2. Roupe G. Skin of the aging human being. Lakartidningen 2001;98(10):1091–1095.
3. Lovell CR, Smolenski KA, Duance VC, Light ND, Young S, Dyson M. Type I and III collagen content and fibre distribution in normal human skin during ageing. Br J Dermatol 1987;117:419–428.
4. Uitto J. Understanding premature skin aging. N Engl J Med 1997;337:1463–1465.
5. Lavker RM. Structural alterations in exposed and unexposed aged skin. J Invest Dermatol 1979;73:59–66.
6. Yaar M, Gilchrest BA. Aging of Skin in Fitzpatrick's Dermatology in General Medicine. New York: McGraw-Hill, p 1700.
7. Geserick C, Blasco MA. Novel roles for telomerase in aging. Mech Ageing Dev 2006;127 (6):579–583.
8. Boukamp P. Ageing mechanisms: the role of telomere loss. Clin Exp Dermatol 2001;26 (7):562–565.
9. Bellon M, Nicot C. Regulation of telomerase and telomeres: human tumor viruses take control. J Natl Cancer Inst 2008;100(2):98–108.
10. Pendino F, Tarkanyi I, Dudognon C, Hillion J, Lanotte M, Aradi J, Segal-Bendirdjian E. Telomeres and telomerase: pharmacological targets for new anticancer strategies? Curr Cancer Drug Targets 2006;(2):147–180.
11. Boukamp P. Skin aging: a role for telomerase and telomere dynamics? Curr Mol Med 2005;5 (2):71–77.

12. Nakamura K, Izumiyama-Shimomura N, Sawabe M, Arai T, Aoyagi Y, Fujiwara M, Tsuchiya E, Kobayashi Y, Kato M, Oshimura M, Sasajima K, Nakachi K, Takubo K. Comparative analysis of telomere lengths and erosion with age in human epidermis and lingual epithelium. J Invest Dermatol 2002;119(5):1014–1019.

13. Bataille V, Kato BS, Falchi M, Gardner J, Kimura M, Lens M, Perks U, Valdes AM, Bennett DC, Aviv A, Spector TD. Nevus size and number are associated with telomere length and represent potential markers of a decreased senescence *in vivo*. Cancer Epidemiol Biomarkers Prev 2007;16(7):1499–1502.

14. Kosmadaki MG, Gilchrest BA. The role of telomeres in skin aging/photoaging. Micron 2004;35(3):155–159.

15. Lebel M, Leder P. A deletion within the murine Werner syndrome helicase induces sensitivity to inhibitors of topoisomerase and loss of cellular proliferative capacity. Proc Natl Acad Sci U S A 1998;95(22):13097–13102.

16. Ahn B, Harrigan JA, Indig FE, Wilson DM III, Bohr VA. Regulation of WRN helicase activity in human base excision repair. J Biol Chem 2004;279(51):53465–53474.

17. Poot M, Gollahon KA, Emond MJ, Silber JR, Rabinovitch PS. Werner syndrome diploid fibroblasts are sensitive to 4-nitroquinoline-*N*-oxide and 8-methoxypsoralen: implications for the disease phenotype. FASEB J 2002;16(7):757–758.

18. Chang S, Multani AS, Cabrera NG, Naylor ML, Laud P, Lombard D, Pathak S, Guarente L, DePinho RA. Essential role of limiting telomeres in the pathogenesis of Werner syndrome. Nat Genet 2004;36(8):877–882.

19. Harman D. Aging: a theory based on free radical and radiation chemistry. J Gerontol 1956;11:298–300.

20. Pelle E, Maes D, Padulo GA, Kim EK, Smith WP. An *in vitro* model to test relative antioxidant potential: ultraviolet-induced lipid peroxidation in liposomes. Arch Biochem Biophys 1990;283:234–240.

21. Werninghaus K. The role of antioxidants in reducing photodamage, in Gilchrest B (ed.) Photodamage. London: Blackwell Science, 1995, p 249.

22. Rikans LE, Hornbrook KR. Lipid peroxidation, antioxidant protection and aging. Biochim Biophys Acta 1997;1362:116–127.

23. Hensley K, Floyd R. Reactive oxygen species and protein oxidation in aging: a look back, a look ahead. Arch Biochem Biophys 2002;397:377–383.

24. Black HS. Potential involvement of free radical reactions in ultraviolet light-mediated cutaneous damage. Photochem Photobiol 1987;46:213–221.

25. Verdier-Sévrain S, Bonté F, Gilchrest B. Biology of estrogens in skin: implications for skin aging. Exp Dermatol 2006;15:83–94.

26. Creidi P, Faivre B, Agache P, Richard E, Haudiquet V, Sauvanet JP. Effect of a conjugated oestrogen (Premarin) cream on ageing facial skin A. comparative study with a placebo cream. Maturitas 1994;19:211–223.

27. Dunn LB, Damesyn M, Moore AA, Reuben DB, Greendale GA. Does estrogen prevent skin aging? Results from the First National Health and Nutritional Examination Survey. Arch Dermatol 1997;133:339–342.

28. Fisher GJ, Kang S, Varani J, Bata-Csorgo Z, Wan Y, Datta S, Voorhees JJ. Mechanisms of photoaging and chronological skin aging. Arch Dermatol 2002;138:1462–1470.

29. Kligman AM, Kligman LH. Photoaging, in Freedberg IM, Eisen AZ, Wolff K, et al. (eds.) Fitzpatrick's Dermatology in General Medicine, 5th Ed., Vol. 1. New York: McGraw-Hill, 1999, pp 1717–1723.

30. Yao W, Malaviya R, Magliocco M, Gottlieb A. Topical treatment of UVB-irradiated human subjects with EGCG, a green tea polyphenol, increases caspase-3 activity in keratinocytes. J Am Acad Dermatol 2005;52:150.

31. Pinnell S, Lin F-Y, Grichnik J, et al. A topical antioxidant solution containing vitamin C, vitamin E, and ferulic acid prevents ultraviolet radiation induced caspase-3 induction in skin. JAAD 2005;2(52):158.

32. Bosset S, Bonnet-Duquennoy M, Barre P, Chalon A, Kurfurst R, Bonte F, Schnebert S, Le Varlet B, Nicolas JF. Photoageing shows histological features of chronic skin inflammation without clinical and molecular abnormalities. Br J Dermatol 2003;149(4):826–835.
33. Kappes UP, Luo D, Potter M, Schulmeister K, Runger TM. Short- and long-wave UV light (UVB and UVA) induce similar mutations in human skin cells. J Invest Dermatol 2006;126 (3):667–675.
34. Marrot L, Belaïdi JP, Meunier JR. Importance of UVA photoprotection as shown by genotoxic related endpoints: DNA damage and p53 status. Mutat Res 2005;571(1–2):175–184.
35. Sugimoto M, Yamashita R, Ueda M. Telomere length of the skin in association with chronological aging and photoaging. J Dermatol Sci 2006;43(1):43–47.
36. Makrantonaki E, Zouboulis CC. Characteristics and pathomechanisms of endogenously aged skin. Dermatology 2007;214:352–360.
37. Moragas A, Castells C, Sans M. Mathematical morphologic analysis of aging-related epidermal changes. Anal Quant Cytol Histol 1993;15:75–82.
38. Lock-Andersen J, Therkildsen P, de Fine Olivarius F, Gniadecka M, Dahlstrom K, Poulsen T, Wulf HC. Epidermal thickness, skin pigmentation and constitutive photosensitivity. Photodermatol Photoimmunol Photomed 1997;13:153–158.
39. Whitton JT, Everall JD. The thickness of the epidermis. Br J Dermatol 1973;89:467–476.
40. Sandby-Møller J, Poulsen T, Wulf HC. Epidermal thickness at different body sites: relationship to age, gender, pigmentation, blood content, skin type and smoking habits. Acta Derm Venereol 2003;83:410–413.
41. El-Domyati M, Attia S, Saleh F, Brown D, Birk DE, Gasparro F, Ahmad H, Uitto J. Intrinsic aging vs. photoaging: a comparative histopathological, immunohistochemical, and ultrastructural study of skin. Exp Dermatol 2002;11(5):398–405.
42. Contet-Audonneau JL, Jeanmaire C, Pauly G. A histological study of human wrinkle structures: comparison between sun-exposed areas of the face, with or without wrinkles, and sun-protected areas. Br J Dermatol 1999;140:1038–1047.
43. Katzberg AA. The area of the dermo-epidermal junction in human skin. Anat Rec 1958;131:717–721.
44. Yaar M, Gilchrest BA. Aging of Skin in Fitzpatrick's Dermatology in General Medicine. New York: McGraw-Hill, pp 1697–1706.
45. Kligman AM. Perspectives and problems in cutaneous gerontology. J Invest Dermatol 1979;73:39–46.
46. Orentreich N, Selmanowitz VJ. Levels of biological functions with aging. Trans NY Acad Sci 1969;31:992–998.
47. Grewe M. Chronological ageing and photoageing of dendritic cells. Clin Exp Dermatol 2001;26:608–612.
48. Fisher GJ, Wang ZQ, Datta SC, Varani J, Kang S, Voorhees JJ. Pathophysiology of premature skin aging induced by ultraviolet light. N Engl J Med 1997;337:1419–1428.
49. Kligman AM, Zheng P, Lavker RM. The anatomy and pathogenesis of wrinkles. Br J Dermatol 1985;113:37–42.
50. Gniadecka M, Nielsen OF, Wessel S, Heidenheim M, Christensen DH, Wulf HC. Water and protein structure in photoaged and chronically aged skin. J Invest Dermatol 1998;111:1129–1133.
51. Oikarinen A. The aging of skin: chronoaging versus photoaging. Photodermatol Photoimmunol Photomed 1990;7:3–4.
52. Shuster S, Black MM, McVitie E. The influence of age and sex on skin thickness, skin collagen and density. Br J Dermatol 1975;93:639–643.
53. Montagna W, Carlisle K. Structural changes in aging human skin. J Invest Dermatol 1979;73:47–53.
54. Griffiths CE, Russman AN, Majmudar G, Singer RS, Hamilton TA, Voorhees JJ. Restoration of collagen formation in photodamaged human skin by tretinoin (retinoic acid). N Engl J Med 1993;329:530–535.

55. Craven NM, Watson RE, Jones CJ, Shuttleworth CA, Kielty CM, Griffiths CE. Clinical features of photodamaged human skin are associated with a reduction in collagen VII. Br J Dermatol 1997;137:344–350.

56. Rittie L, Fisher GJ. UV-light-induced signal cascades and skin aging. Ageing Res Rev 2002;1(4):705–720.

57. Varani J, Warner RL, Gharaee-Kermani M, Phan SH, Kang S, Chung JH, Wang ZQ, Datta SC, Fisher GJ, Voorhees JJ. Vitamin A antagonizes decreased cell growth and elevated collagen-degrading matrix metalloproteinases and stimulates collagen accumulation in naturally aged human skin. J Invest Dermatol 2000;114:480–486.

58. Fisher GJ, Datta SC, Talwar HS, Wang ZQ, Varani J, Kang S, Voorhees JJ. Molecular basis of sun-induced premature skin ageing and retinoid antagonism. Nature 1996;379:335–339.

59. Mitchel RE. Chronic solar dermatosis: a light and electron microscopic study of the dermis. J Invest Dermatol 1967;48:203–211.

60. Tsuji T, Hamada T. Age-related changes in human dermal elastic fibers. Br J Dermatol 1981;105:57–63.

61. Scharffetter-Kochanek K, Brenneisen P, Wenk J, Herrmann G, Ma W, Kuhr L, Meewes C, Wlaschek M. Photoaging of the skin from phenotype to mechanisms. Exp Gerontol 2000;35:307–316.

62. Matsuoka L, Uitto J. Alterations in the elastic fibers in cutaneous aging and solar elastosis, in Balin A, Kligman AM (eds.) Aging and the Skin. New York: Raven Press, 1989, pp 141–151.

63. Lavker RM. Cutaneous aging: chronologic versus photoaging, in Gilchrest BA (eds.) Photodamage, 1st Ed. Cambridge, MA: Blackwell Science, 1995, p 128.

64. Escoffier C, de Rigal J, Rochefort A, Vasselet R, Lévêque JL, Agache PG. Age-related mechanical properties of human skin: an *in vivo* study. J Invest Dermatol 1989;93:353–357.

65. Ghersetich I, Lotti T, Campanile G, Grappone C, Dini G. Hyaluronic acid in cutaneous intrinsic aging. Int J Dermatol 1994;33:119–122.

66. Pearce RH, Grimmer BJ. Age and the chemical constitution of normal human dermis. J Invest Dermatol 1972;58:347–361.

67. Elsner P, Maibach HI. Cosmeceuticals and Active Cosmetics: Drugs versus Cosmetics. 2nd Ed. Dekker: New York, 2005.

68. Bernstein EF, Underhill CB, Hahn PJ, Brown DB, Uitto J. Chronic sun exposure alters both the content and distribution of dermal glycosaminoglycans. Br J Dermatol 1996;135:255–262.

69. Tammi R, Säämänen AM, Maibach HI, Tammi M. Degradation of newly synthesized high molecular mass hyaluronan in the epidermal and dermal compartments of human skin in organ culture. J Invest Dermatol 1991;97(1):126–130.

70. Sakai S, Yasuda R, Sayo T, Ishikawa O, Inoue S. Hyaluronan exists in the normal stratum corneum. J Invest Dermatol 2000;114(6):1184–1187.

71. Rieger M. Hyaluronic acid in cosmetics. Cosm Toil 1998;113(3):35–42.

72. Ortonne JP. Pigmentary changes of the ageing skin. Br J Dermatol 1990;122:21–28.

73. Gilchrest BA, Stoff JS, Soter NA. Chronologic aging alters the response to ultraviolet-induced inflammation in human skin. J Invest Dermatol 1982;79:11–15.

74. Ghadially R, Brown BE, Sequeira-Martin SM, Feingold KR, Elias PM. The aged epidermal permeability barrier. Structural, functional, and lipid biochemical abnormalities in humans and a senescent murine model. J Clin Invest 1995;95:2281–2290.

75. Tezuka T, Qing J, Saheki M, Kusuda S, Takahashi M. Terminal differentiation of facial epidermis of the aged: immunohistochemical studies. Dermatology 1994;188:21–24.

76. Nelson BR, Majmudar G, Griffiths CE, Gillard MO, Dixon AE, Tavakkol A, Hamilton TA, Woodbury RA, Voorhees JJ, Johnson TM. Clinical improvement following dermabrasion of photoaged skin correlates with synthesis of collagen I. Arch Dermatol 1994;130:1136–1142.

77. Ostler EL, Wallis CV, Aboalchamat B, Faragher RG. Telomerase and the cellular lifespan: implications of the aging process. J Pediatr Endocrinol Metab 2000;6:1467–1476.

78. Kang S, Voorhees JJ. Photoaging therapy with topical tretinoin: an evidence-based analysis. J Am Acad Dermatol 1998;39(2 pt 3):S55–S61.

79. Gilchrest BA. Treatment of photodamage with topical tretinoin: an overview. J Am Acad Dermatol 1997;36(3 pt 2):S27–S36.
80. Fisher GJ, Voorhees JJ. Molecular mechanisms of photoaging and its prevention by retinoic acid: ultraviolet irradiation induces MAP kinase signal transduction cascades that induce AP-1-regulated matrix metalloproteinases that degrade human skin *in vivo*. J Investig Dermatol Symp Proc 1998;3:61–68.
81. Baumann L. How to prevent photoaging? J Invest Dermatol 2005;125(4):xii–xiii.
82. Nusgens BV, Humbert P, Rougier A, Colige AC, Haftek M, Lambert CA, Richard A, Creidi P, Lapiere CM. Topically applied vitamin C enhances the mRNA level of collagens I and III, their processing enzymes and tissue inhibitor of matrix metalloproteinase 1 in the human dermis. J Invest Dermatol 2001;116(6):853–859.
83. Kockaert M, Neumann M. Systemic and topical drugs for aging skin. J Drugs Dermatol 2003;2(4):435–441.
84. Margelin D, Medaisko C, Lombard D, Picard J, Fourtanier A. Hyaluronic acid and dermatan sulfate are selectively stimulated by retinoic acid in irradiated and nonirradiated hairless mouse skin. J Invest Dermatol 1996;106(3):505–509.
85. Tajima S, Hayashi A, Suzuki T. Elastin expression is up-regulated by retinoic acid but not by retinol in chick embryonic skin fibroblasts. J Dermatol Sci 1997;15(3):166–172.
86. Matheson AJ, Perry CM. Glucosamine: a review of its use in the management of osteoarthritis. Drugs Aging 2003;20(14):1041–1060.
87. Fitzpatrick RE. Endogenous growth factors as cosmeceuticals. Dermatol Surg 2005;31(7 pt 2):827–831; discussion 831.
88. Kang S, Chung JH, Lee JH, Fisher GJ, Wan YS, Duell EA, Voorhees JJ. Topical *N*-acetyl cysteine and genistein prevent ultraviolet-light-induced signaling that leads to photoaging in human skin *in vivo*. J Invest Dermatol 2003;120(5):835–841.
89. Greul AK, Grundmann JU, Heinrich F, Pfitzner I, Bernhardt J, Ambach A, Biesalski HK, Gollnick H. Photoprotection of UV-irradiated human skin: an antioxidative combination of vitamins E and C, carotenoids, selenium and proanthocyanidins. Skin Pharmacl Appl Skin Physiol 2002;15(5):307–315.
90. Passi S, De Pita O, Grandinetti M, Simotti C, Littaru GP. The combined use of oral and topical lipophilic antioxidants increases their levels both in sebum and stratum corneum. Biofactors 2003;18(1–4):289–297.
91. Lin FH, Lin JY, Gupta RD, Tournas JA, Burch JA, Selim MA, Monteiro-Riviere NA, Grichnik JM, Zielinski J, Pinnell SR. Ferulic acid stabilizes a solution of vitamins C and E and doubles its photoprotection of skin. J Invest Dermatol 2005;125(4):826–832.
92. Conney AH, Lu YP, Lou YR, Huang MT. Inhibitory effects of tea and caffeine on UV-induced carcinogenesis: relationship to enhanced apoptosis and decreased tissue fat. Eur J Cancer Prev 2002;11:S28–S36.
93. Lu YP, Lou YR, Xie JG, Peng QY, Liao J, Yang CS, Huang MT, Conney AH. Topical applications of caffeine or (−)-epigallocatechin gallate (EGCG) inhibit carcinogenesis and selectively increase apoptosis in UVB-induced skin tumors in mice. Proc Natl Acad Sci USA 2002;99:12455–12460.
94. Koo SW, Hirakawa S, Fujii S, Kawasumi M, Nghiem P. Protection from photodamage by topical application of caffeine after ultraviolet irradiation. Br J Dermatol 2007;156: 957–964.
95. Papucci L, Schiavone N, Witort E, Donnini M, Lapucci A, Tempestini A, Formigli L, Zecchi-Orlandini S, Orlandini G, Carella G, Brancato R, Capaccioli S. Coenzyme q10 prevents apoptosis by inhibiting mitochondrial depolarization independently of its free radical scavenging property. J Biol Chem 2003;278(30):28220–28228.
96. Beyer RE, Ernster L. The antioxidant role of coenzyme Q, in Lenaz G, et al. (eds.) Highlights in Ubiquinone Research. London: Taylor and Francis, 1990, pp 191–213.

97. Bourne LC, Rice-Evans C. Bioavailability of ferulic acid. Biochem Biophys Res Commun 1998;253:222–227.
98. Svobodova A, Psotova J, Walterova D. Natural phenolics in the prevention of UV-induced skin damage. A review. Biomed Pap Med Fac Univ Palacky Olomouc Czech Repub 2003;147: 137–145.
99. Graf E. Antioxidant potential of ferulic acid. Free Radic Biol Med 1992;13:435–448.
100. Bonina F, Puglia C, Ventura D, Aquino R, Tortora S, Sacchi A, Saija A, Tomaino A, Pellegrino ML, de Caprariis P. *In vitro* antioxidant and *in vivo* photoprotective effects of a lyophilized extract of *Capparis spinosa* L buds. J Cosmet Sci 2002;53:321–335.
101. Saija A, Tomaino A, Trombetta D, De Pasquale A, Uccella N, Barbuzzi T, Paolino D, Bonina F. *In vitro* and *in vivo* evaluation of caffeic and ferulic acids as topical photoprotective agents. Int J Pharm 2000;199:39–47.
102. Tournas JA, Lin FH, Burch JA, Selim MA, Monteiro-Riviere NA, Zielinski JE, Pinnell SR. Ubiquinone, idebenone, and kinetin provide ineffective photoprotection to skin when compared to a topical antioxidant combination of vitamins C and E with ferulic acid. J Invest Dermatol 2006;126:1185–1187.
103. Mills S, Bone K. Principles and Practice of Phytotherapy: Modern Herbal Medicine. London: Churchill Livingstone, 2000.
104. Won YK, Ong CN, Shi X, Shen HM. Chemopreventive activity of parthenolide against UVB-induced skin cancer and its mechanisms. Carcinogenesis 2004;25:1449–1458.
105. Herrera F, Martin V, Rodriguez-Blanco J, García-Santos G, Antolín I, Rodriguez C. Intracellular redox state regulation by parthenolide. Biochem Biophys Res Commun 2005; 332:321–325.
106. Sweeney CJ, Mehrotra S, Sadaria MR, Kumar S, Shortle NH, Roman Y, Sheridan C, Campbell RA, Murry DJ, Badve S, Nakshatri H. The sesquiterpene lactone parthenolide in combination with docetaxel reduces metastasis and improves survival in a xenograft model of breast cancer. Mol Cancer Ther 2005;4:1004–1012.
107. Tanaka K, Hasegawa J, Asamitsu K, Okamoto T. Prevention of the ultraviolet B-mediated skin photoaging by a nuclear factor kappaB inhibitor, parthenolide. J Pharmacol Exp Ther 2005; 315:624–630.
108. Katiyar SK, Ahmad N, Mukhtar H. Green tea and skin. Arch Dermatol 2000;136:989–994.
109. Wright TI, Spencer JM, Flowers FP. Chemoprevention of nonmelanoma skin cancer. J Am Acad Dermatol 2006;54:933–946.
110. Yusuf N, Irby C, Katiyar SK, Elmets CA. Photoprotective effects of green tea polyphenols. Photodermatol Photoimmunol Photomed 2007;23:48–56.
111. Middlekamp-Hup MA, Pathak MA, Parrado C, Garcia-Caballero T, Rius-Diaz F, Fitzpatrick TB, Gonzalez S. Orally administered *Polypodium leucotomos* extract decreases psoralen-UVA-induced phototoxicity, pigmentation, and damage of human skin. J Am Acad Dermatol 2004;50(1):41–49.
112. Middlekamp-Hup MA, Pathak MA, Parrado C, Goukassian D, Rius-Diaz F, Mihm MC, Fitzpatrick TB, Gonzalez S. Oral Polypodium leucotomos extract decreases ultraviolet-induced damage of human skin. J Am Acad Dermatol 2004;51(6):910–918.
113. Philips N, Smith J, Keller T, Gonzalez S. Predominant effects of *Polypodium leucotomos* on membrane integrity, lipid peroxidation, and expression of elastin and matrixmetalloproteinase-1 in ultraviolet radiation exposed fibroblasts, and keratinocytes. J Dermatol Sci 2003;32 (1):1–9.
114. Sime S, Reeve VE. Protection from inflammation, immunosuppression and carcinogenesis induced by UV radiation in mice by topical. Pycnogenol Photochem Photobiol 2004;79 (2):193–198.
115. Saliou C, Rimbach G, Moini H, McLaughlin L, Hosseini S, Lee J, Watson RR, Packer L. Solar ultraviolet-induced erythema in human skin and nuclear factor-kappa-B-dependent

gene expression in keratinocytes are modulated by a French maritime pine bark extract. Free Radic Biol Med 2001;30(2):154–160.

116. Bito T, Roy S, Sen CK, Packer L. Pine bark extract pycnogenol downregulates IFN-gamma-induced adhesion of T cells to human keratinocytes by inhibiting inducible ICAM-1 expression. Free Radic Biol Med 2000;28(2):219–227.

117. Chen CY, Jang JH, Li MH, Surh YJ. Resveratrol upregulates heme oxygenase-1 expression via activation of NF-E2-related factor 2 in PC12 cells. Biochem Biophys Res Commun 2005;331:993–1000.

118. She QB, Bode AM, Ma WY, Chen NY, Dong Z. Resveratrol-induced activation of p53 and apoptosis is mediated by extracellular-signal-regulated protein kinases and p38 kinase. Cancer Res 2001;61:1604–1610.

119. Jang M, Cai L, Udeani GO, Slowing KV, Thomas CF, Beecher CW, Fong HH, Farnsworth NR, Kinghorn AD, Mehta RG, Moon RC, Pezzuto JM. Cancer chemopreventive activity of resveratrol, a natural product derived from grapes. Science 1997;275:218–220.

120. Afaq F, Adhami VM, Ahmad N. Prevention of short-term ultraviolet B radiation-mediated damages by resveratrol in SKH-1 hairless mice. Toxicol Appl Pharmacol 2003;186:28–37.

121. Chan MM. Antimicrobial effect of resveratrol on dermatophytes and bacterial pathogens of the skin. Biochem Pharmacol 2002;63:99–104.

122. Ding XZ, Adrian TE. Resveratrol inhibits proliferation and induces apoptosis in human pancreatic cancer cells. Pancreas 2002;25:e71–e76.

123. Delmas D, Rébé C, Lacour S, Filomenko R, Athias A, Gambert P, Cherkaoui-Malki M, Jannin B, Dubrez-Daloz L, Latruffe N, Solary E. Resveratrol-induced apoptosis is associated with Fas redistribution in the rafts and the formation of a death-inducing signaling complex in colon cancer cells. J Biol Chem 2003;278:41482–41490.

124. Aziz MH, Afaq F, Ahmad N. Prevention of ultraviolet-B radiation damage by resveratrol in mouse skin is mediated via modulation in survivin. Photochem Photobiol 2005;81:25–31.

125. Aziz MH, Reagan-Shaw S, Wu J, Longley BJ, Ahmad N. Chemoprevention of skin cancer by grape constituent resveratrol: relevance to human disease? FASEB J 2005;19:1193–1195.

126. Darshan S, Doreswamy R. Patented antiinflammatory plant drug development from traditional medicine. Phytother Res 2004;18:343–357.

127. Aburjai T, Natsheh FM. Plants used in cosmetics. Phytother Res 2003;17:987–1000.

128. Saito Y, Shiga A, Yoshida Y, Furuhashi T, Fujita Y, Niki E. Effects of a novel gaseous antioxidative system containing a rosemary extract on the oxidation induced by nitrogen dioxide and ultraviolet radiation. Biosci Biotechnol Biochem 2004;68:781–786.

129. Ho CT, Wang M, Wei GJ, Huang TC, Huang MT. Chemistry and antioxidative factors in rosemary and sage. Biofactors 2000;13:161–166.

130. Sancheti G, Goyal P. Modulatory influence of *Rosemarinus officinalis* on DMBA-induced mouse skin tumorigenesis. Asian Pac J Cancer Prev 2006;7:331–335.

131. Sancheti G, Goyal PK. Effect of *Rosmarinus officinalis* in modulating 7,12-dimethylbenz(a) anthracene induced skin tumorigenesis in mice. Phytother Res 2006;20:981–986.

132. Offord EA, Gautier JC, Avanti O, Scaletta C, Runge F, Krämer K, Applegate LA. Photoprotective potential of lycopene, beta-carotene, vitamin E, vitamin C and carnosic acid in UVA-irradiated human skin fibroblasts. Free Radic Biol Med 2002;32:1293–1303.

133. Chiu A, Kimball AB. Topical vitamins, minerals and botanical ingredients as modulators of environmental and chronological skin damage. Br J Dermatol 2003;149:681–691.

134. Calabrese V, Scapagnini G, Catalano C, Dinotta F, Geraci D, Morganti P. Biochemical studies of a natural antioxidant isolated from rosemary and its application in cosmetic dermatology. Int J Tissue React 2000;22:5–13.

135. Calabrese V, Scapagnini G, Catalano C, Bates TE, Dinotta F, Micali G, Giuffrida Stella AM. Induction of heat shock protein synthesis in human skin fibroblasts in response to oxidative stress: regulation by a natural antioxidant from rosemary extract. Int J Tissue React 2001;23:51–58.

136. Katiyar SK. Silymarin and skin cancer prevention: anti-inflammatory, antioxidant and immunomodulatory effects (Review). Int J Oncol 2005;26(1):169–176.
137. Zhao J, Agarwal R. Tissue distribution of silibinin, the major active constituent of silymarin, in mice and its association with enhancement of phase II enzymes: implications in cancer chemoprevention. Carcinogenesis 1999;20(11):2101–2108.
138. Dhanalakshmi S, Mallikarjuna GU, Singh RP, Agarwal R. Silibinin prevents ultraviolet radiation-caused skin damages in SKH-1 hairless mice via a decrease in thymine dimer positive cells and an up-regulation of p53–p21/Cip1 in epidermis. Carcinogenesis 2004;25 (8):1459–1465.
139. Gallagher RP, Rivers JK, Lee TK, Bajdik CD, McLean DI, Coldman AJ. Broad-spectrum sunscreen use and the development of new nevi in white children: a randomized controlled trial. JAMA 2000;283:2955.
140. Schröder JM, Harder J. Innate antimicrobial peptides in the skin. Med Sci Paris 2006;22 (2):153–157.
141. Nizet V, Ohtake T, Lauth X, Trowbridge J, Rudisill J, Dorschner RA, Pestonjamasp V, Piraino J, Hutter K, Gallo RL. Innate antimicrobial peptide protects the skin from invasive bacterial infection. Nature 2001;414:454–457.
142. Elsner P. Antimicrobials and the skin physiological and pathological flora. Curr Probl Dermatol 2006;33:35–41.
143. Harder J, Schröder JM. Antimicrobial peptides in human skin. Chem Immunol Allergy 2005;86:22–41.
144. Ehlers C, Ivens UI, Møller ML, Senderovitz T, Serup J. Females have lower skin surface pH than men: a study on the influence of gender, forearm site variation, right/left difference and time of the day on the skin surface pH. Skin Res Technol 2001;7(2):90–94.
145. Noble WC. Carriage of micro-organisms on the skin, in Newsom SWB, Caldwell ADS (eds.) Problems in the Control of Hospital Infection. London: Royal Society of Medicine, 1980, pp 7–10.
146. Mackowiak PA. The normal microbial flora. N Engl J Med 1982;307:83–93.
147. Price PB. The bacteriology of normal skin; a new quantitative test applied to a study of the bacterial flora and disinfectant action of mechanical cleansing. J Infect Dis 1938;63: 301–318.
148. Williamson P, Kligman AM. A new method for the quantitative investigation of cutaneous bacteria. J Invest Dermatol 1965;45(6):498–503.
149. Marples MJ. The Ecology of Human Skin. Springfield, IL: Thomas CC Publisher, 1965.
150. Noble WC, Somerville CA. Microbiology of Human Skin. Philadelphia: Saunders, 1974, pp 50–76, 131, 212.
151. Kligman AM. The bacteriology of normal skin, in Maibach HI, Hildick-Smith G (eds.) Skin Bacteria and Their Role in Infection. New York: McGraw-Hill, 1965, pp 13–31.
152. Hartmann AA. A comparative investigation of methods for sampling skin flora. Arch Dermatol Res 1982;274:381–385.
153. Marples RR. Sex, constancy, and skin bacteria. Arch Dermatol 1982;272:317–320.
154. Wilburg J, Kasprowicz A, Heczko PB. Composition of normal bacterial flora of human skin in relation to the age and sex of examined persons. Przegl Dermatol 1984;71(6):551–557.
155. Larson EL, Cronquist AB, Whittier S, Lai L, Lyle CT, Latta PD. Differences in skin flora between inpatients and chronically ill outpatients. Heart Lung 2000;29:298–305.
156. Rebel G, Pillsbury DM, Phalle G, de Saint M, Ginsberg D. Factors affecting the rapid disappearance of bacteria placed on the normal flora. J Invest Dermatol 1950;14:247–263.
157. Aly R, Shirley C, Cunico B, Maibach HI. Effect of prolonged occlusion on the microbial flora, pH, C02 and transepidermal water loss. J Invest Dermatol 1978;71:378–381.
158. Sarkany I, Gaylarde CC. Bacterial colonisation of the skin of the newborn. J Pathol Bacteriol 1968;95:115–122.
159. Thestrup-Pedersen K. Bacteria and the skin: clinical practice and therapy update. Br J Dermatol 1998;13953:1–3.

160. Medves JM, O'Brien B. Does bathing newborns remove potentially harmful pathogens from the skin? Birth 2001;28(3):161–165.
161. Ashbee HR, Leck AK, Puntis JW, Parsons WJ, Evans EG. Skin colonisation by *Malassezia* in neonates and infants Infect Control Hosp Epidemiol 2002;23:212–216.
162. Juncosa Morros T, González-Cuevas A, Alayeto Ortega J, Muñoz Almagro C, Moreno Hernando J, Gené Giralt A, Latorre Otín C. Cutaneous colonization by *Malassezia* spp. in neonates. An Esp Pediatr 2002;57(5):452–456.
163. Venkatesh MP, Placencia F, Weisman LE. Coagulase-negative staphylococcal infections in the neonate and child: an update. Semin Pediatr Infect Dis 2006;17(3):120–127.
164. Leyden JJ, McGinley KJ, Mills OH, Kligman AM. Age-related changes in the resident bacterial flora of the human face. J Invest Dermatol 1975;65(4):379–381.
165. Sultana B, Cimiotti J, Aiello AE, Sloan D, Larson E. Effects of age and race on skin condition and bacterial counts on hands of neonatal ICU nurses. Heart Lung 2003;32 (4):283–289.
166. Foca K, Jakob S, Whittier P, Della-Latta S, Factor D, Rubenstein, Saiman L. Endemic *Pseudomonas aeruginosa* infection in a neonatal intensive care unit. N Engl J Med 2000;343:695–700.
167. Lindberg E, Ingegerd Adlerberth I, Hesselmar B, Saalman R, Inga-Lisa Strannegård I-L, Åberg N, Wold AE. High rate of transfer of *Staphylococcus aureus* from parental skin to infant gut flora. Clin Microbiol 2004;42(2):530–534.
168. Webster GF. Skin microecology: the old and the new. Arch Dermatol 2007;143(1):105–106.
169. Kloos WE, Schleifer KH. Simplified scheme for routine identification of human *Staphylococcus* species. J Clin Microbiol 1975;1(1):82–88.
170. Frank DN, Spiegelman GB, Davis W, Wagner E, Lyons E, Pace NR. Culture-independent molecular analysis of microbial constituents of the healthy human outer ear. J Clin Microbiol 2003;41:295–303.
171. Dekio I, Hayashi H, Sakamoto M, Kitahara M, Nishikawa T, Suematsu M, Benno Y. Detection of potentially novel bacterial components of the human skin microbiota using culture-independent molecular profiling. J Med Microbiol 2005;54:1231–1238.
172. Gao Z, Tseng CH, Pei Z et al. Molecular analysis of human forearm superficial skin bacterial biota. Proc Natl Acad Sci USA 2007;104:2927–2932.
173. Vuong C, Otto M. *Staphylococcus epidermidis* infections. Microbes Infect 2002;4:481–489.
174. Harmory BH, Parisi JT. *Staphylococcus epidermidis*: a significant nosocomial pathogen. J Infect Control 1987;15:59–74.
175. Fekety FR Jr. The epidemiology and prevention of staphylococcal infection. Medicine 1964;43:593–613.
176. Nagase N, Sasaki A, Yamashita K, Shimizu A, Wakita Y, Kitai S, Kawano J. Isolation and species distribution of staphylococci from animal and human skin. J Vet Med Sci 2002;64 (3):245–250.
177. Barth JH. Nasal carriage of staphylococci and streptococci. Int J Dermatol 1987;26:24–26.
178. Solberg CO. Spread of *Staphylococcus aureus* in hospitals: causes and prevention. Scand J Infect Dis 2000;32:587–595.
179. Kloos WE, Musselwhite MS. Distribution and persistence of *Staphylococcus* and *Micrococcus* species and other aerobic bacteria on human skin. Appl Microbiol 1975; 30:381–395.
180. Nobel WC. Microbiology of Human Skin. London: Lloyd-Luke, 1981, p 433.
181. Seifert H, Dijkshoorn L, Gerner-Smidt P, Pelzer N, Tjernberg I, Vaneechoutte M. Distribution of *Acinetobacter* species on human skin: comparison of phenotypic and genotypic identification methods. J Clin Microbiol 1997;53:2819–2825.
182. Berlau J, Aucken H, Malnick H, Pitt T. Distribution of *Acinetobacter* species on skin of healthy humans. Eur J Clin Microbiol Infect Dis 1999;18:179–183.
183. Ashbee HR. Update on the genus *Malassezia*. Med Mycol 2007;45(4):287–303.

184. Paulino LC, Tseng C-H, Strober BE, Blaser MJ. Molecular analysis of fungal microbiota in samples from healthy human skin and psoriatic lesions. J Clin Microbiol 2006; 44:2933–2941.
185. Gupta AK, Kohli Y. Prevalence of *Malassezia* species on various body sites in clinically healthy subjects representing different age groups. Med Mycol 2004;10:125–159.
186. Lee YW, Yim SM, Lim SH, Choe YB, Ahn KJ. Quantitative investigation on the distribution of *Malassezia* species on healthy human skin in Korea. Mycoses 2006;49(5):405–410.
187. Leyden JJ, McGinley KJ, Nordstrom KM, Webster GF. Skin microflora. J Invest Dermatol 1987;88:65s–72s.
188. McGinley KJ, Leyden JJ, Marples RR, Kligman AM. Quantitative microbiology of the scalp in non-dandruff, dandruff, and seborrheic dermatitis. J Invest Dermatol 1975;64(6):401–405.
189. Chamberlain AN, Halablab MA, Gould DJ, Miles RJ. Distribution of bacteria on hands and the effectiveness of brief and thorough decontamination procedures using non-medicated soap. Zentralbl Bakteriol 1997;285(4):565–575.
190. Aly R, Maibach HI. Aerobic microbial flora of intertrigenous skin. Appl Environ Microbiol 1977;33(1):97–100.
191. Bojar RA, Holland KT. The human cutaneous microbiota and factors controlling colonisation. World J Microbiol Biotechnol 2002;18:889–903.
192. Somerville DA. The normal flora of the skin in different age groups. Br J Dermatol 1980;81:248–258.
193. Selwyn S. Microbiology and ecology of human skin. Practitioner 1980;224:1059–1062.
194. LeFrock JL, Ellis CA, Weinstein L. The impact of hospitalization on the aerobic fecal microflora. Am J Med Sci 1979;277:269–274.
195. Larson EL. Persistent carriage of Gram-negative bacteria on hands. Am J Infect Control 1981;9:112–119.
196. Larson EL, McGinley KJ, Foglia AR, Talbot GH, Leyden JJ. Composition and antimicrobial resistance of skin flora in hospitalized and healthy adults. J Clin Microbiol 1986;23:604–608.
197. Bickers DR, Athar M. Oxidative stress in the pathogenesis of skin disease. J Invest Dermatol 2006;126(12):2565–2575.
198. Platzek T, Lang C, Grohmann G, Gi US, Baltes W. Formation of a carcinogenic aromatic amine from an azo dye by human skin bacteria *in vitro*. Hum Exp Toxicol 1999;18(9):552–559.
199. Papacostas G, Gate J eds. Les associations microbiennes, leurs applications therapeutiques. Paris: Doin, 1928.
200. Barak O, Treat JR, James WD. Antimicrobial peptides: effectors of innate immunity in the skin. Adv Dermatol 2005;21:357–374.
201. Chiller K, Selkin BA, Murakawa GJ. Skin microflora and bacterial infections of the skin. J Investig Dermatol Symp Proc 2001;6:170–174.
202. Fredricks DN. Microbial ecology of human skin in health and disease. J Investig Dermatol Symp Proc 2001;6:167–169.
203. Hadaway LC. Skin flora and infection. J Infus Nurs 2003;26:44–48.
204. Hadaway LC. Skin flora: unwanted dead or alive. Nursing 2005;35(7):20.
205. Roth RR, James WD. Microbiology of the skin: resident flora, ecology, infection. J Am Acad Dermatol 1989;20:367–390.
206. Laube S, Farrell AM. Bacterial skin infections in the elderly: diagnosis and treatment. Drugs Aging 2002;19:331–342.
207. http://www.ncbi.nlm.nih.gov/pubmed/18603682?ordinalpos=1&itool=EntrezSystem2.PEntrez.   Pubmed.Pubmed_ResultsPanel.Pubmed_DefaultReportPanel.Pubmed_RVDocSum" Bansal E, Garg A, Bhatia S, Attri AK, Chander J. Spectrum of microbial flora in diabetic foot ulcers. Indian J Pathol Microbiol. 2008;51(2):204–208.

208. Cogen AL, Nizet V, Gallo RL. *Staphylococcus epidermidis* functions as a component of the skin innate immune system by inhibiting the pathogen Group A Streptococcus. J Invest Dermatol 2007;127:S131.
209. Lyon GJ, Novick RP. Peptide signaling in *Staphylococcus aureus* and other Gram-positive bacteria. Peptides 2004;25:1389–1403.
210. von Eiff C, Becker K, Machka K, Stammer H, Peters G. Nasal carriage as a source of *Staphylococcus aureus* bacteremia. Study Group. N Engl J Med 2001;344:11–16.
211. Von Eiff C, Peters G, Heilmann C. Pathogenesis of infections due to coagulase negative staphylococci. Lancet Infect Dis 2002;2:677–685.
212. Mainous AG III, Hueston WJ, Everett CJ, Diaz VA. Nasal carriage of *Staphylococcus aureus* and methicillin-resistant *S. aureus* in the United States, 2001–2002. Ann Fam Med 2006;4:132–137.
213. Iwatsuki K, Yamasaki O, Morizane S, Oono T. Staphylococcal cutaneous infections: invasion, evasion and aggression. J Dermatol Sci 2006;42:203–214.
214. Bokarewa MI, Jin T, Tarkowski A. *Staphylococcus aureus*: Staphylokinase. Int J Biochem Cell Biol 2006;38(4):504–509.
215. Wichmann S, Wirsing von Koenig CH, Becker-Boost E, Finger H, Group JK. Corynebacteria in skin flora of healthy persons and patients. Eur J Clin Microbiol 1985;4:502–504.
216. Kaźmierczak AK, Szewczyk EM. Bacteria forming a resident flora of the skin as a potential source of opportunistic infections. Pol J Microbiol 2005;54(1):27–35.
217. Kaźmierczak AK, Szarapińska-Kwaszewska JK, Szewczyk EM. Opportunistic coryneform organisms–residents of human skin. Pol J Microbiol 2005;54(1):27–35.
218. Brüggemann H, Henne A, Hoster F, Liesegang H, Wiezer A, Strittmatter A, Hujer S, Dürre P, Gottschalk G. The complete genome sequence of *Propionibacterium acnes*, a commensal of human skin. Science 2004;305:671–673.
219. Mowad CM, McGinley KJ, Foglia A, Leyden JJ. The role of extracellular polysaccharide substance produced by *Staphylococcus epidermidis* in miliaria. J Am Acad Dermatol 1995;33:729–733.
220. Goodyear HM, Watson PJ, Egan SA, Price EH, Kenny PA, Harper JI. Skin microflora of atopic eczema in first time hospital attenders. Clin Exp Dermatol 1993;18(4):300–304.
221. Spielman AI, Zeng XN, Leyden JJ, Preti G. Proteinaceous precursors of human axillary odor: isolation of two novel odor-binding proteins. Experientia 1995;51(1):40–47.
222. Cogen AL, Nizet V, Gallo RL. Skin microbiota: a source of disease or defence? Br J Dermatol 2008;158:442–455.

Chapter 5
Lung Infections and Aging

Sameer K. Mathur and Keith C. Meyer

Introduction

On the basis of US Census data and projections, the fastest growing segment of the US population is >65 years old. As the demographics in the United States change, there are projections for a doubling of the elderly population (>65 years old) within the next 20–30 years. It is recognized that respiratory infections comprise a significant cause of morbidity and mortality in this population, and many factors have been identified that contribute to increased incidence as well as increased severity of respiratory infections in the elderly (Table 5.1).

Age-Associated Changes in Lung Structure and Function

It is well recognized that the normal aging process results in changes in the structural properties of the lung as well as airway protective mechanisms. These changes alter lung physiology and function and may contribute to the increased propensity of elderly individuals to develop respiratory infections.

Lung Tissue

As a consequence of aging, the diameter of bronchioles decreases owing to diminished tethering that would normally maintain patency at a given lung volume, alveolar ducts increase in diameter, and the elastic recoil of the lung declines. Airways tend to close prematurely and lead to ventilation–perfusion mismatching, air-trapping, and an increase in the alveolar-to-arterial gradient for oxygen. In addition, the total gas-exchange surface area declines.

S.K. Mathur and K.C. Meyer
University of Wisconsin School of Medicine and Public Health, Department of Medicine Section of Allergy, Pulmonary and Critical Care Medicine, 600 Highland Ave. K4/910 CSC, Madison, WI, 53792, USA

S.L. Percival (ed.), *Microbiology and Aging.*
DOI: 10.1007/978-1-59745-327-1_5; © Springer Science + Business Media, LLC 2009

Table 5.1 Factors predisposing the elderly to lung infections

- Changes in airway structure and physiology
  - Diminished airway tethering and early closure in expiration
  - Diminished mucociliary clearance
- Chest wall changes
  - Altered contour and composition
  - Decreased compliance
- Declining airway protective reflexes
- Immune dysfunction
  - Innate immunity
  - Adaptive immunity

Studies have demonstrated an age-related decrease in the static elastic recoil pressures, which is most evident at higher lung volumes.[1,2] This increase in lung compliance with aging is thought to be, in part, due to structural changes in the lung tissue, particularly the expression or modification of extracellular matrix proteins responsible for supporting the airway, such as elastin and collagen. In the presence of comorbid conditions, such as chronic obstructive pulmonary disease (COPD), a net increase in collagen mass was reported, while the collagen content of lungs from nonsmokers did not significantly decline with advancing age.[3] Individuals with glucose intolerance or diabetes may be particularly prone to altered collagen modification due to increased cross-linking by glucose adducts.[4] It has been observed that airspaces do become dilated in healthy older lungs, a feature that has been referred to as "senile lung."[5,6] Nonetheless, although extracellular matrix changes have been noted for age-related comorbid conditions, it remains somewhat unclear as to whether the aging of the normal healthy lung in humans is associated with clear-cut changes in extracellular matrix composition. Moreover, some investigators have quantitated extracellular components, such as elastin levels, and reported an increase rather than decline with aging.[7,8] Thus, it is likely that the age-related changes in extracellular matrix composition are quite complex and involve changes in both the levels of matrix proteins and age-associated modifications of matrix constituents.

Chest Wall

In addition to changes in lung matrix, the chest wall becomes less compliant because of altered costovertebral articulations and calcification of rib cartilage, narrowing of intervertebral disc spaces, and changes in the contour of the chest, which can be greatly exacerbated by the presence of kyphoscoliosis or vertebral compression fractures.[9] A decrease in diaphragmatic muscle strength has also been observed in elderly individuals,[10,11] which may be due to a general decline in muscle mass associated with aging.[12] Furthermore, several comorbidities such as poor nutritional status, cardiac dysfunction (e.g., congestive heart failure), and neurological dysfunction (e. g., cerebral vascular disease) can also affect respiratory muscle strength.[13–17]

Ventilatory responses to hypoxic or hypercapneic stimuli also become blunted as part of the aging process in clinically healthy individuals who have no evidence of pulmonary disease. Although often mild, the age-associated structural and functional changes that affect both the chest wall and the lung itself may significantly limit an elderly individual's ability to cope with a severe stress such as pneumonia, especially in patients who already have entered an age-associated "frail" state.[18]

Airway Protection

Intact and well-functioning protective reflexes to prevent the aspiration of upper airway contents are essential for preventing lower respiratory tract infections. It has been shown that larger volumes of liquid are required to stimulate the pharyngo-glottal closure reflex in elderly individuals without neurologic dysfunction, as compared to younger subjects.[19] Furthermore, there are data to suggest that small amounts of aspirated gastric secretions with moderate acid exposure of human tracheal epithelial cells (pH 3.0–5.0) can inhibit the production of bactericidal molecules such as human beta-defensin-2 and are associated with reduced bactericidal activity in epithelial surface liquid.[20] Therefore, the reduced airway protection in the elderly can increase the risk of potential pathogens gaining access to the lower respiratory tract. Furthermore, innate antibacterial defenses may be blunted if aspiration of upper airway contents is accompanied by refluxed acidic gastric secretions, increasing the risk of lower-tract bacterial infection occurring. A predisposition to aspirate is especially problematic for individuals with neurologic dysfunction. Pneumonia is a major cause of morbidity and mortality in patients with Alzheimer disease or other forms of central nervous system disorders such as stroke, and the majority of these episodes of pneumonia are initiated by aspiration of contaminated material from the upper airway into the lung.[21,22]

Mucociliary Clearance

If aspirated secretions with associated pathogens gain access to the lower respiratory tract because of insufficient glottic protective mechanisms and cough reflex, the mucociliary clearance mechanism can reduce the likelihood of establishing an infection by transporting the infectious organisms proximally to the glottis. Mucociliary clearance is accomplished through a rhythmic movement of ciliary structures on the apical surface of epithelial cells, and the function of these ciliary structures appears to decline with advancing age.[23] Ho and colleagues reported that the cilia of nasal epithelial cells in elderly individuals had a lower ciliary beat frequency, and increased microtubular abnormalities in cilia were found and associated with depressed nasal mucociliary clearance times.[24] Because nasal ciliary beat frequency correlates with that of tracheal epithelium,[25] this study suggests that ciliary abnormalities appear with advancing age and may play a role in increased susceptibility to respiratory infection by depressing the mucociliary clearance rate.

However, this may not provide the entire explanation for deficient mucociliary clearance, as it has also been noted that ciliary beat frequency and clearance time did not necessarily correlate with each other.[25]

Immunological Changes Associated with Advancing Age

It is recognized that immune function changes with aging, often but not always, resulting in a decline in function. The change in immune function with aging is often referred to as "immunosenescence" and has also been termed "immune remodeling." Studies of the effects of aging on the various components of the immune system have defined features of immunosenescence as detailed below, although there is considerable interindividual difference in these findings among the elderly, and centenarians can have fairly robust, preserved immune responses.

Systemic Immunity

The immune system is generally described as having two interacting major components, innate and adaptive immunity. Innate immunity has been highly conserved among organisms that range from invertebrates to primates and is composed of several different cell types, including immune cells (e.g., macrophage and neutrophils) and nonimmune cells (e.g., epithelial cells).[26] These innate immune cells employ numerous receptors, cytokines, and chemokines, some of which are common to the adaptive immune system. However, innate immune cells respond in a nonspecific manner to broad classes of foreign stimuli. In contrast, adaptive immunity is antigen specific and coordinated by lymphocytes derived from fetal liver and bone marrow precursors in the developing embryo, and the thymus gland and other collections of lymphoid tissue (spleen, lymph nodes, and mucosa-associated lymphoid tissue) play key roles in generating adaptive responses.[27,28] Adaptive immunity can be considered a more sophisticated form of defense that also has a component of memory such that responses to a repeat offender occur more quickly and more effectively.

Other important modulators of immune function that can have a significant effect on the elderly include neuroendocrine system responses to stress.[29] Elderly individuals display a gradual increase in endogenous glucocorticoids with age, and a dysfunctional hypothalamus–pituitary–adrenal axis can impair immune function yet cause an exaggerated response to stressors such as infection.

Innate Immunity

The innate immune system can respond immediately to a microbial challenge via pattern-recognition receptors (PRR), now recognized to be part of a group of receptors referred to as the *Toll-like receptor* (TLR) family, that bind determinants (e.g., lipopolysaccharide, lipoteichoic acids, mannans, peptidoglycans, glucans, or bacterial DNA) borne by infectious agents. Stimulation of these receptors triggers the production and release of cytokines and costimulatory molecules. The pathogen-associated molecular patterns (PAMPs) recognized by TLRs are shared by large classes of microorganisms, and these PAMPs are highly conserved and absent from mammalian tissues.[30,31] Although innate immune responses alone may be adequate to deal with a microbial challenge, a significant innate response can trigger and augment adaptive immune responses (e.g., via costimulatory molecules) as needed to meet an immediate infectious challenge and to prepare for future challenges.

Other important components of the innate immune response include dendritic cells, phagocytic cells, the alternate complement pathway, and antimicrobial molecules such as nitric oxide, defensins, and collectins. Indeed, dendritic cells, and to a lesser extent macrophages, play a major immunoregulatory role and provide a key link between innate and adaptive immune responses. As antigen-presenting cells, they can stimulate primary T-cell responses and T-cell differentiation via production of costimulatory molecules and cytokine production.

Interestingly, the Leiden 85-plus study demonstrated that impaired production of both proinflammatory and anti-inflammatory cytokines by ex vivo whole blood samples from 85-year-old subjects predicted a greater than twofold increase in overall mortality risk that was independent of the presence of chronic illnesses.[32] These authors speculated that impaired innate immunity, as reflected by impaired production of cytokines produced by cellular components of the innate immune system, is predictive of frailty and increased risk of mortality in the elderly.

Neutrophils

This phagocytic cell is often recruited very early into areas of inflammation. Many neutrophil functions are unchanged with aging, including adhesion, migration into inflammatory tissue, and phagocytosis. However, the ability of neutrophils to kill phagocytosed organisms is diminished in the elderly compared to younger individuals,[33] a defect that is attributed to a decrease in the production of reactive oxygen species (ROS).[34,35] In addition, it has been observed that neutrophils in the elderly are more prone to undergoing apoptosis, because the cytokine-mediated signaling pathways to protect the neutrophils are deficient.[36,37] Therefore, neutrophils may be less abundant because of greater apoptosis, and those that remain have diminished antibacterial activity. Both of these changes with aging may contribute to more frequent and more severe respiratory infections.

Dendritic Cells

The primary function of dendritic cells is to serve as "professional" antigen-presenting cells. Because they are able to interact with both T cells and B cells to facilitate their activation, enhancement of cytolytic T-cell activity, and production of antibodies, dendritic cells represent an important link between the innate and adaptive arms of the immune system.

Dendritic cells that are localized to lymphoid tissue are termed *follicular dendritic cells*, and these cells are particularly important for the production of antibodies. The ability of follicular dendritic cells to accumulate antigen and organize into germinal centers within lymphoid tissue diminishes with age in mice.[38]

There is some evidence that dendritic cells localized to non-lymphoid tissues display diminished antigen-presenting activity, which may be related to decreased major histocompatibility complex (MHC) II expression.[39] Interestingly, there have been other studies with opposing results, showing no age-related changes in MHC II and no deficiency in antigen presentation to T cells.[40,41] These conflicting results have been attributed to variations arising from the use of different mouse strains and differences in the in vitro stimuli used in the respective protocols. A recently published study in human subjects showed that circulating levels of a specific subtype of dendritic cells, the plasmacytoid dendritic cells, were 50% less in the elderly vs. younger subjects.[42]

Macrophage

Macrophages can act as antigen-presenting cells and can also efficiently phagocytose microbes and foreign particles. There are multiple mechanisms by which the macrophage can perform intracellular killing of bacteria, including the production of superoxide anion with its downstream reactive oxygen intermediates as well as the production of reactive nitrogen intermediates. Analyses of macrophage effector functions in aged mice and rats have demonstrated a decrease in the production of superoxide anion.[43–45] However, there were conflicting findings of both increases and decreases in the production of reactive nitrogen intermediates.[46,47] The conflicting findings were most likely due to differences in the experimental protocols and may reflect the possibility that only specific signaling pathways for the generation of reactive nitrogen species are affected under these experimental conditions.

The production of cytokines by macrophages stimulated in vitro has been shown to diminish with age.[48,49] Additionally, in vivo assays of macrophage function have assessed recruitment to sites of injury and participation in wound healing. Although an age-associated increased infiltration of macrophages to sites of injury was observed in mice,[50] decreased macrophage infiltration occurred in humans in association with advanced age.[51] Collectively, these age-related changes in macrophage function suggest that a diminished capacity to eradicate infection may appear with advancing age and contribute to more frequent and more severe respiratory infections.

NK Cells

Natural killer (NK) cells are important for the destruction of tumor cells and cells with intracellular pathogens, such as virus-infected cells. Interestingly, the numbers of NK cells increase with aging.[52] However, the functional activities of these cells appear to diminish in association with a tendency for NK cells to become more agranular in appearance and less capable of cytolytic activity towards tumor cells.[53]

There has also been recent interest in NKT cells, which, like NK cells, exhibit an increase in circulating levels with aging.[54] Furthermore, NKT cells exhibit decreased Th1 cytokine production with aging, although changes in Th2 cytokine production by NKT cells with aging remain controversial.[55,56]

Adaptive Immunity

The adaptive immune system exhibits specificity for molecular moieties of target pathogens and is able to generate a memory of previous responses. The T and B lymphocytes are the cells that mediate the adaptive arm of immune function. T-cell antigen specificity is localized to the T-cell receptor (TCR), and T cells undergo selective expansion of appropriate T-cell clones with the requisite antigen specificity upon stimulation. B-cell antigen specificity is localized to surface antibody receptors and secreted antibody, and B cells contribute to antigen specificity by selective activation of B-cell clones that have antibody specificity for the target pathogen and display "editing" of the antibody upon repeat exposures to enhance future specificity.

T Cells

With regard to the effects of aging on the adaptive immune system, the T-cell population has been most extensively studied. It is clear that the thymus gland begins to gradually involute shortly after birth and undergoes replacement by fatty tissue that is nearly complete by the age of 60 years. As a result, the numbers of CD3+, CD4+, and CD8+ T cells decrease with advancing age. A decline in naïve T-cell populations gradually occurs, and memory T cells (CD45RO+) eventually predominate, although memory cell responses also gradually wane with aging.[57] T-cell receptor repertoire diversity appears to diminish, and T helper cell activity declines.[58] Reduced proliferative responses,[59] a shift of Th1 to Th2 cytokine profiles,[60] a decline in Fas-mediated T-cell apoptosis,[61] and increased DR expression on T-cells[62] have also been observed.

Interestingly, some observations suggest that as many components of immunity decline with advanced age owing to sustained antigenic stress over an individual's lifespan, there is a shift to a chronic, proinflammatory state as effector/memory cells gradually replace naïve cells, and expanded effector/memory T cells secrete increased amounts of proinflammatory cytokines such as IL-6.[63] Also, prolonged survival appears to correlate with fairly well-preserved immune responses in the very old,[64] while decreased survival in a longitudinal study in a Swedish population was associated with the "immune cluster parameter" of impaired T-cell proliferative response to mitogenic stimulation, increased numbers of CD8+ cytotoxic/suppressor cells, and low numbers of CD4+ T cells and CD19+ B cells.[65]

B Cells

A decreased production of B cells with aging is well established in mice and likely to be true for humans.[66,67] This supports the notion that the distribution of B-cell subsets present in the elderly differs from that of younger individuals. More specifically, there is a transition from the presence of naïve B cells to "antigen-experienced" B cells.[68] In mice, it appears that the functional ability to produce antibody remains intact with aging.[69] However, the quality of antibody produced with aging is lower; i.e., the antibodies exhibit lower affinity and avidity for antigen.[70] This observation is likely explained by deficient somatic hypermutation, which is the typical mechanism for enhancement of antibody specificity for antigen.[71]

Pulmonary

Although there is considerable information concerning systemic immune responses and how these change with aging, relatively little is known about compartmentalized immune surveillance and innate immune responses in the lung. Studies in normal human volunteers have shown a modestly increased number of lymphocytes and neutrophils in bronchoalveolar lavage (BAL) fluid for healthy, never-smoking elderly subjects vs. younger individuals.[72-74] This was accompanied by a shift in T-cell subsets and activation markers, increased immunoglobulin and IL-6 concentrations, increased alveolar macrophage oxyradical production, and a decline in vascular endothelial growth factor concentrations.[74-76] These changes may be beneficial for immune surveillance and resisting infection, but they may also reflect dysfunctional immunoregulation. Furthermore, these immunoregulatory changes may contribute to age-associated changes in matrix components and the decrease in elastic recoil and structural changes observed in the aging human lung.

Because the alveolar macrophage (AM) figures prominently in inflammatory responses and pulmonary host defense, various aspects of AM function have been evaluated in elderly populations and animal models. Examination of macrophage populations in aged animals and in humans have suggested that aging is associated with a decline in numerous macrophage functions that include the expression of certain pattern recognition receptors such as TLRs, a reduced capacity for phagocytosis, decreased generation of nitric oxide, and impaired secretion of certain cytokines and chemokines.[77] Because TLRs are key receptors for macrophage responses to pathogens and for the initiation of both innate and adaptive immune responses, impaired TLR expression and function by the AM may play a key role in susceptibility to respiratory infections in the elderly. In addition to the demonstration that macrophages from aged mice have reduced TLR expression,[49] AM from aged rats have been shown to have impaired NO production in response to concanavalin A as well as impaired TNF-α release upon stimulation by LPS that appeared to be linked to altered protein kinase C activation and translocation.[78,79] Although little is known about the effects of advanced age on AM function in humans, Zissel et al. have shown a decrease in human AM accessory cell function that correlated with advanced age but could not demonstrate an effect of age on spontaneous release of TNF-α, TGF-β, or IL-6.[80] Anti-inflammatory cytokine production by AM in response to proinflammatory stimuli may also be impaired and may have important consequences for resolution of inflammation induced by infection or noninfectious injurious agents. Corsini et al. recently demonstrated that AM from aged rats that were exposed to carrageenan displayed impaired production of IL-10, which correlated with an accentuated inflammatory response in the lungs of aged rats following carrageenan challenge when compared to young rats.[81]

Lung Infections in the Elderly

The above-mentioned changes in the structural properties of the lung plus alterations in immune function with aging are thought to contribute to the increased susceptibility and increased severity of respiratory infections caused by bacteria and/or viruses in the elderly (Table 5.2).

Community-Acquired Pneumonia

Pneumonia is a leading cause of morbidity and mortality in the elderly population. Bacteria, especially *Streptococcus pneumoniae*, remain the pathogens that most commonly cause pneumonia in the elderly; and community-acquired pneumonia (CAP) caused by *S. pneumoniae*, *H. influenzae*, *S. aureus*, and enteric Gram-negative bacilli occur more frequently in the elderly than in younger age groups.[82] Aspiration pneumonia is often associated with *S. pneumoniae*, *H. influenzae*, or *S. aureus* unless poor dentition is present, which increases the possibility of pneumonia caused by anaerobic bacteria. Additionally, the elderly are more likely to have colonization with Gram-negative bacilli, particularly if they reside in long-term care facilities, and develop pneumonia associated with these organisms. The presence of diseases that alter lung structure such as COPD or bronchiectasis also increase the likelihood of Gram-negative rods as a cause of bacterial pneumonia. Viral pneumonias, although comprising a smaller proportion of lower respiratory tract infections in the elderly, can have significant morbidity and mortality and predispose the elderly individual to subsequent serious bacterial pneumonia.[83]

Table 5.2 Pathogens associated with lung infections in the elderly

- Bacterial
  - *Streptococcus pneumoniae*
  - *Hemophilus influenzae*
  - *Staphylococcus aureus*
  - *Pseudomonas aeruginosa*
  - *Legionella* spp.
  - Enteric gram negative spp.
  - *Mycobacterium tuberculosis*
- Viral
  - Influenza
  - Respiratory syncytial virus (RSV)
  - Rhinovirus

Making the diagnosis of pneumonia may prove particularly difficult in the elderly patient. Prominent respiratory symptoms and fever are frequently absent, although mental status changes are relatively common.[84] A chest radiograph, which can be unremarkable in earlier phases of pneumonia, is nonetheless the most helpful diagnostic test and may yield clues that suggest the more likely causative pathogens. Other tests such as blood cultures or sputum Gram stain and culture may prove useful in patients who are ill enough to require hospital admission, but an empiric approach to antibiotic therapy without extensive diagnostic testing is currently advocated.[85] Two key actions that can optimize outcome when treating pneumonia in the elderly are recognizing which patients should be hospitalized and expeditiously giving adequate antibiotic therapy with minimal time elapsing between diagnosis and the administration of an effective antibiotic.[86,87] Extensive diagnostic testing fails to reveal a specific etiology for CAP in approximately half or more of patients, and delays in the initiation of appropriate therapy for diagnostic studies may have an adverse effect on outcome. Diagnostic testing should be done rapidly and not delay the initiation of empiric antibiotic therapy, and treating physicians should always keep in mind the possibility of an atypical agent, such as *Mycobacterium tuberculosis* or endemic fungi, as a cause of CAP.

Viral Infection

It is increasingly recognized that viral lower respiratory infections represent a source of significant morbidity and mortality in the elderly, and estimates range from 1 to 23% that CAP cases have a viral etiology.[88] Furthermore, several viruses have been identified as frequent or severe respiratory pathogens, including influenza, respiratory syncytial virus (RSV), and rhinovirus.

Influenza has a typical seasonal peak in early winter and a milder peak in early spring. Influenza infection has a much greater impact on the elderly relative to other age groups, and estimates indicate that 85% of influenza-related deaths and 63% of influenza-related hospitalizations in the US involve the elderly.[89] Furthermore, it has also been documented that influenza virus has been the cause of multiple severe infectious outbreaks in long-term care facilities.[90]

RSV has traditionally been considered a pathogen for children. However, it is now recognized as an important pathogen in the elderly as well, and surveillance data indicate that RSV infection occurs in 3–7% of healthy elderly individuals which can progress to a pneumonia in 2–7% of infected individuals.[91] It has been shown in vitro that RSV infection of cells derived from elderly subjects is associated with diminished Th1 cytokine production, suggesting an impaired ability to eradicate an RSV infection in the elderly.[92]

Rhinovirus is the most common cause for the common cold in all age groups, and rhinoviruses account for 25–50% of respiratory illnesses in the elderly. Interestingly, there have been documented outbreaks of rhinovirus infections in long-term care facilities resulting in significant morbidity.[93,94] Although rhinovirus is typically considered an upper-airway pathogen, there are studies documenting the migration of rhinovirus into the lung.[95] However, lower respiratory tract rhinovirus infection has not been systematically evaluated, and the prevalence of pneumonia in the elderly caused by rhinovirus remains unclear.

Approach to Treatment and Prevention

Pneumonia

Antibacterial therapy for CAP is generally similar to that for younger individuals and should be administered empirically on the basis of the presence of cardiopulmonary disease (COPD, congestive heart failure), the presence of modifying factors (nursing home residence, risk factors for drug-resistant *S. pneumoniae*, risk factors for *P. aeruginosa*), and place of therapy (outpatient vs. hospital ward vs. intensive care unit), which generally reflects pneumonia severity.[85] Antibiotics should cover *S. pneumoniae*, *H. influenzae*, *S. aureus*, and Gram-negative bacilli, and coverage of atypical organisms such as *Legionella* must be seriously considered, especially in patients with COPD and during summer. Additionally, the elderly are at increased risk for drug-resistant *S. pneumoniae* as an etiology of CAP, especially if other risk factors are present such as alcoholism, multiple medical comorbidities, treatment with a β-lactam antibiotic within the previous 3 months, or immunosuppression.

The most common agent causing CAP remains *S. pneumoniae*, and isolates of this bacterium have become increasingly resistant to various antibiotics on in vitro testing.[96] Drug-resistant *S. pneumoniae* (DRSP) are identified on the basis of resistance to penicillin in vitro and can display in vitro resistance to many antibiotics including doxycycline, trimethoprim/sulfmethoxizole, macrolides, and cephalosporins.[97] However, antipneumococcal fluoroquinolones, vancomycin, ketolides, and linezolid are all active, although quinolone resistance may be increasing.[97,98] Although high-dose β-lactam therapy is unlikely to result in clinical failure in individuals with CAP without meningitis, CAP caused by DRSP been associated with an increased incidence of suppurative complications such as empyema.[99]

The emergence of resistance in other CAP bacterial pathogens is a major concern.[100,101] Nearly all isolates of *Moraxella catarrhalis* are now ampicillin resistant, and up to half of *Hemophilus influenzae* isolates have become ampicillin resistant. Infections with other agents such as Gram-negative bacilli or *S. aureus* tend not to occur in community-dwelling elderly individuals who lack significant comorbid diseases, but these organisms frequently cause severe infection in institutionalized or hospitalized elderly, who typically have significant comorbid illness and are increasingly resistant to various antibiotics.

Antivirals

When infection with influenza A or B is considered as a cause of infection, antineuraminidase drugs can be given such as amantadine and rimantidine, which are effective for both chemoprophylaxis and treatment if such therapy can be started within 36–48 h of the onset of symptoms.[83,102] More recent data, however, suggest that alternative antiviral therapy with oseltamavir or zanamivir, which only have efficacy for influenza A and are more effective for treatment of influenza A but must be initiated within 48 h of the onset of symptoms. Since influenza A is the predominant component of the fall peak of influenza, and generally accounts for a majority of influenza infections, the use of oseltamavir or zanamivir may be appropriate at any time during "influenza season."

Vaccinations

Interventions that prevent pneumonia are without doubt preferable to treatment of pneumonia once established. Immune stimulation with vaccines to prevent respiratory infections caused by common pathogens can be safe, protective, and cost effective. However, vaccine responses unfortunately tend to be attenuated in the elderly because of waning humoral and cell-mediated immune responses.[103] Nonetheless, vaccination of patients at risk for CAP with both influenza and pneumococcal vaccines has been demonstrated to be both safe and effective,[104,105] and other interventions such as cessation of cigarette smoking are also important. Pneumococcal vaccine has been shown to diminish the risk of bacteremia in elderly patients,[106] and efficacy has been demonstrated in immunocompetent individuals over age 65 years as well as in populations with increased risk (COPD, diabetes, congestive heart failure, anatomic asplenia) for pneumococcal pneumonia.[107,108]

However, vaccine-induced antibodies to pneumococcal capsular polysaccharides tend to wane with time, particularly in the elderly,[104] and revaccination with polysaccharide pneumococcal vaccine, which appears to be safe, has been advocated 5 years after the first dose for elderly individuals.[109] Although guidelines issued by various societies advocate for the administration of pneumococcal vaccine, the efficacy of currently used pneumococcal vaccines for the prevention of CAP remains controversial.[110]

The influenza vaccine has been demonstrated to be effective in attenuating or preventing illness in both elderly and younger populations and can prevent illness in up to 90% of individuals under 65 years of age when the vaccine and circulating influenza virus strain are matched.[105,111] Although somewhat less effective in the elderly, particularly in those with chronic illness, the influenza vaccine can still attenuate influenza infection and prevent severe illness and death or subsequent bacterial lower respiratory tract infections. Interestingly, there are data from multiple studies to suggest that wide-scale influenza vaccination, particularly if children in a given community are immunized, can have measurable benefit for the elderly in preventing illness due to influenza.[112,113]

Conclusion

Elderly individuals are at increased risk for developing respiratory infections, and this susceptibility has been linked to changes in lung structure and function that occur with normal aging as well as changes in immune function. The presence of comorbid conditions, such as congestive heart failure or neurologic dysfunction that predisposes to aspiration, can greatly increase this risk. Empiric therapies to treat suspected CAP in elderly patients should be instituted rapidly and cover potentially resistant organisms. Vaccination, especially the administration of the influenza vaccine, should be given to all elderly patients to protect against CAP.

References

1. Mittman C, Edelman NH, Norris AH, Shock NW. Relationship between chest wall and pulmonary compliance and age. J Appl Physiol 1965;20(6):1211–1216.
2. Turner JM, Mead J, Wohl ME. Elasticity of human lungs in relation to age. J Appl Physiol 1968;25(6):664–671.
3. Lang MR, Fiaux GW, Gillooly M, Stewart JA, Hulmes DJ, Lamb D. Collagen content of alveolar wall tissue in emphysematous and non-emphysematous lungs. Thorax 1994;49 (4):319–326.
4. Reiser KM. Nonenzymatic glycation of collagen in aging and diabetes. Proc Soc Exp Biol Med 1998;218(1):23–37.

5. Verbeken EK, Cauberghs M, Mertens I, Clement J, Lauweryns JM, Van de Woestijne KP. The senile lung. Comparison with normal and emphysematous lungs. 1. Structural aspects. Chest 1992;101(3):793–799.

6. Fishman AP. One hundred years of chronic obstructive pulmonary disease. Am J Respir Crit Care Med 2005;171(9):941–948.

7. Briscoe AM, Loring WE. Elastin content of the human lung. Proc Soc Exp Biol Med 1958;99 (1):162–164.

8. Pierce JA, Hocott JB. Studies on the collagen and elastin content of the human lung. J Clin Invest 1960;39:8–14.

9. Edge JR, Millard FJ, Reid L, Simon G. The radiographic appearances of the chest in persons of advanced age. Br J Radiol 1964;37:769–774.

10. Tolep K, Kelsen SG. Effect of aging on respiratory skeletal muscles. Clin Chest Med 1993;14 (3):363–378.

11. Polkey MI, Harris ML, Hughes PD, Hamnegard CH, Lyons D, Green M et al. The contractile properties of the elderly human diaphragm. Am J Respir Crit Care Med 1997;155(5): 1560–1564.

12. Evans WJ, Campbell WW. Sarcopenia and age-related changes in body composition and functional capacity. J Nutr 1993;123(2 Suppl):465–468.

13. Evans SA, Watson L, Hawkins M, Cowley AJ, Johnston ID, Kinnear WJ. Respiratory muscle strength in chronic heart failure. Thorax 1995;50(6):625–628.

14. Mancini DM, Henson D, LaManca J, Levine S. Respiratory muscle function and dyspnea in patients with chronic congestive heart failure. Circulation 1992;86(3):909–918.

15. Nishimura Y, Maeda H, Tanaka K, Nakamura H, Hashimoto Y, Yokoyama M. Respiratory muscle strength and hemodynamics in chronic heart failure. Chest 1994;105(2):355–359.

16. Arora NS, Rochester DF. Respiratory muscle strength and maximal voluntary ventilation in undernourished patients. Am Rev Respir Dis 1982;126(1):5–8.

17. Peterson DD, Pack AI, Silage DA, Fishman AP. Effects of aging on ventilatory and occlusion pressure responses to hypoxia and hypercapnia. Am Rev Respir Dis 1981;124(4):387–391.

18. Verdery RB. Malnutrition and chronic inflammation – causes or effects of frailty. Aging-Clin Exp Res 1992;4(3):262–263.

19. Shaker R, Ren JL, Bardan E, Easterling C, Dua K, Xie PY et al. Pharyngoglottal closure reflex: characterization in healthy young, elderly and dysphagic patients with predeglutitive aspiration. Gerontology 2003;49(1):12–20.

20. Nakayama K, Jia YX, Hirai H, Shinkawa M, Yamaya M, Sekizawa K et al. Acid stimulation reduces bactericidal activity of surface liquid in cultured human airway epithelial cells. Am J Respir Cell Mol Biol 2002;26(1):105–113.

21. Chouinard J. Dysphagia in Alzheimer disease: a review. J Nutr Health Aging 2000;4(4): 214–217.

22. Ruiz M, Ewig S, Marcos MA, Martinez JA, Arancibia F, Mensa J et al. Etiology of community-acquired pneumonia: impact of age, comorbidity, and severity. Am J Respir Crit Care Med 1999;160(2):397–405.

23. Puchelle E, Zahm JM, Bertrand A. Influence of age on bronchial mucociliary transport. Scand J Respir Dis 1979;60(6):307–313.

24. Ho JC, Chan KN, Hu WH, Lam WK, Zheng L, Tipoe GL et al. The effect of aging on nasal mucociliary clearance, beat frequency, and ultrastructure of respiratory cilia. Am J Respir Crit Care Med 2001;163(4):983–988.

25. Rutland J, Cox T, Dewar A, Cole P, Warner JO. Transitory ultrastructural abnormalities of cilia. Br J Dis Chest 1982;76(2):185–188.

26. Medzhitov R, Janeway CJ. Advances in immunology: innate immunity. N Engl J Med 2000;343(5):338–344.

27. Delves PJ, Roitt IM. The immune system – first of two parts. N Eng J Med 2000;343(1):37–49.

28. Delves PJ, Roitt IM. Advances in immunology: the immune system – second of two parts. N Engl J Med 2000;343(2):108–117.

29. Butcher SK, Lord JM. Stress responses and innate immunity: aging as a contributory factor. Aging Cell 2004;3(4):151–160.

30. Medzhitov R, Janeway C. Innate immune recognition: mechanisms and pathways. Immunol Rev 2000;173:89–97.

31. Zhang P, Summer WR, Bagby GJ, Nelson S. Innate immunity and pulmonary host defense. Immunol Rev 2000;173:39–51.

32. van den Biggelaar AHJ, Huizinga TWJ, de Craen AJM, Gussekloo J, Heijmans BT, Frolich M et al. Impaired innate immunity predicts frailty in old age. The Leiden 85-plus study. Exp Gerontol 2004;39(9):1407–1414.

33. Corberand J, Ngyen F, Laharrague P, Fontanilles AM, Gleyzes B, Gyrard E et al. Polymorphonuclear functions and aging in humans. J Am Geriatr Soc 1981;29(9):391–397.

34. Fu YK, Arkins S, Li YM, Dantzer R, Kelley KW. Reduction in superoxide anion secretion and bactericidal activity of neutrophils from aged rats – reversal by the combination of gamma-interferon and growth-hormone. Infect Immun 1994;62(1):1–8.

35. Tortorella C, Ottolenghi A, Pugliese P, Jirillo E, Antonaci S. Relationship between respiratory burst and adhesiveness capacity in elderly polymorphonuclear cells. Mech Ageing Dev 1993;69(1–2):53–63.

36. Fulop T, Fouquet C, Allaire P, Perrin N, Lacombe G, Stankova J et al. Changes in apoptosis of human polymorphonuclear granulocytes with aging. Mech Ageing Dev 1997;96(1–3):15–34.

37. Tortorella C, Piazzolla G, Spaccavento F, Pece S, Jirillo E, Antonaci S. Spontaneous and fas-induced apoptotic cell death in aged neutrophils. J Clin Immunol 1998;18(5):321–329.

38. Szakal AK, Kapasi ZF, Masuda A, Tew JG. Follicular dendritic cells in the alternative antigen transport pathway: microenvironment, cellular events, age and retrovirus related alterations. Semin Immunol 1992;4(4):257–265.

39. Pietschmann P, Hahn P, Kudlacek S, Thomas R, Peterlik M. Surface markers and transendothelial migration of dendritic cells from elderly subjects. Exp Gerontol 2000;35(2): 213–224.

40. Steger MM, Maczek C, GrubeckLoebenstein B. Morphologically and functionally intact dendritic cells can be derived from the peripheral blood of aged individuals. Clin Exp Immunol 1996;105(3):544–550.

41. Lung TL, Saurwein-Teissl M, Parson W, Schonitzer D, Grubeck-Loebenstein B. Unimpaired dendritic cells call be derived from monocytes in old age and can mobilize residual function in senescent T cells. Vaccine 2000;18(16):1606–1612.

42. Shodell M, Siegal FP. Circulating, interferon-producing plasmacytoid dendritic cells decline during human ageing. Scand J Immunol 2002;56(5):518–521.

43. Davila DR, Edwards CK, III, Arkins S, Simon J, Kelley KW. Interferon-gamma-induced priming for secretion of superoxide anion and tumor necrosis factor-alpha declines in macrophages from aged rats. FASEB J 1990;4(11):2906–2911.

44. Alvarez E, Machado A, Sobrino F, Santa MC. Nitric oxide and superoxide anion production decrease with age in resident and activated rat peritoneal macrophages. Cell Immunol 1996;169(1):152–155.

45. Lavie L, Weinreb O, Gershon D. Age-related alterations in superoxide anion generation in mouse peritoneal macrophages studied by repeated stimulations and heat shock treatment. J Cell Physiol 1992;152(2):382–388.

46. Khare PD, Dhawan R, Chaturvedi UC. Identification and characterization of receptor for dengue virus-induced macrophage cytotoxin. Indian J Exp Biol 1996;34(7):652–657.

47. Chen LC, Pace JL, Russell SW, Morrison DC. Altered regulation of inducible nitric oxide synthase expression in macrophages from senescent mice. Infect Immun 1996;64(10): 4288–4298.

48. Renshaw M, Rockwell J, Engleman C, Gewirtz A, Katz J, Sambhara S. Cutting edge: impaired Toll-like receptor expression and function in aging. J Immunol 2002;169(9):4697–4701.

49. Boehmer ED, Goral J, Faunce DE, Kovacs EJ. Age-dependent decrease in Toll-like receptor 4-mediated proinflammatory cytokine production and mitogen-activated protein kinase expression. J Leukoc Biol 2004;75(2):342–349.

50. Swift ME, Burns AL, Gray KL, DiPietro LA. Age-related alterations in the inflammatory response to dermal injury. J Invest Dermatol 2001;117(5):1027–1035.
51. Ashcroft GS, Horan MA, Ferguson MW. Aging alters the inflammatory and endothelial cell adhesion molecule profiles during human cutaneous wound healing. Lab Invest 1998;78 (1):47–58.
52. McNerlan SE, Rea IM, Alexander HD, Morris TC. Changes in natural killer cells, the CD57CD8 subset, and related cytokines in healthy aging. J Clin Immunol 1998;18(1):31–38.
53. Ogata K, Yokose N, Tamura H, An E, Nakamura K, Dan K et al. Natural killer cells in the late decades of human life. Clin Immunol Immunopathol 1997;84(3):269–275.
54. Miyaji C, Watanabe H, Toma H, Akisaka M, Tomiyama K, Sato Y et al. Functional alteration of granulocytes, NK cells, and natural killer T cells in centenarians. Hum Immunol 2000;61 (9):908–916.
55. Poynter ME, Mu HH, Chen XP, Daynes RA. Activation of NK1.1+ T cells in vitro and their possible role in age-associated changes in inducible IL-4 production. Cell Immunol 1997;179 (1):22–29.
56. Dubey DP, Husain Z, Levitan E, Zurakowski D, Mirza N, Younes S et al. The MHC influences NK and NKT cell functions associated with immune abnormalities and lifespan. Mech Ageing Dev 2000;113(2):117–134.
57. Flurkey K, Stadecker M, Miller RA. Memory T lymphocyte hyporesponsiveness to non-cognate stimuli: a key factor in age-related immunodeficiency. Eur J Immunol 1992;22 (4):931–935.
58. Naylor K, Li G, Vallejo AN, Lee WW, Koetz K, Bryl E et al. The influence of age on T cell generation and TCR diversity. J Immunol 2005;174(11):7446–7452.
59. Swain S, Clise-Dwyer K, Haynes L. Homeostasis and the age-associated defect of CD4 T cells. Semin Immunol 2005;17(5):370–377.
60. Cakman I, Rohwer J, Schutz RM, Kirchner H, Rink L. Dysregulation between TH1 and TH2 T cell subpopulations in the elderly. Mech Ageing Dev 1996;87(3):197–209.
61. Zhou T, Edwards CK, III, Mountz JD. Prevention of age-related T cell apoptosis defect in CD2-fas-transgenic mice. J Exp Med 1995;182(1):129–137.
62. Jackola DR, Ruger JK, Miller RA. Age-associated changes in human T cell phenotype and function. Aging (Milano) 1994;6(1):25–34.
63. Franceschi C, Bonafe M. Centenarians as a model for healthy aging. Biochem Soc Trans 2003;31(2):457–461.
64. Franceschi C, Monti D, Sansoni P, Cossarizza A. The immunology of exceptional individuals: the lesson of centenarians. Immunol Today 1995;16(1):12–16.
65. Ferguson FG, Wikby A, Maxson P, Olsson J, Johansson B. Immune parameters in a longitudinal study of a very old population of Swedish people: a comparison between survivors and nonsurvivors. J Gerontol A Biol Sci Med Sci 1995;50(6):B378–B382.
66. Johnson SA, Cambier JC. Ageing, autoimmunity and arthritis: Senescence of the B cell compartment – implications for humoral immunity. Arthritis Res Ther 2004;6(4):131–139.
67. McKenna RW, Washington LT, Aquino DB, Picker LJ, Kroft SH. Immunophenotypic analysis of hematogones (B-lymphocyte precursors) in 662 consecutive bone marrow specimens by 4-color flow cytometry. Blood 2001;98(8):2498–2507.
68. Johnson SA, Rozzo SJ, Cambier JC. Aging-dependent exclusion of antigen-inexperienced cells from the peripheral B cell repertoire. J Immunol 2002;168(10):5014–5023.
69. Dailey RW, Eun SY, Russell CE, Vogel LA. B cells of aged mice show decreased expansion in response to antigen, but are normal in effector function. Cell Immunol 2001;214(2):99–109.
70. Doria G, Dagostaro G, Poretti A. Age-dependent variations of antibody avidity. Immunology 1978;35(4):601–611.
71. Miller C, Kelsoe G. Ig V-H hypermutation is absent in the germinal-centers of aged mice. J Immunol 1995;155(7):3377–3384.
72. Meyer KC, Ershler W, Rosenthal NS, Lu XC, Peterson K. Immune dysregulation in the aging human lung. Am J Respir Crit Care Med 1996;153(3):1072–1079.

73. Meyer KC, Rosenthal NS, Soergel P, Peterson K. Neutrophils and low-grade inflammation in the seemingly normal aging human lung. Mech Ageing Dev 1998;104(2):169–181.

74. Meyer KC, Soergel P. Variation of bronchoalveolar lymphocyte phenotypes with age in the physiologically normal human lung. Thorax 1999;54(8):697–700.

75. Thompson AB, Scholer SG, Daughton DM, Potter JF, Rennard SI. Altered epithelial lining fluid parameters in old normal individuals. J Gerontol 1992;47(5):M171–M176.

76. Meyer KC, Cardoni A, Xiang ZZ. Vascular endothelial growth factor in bronchoalveolar lavage from normal subjects and patients with diffuse parenchymal lung disease. J Lab Clin Med 2000;135(4):332–338.

77. Plowden J, Renshaw-Hoelscher M, Engleman C, Katz J, Sambhara S. Innate immunity in aging: impact on macrophage function. Aging Cell 2004;3(4):161–167.

78. Koike E, Kobayashi T, Mochitate K, Murakami M. Effect of aging on nitric oxide production by rat alveolar macrophages. Exp Gerontol 1999;34(7):889–894.

79. Corsini E, Battaini F, Lucchi L, Marinovich M, Racchi M, Govoni S et al. A defective protein kinase C anchoring system underlying age-associated impairment in TNF-alpha production in rat macrophages. J Immunol 1999;163(6):3468–3473.

80. Zissel G, Schlaak M, Muller-Quernheim J. Age-related decrease in accessory cell function of human alveolar macrophages. J Investig Med 1999;47(1):51–56.

81. Corsini E, Di Paola R, Viviani B, Genovese T, Mazzon E, Lucchi L et al. Increased carrageenan-induced acute lung inflammation in old rats. Immunology 2005;115(2):253–261.

82. Woodhead M. Pneumonia in the elderly. J Antimicrob Chemother 1994;34(Suppl A):85–92.

83. Treanor J, Falsey A. Respiratory viral infections in the elderly. Antiviral Res 1999;44(2): 79–102.

84. Metlay JP, Schulz R, Li YH, Singer DE, Marrie TJ, Coley CM et al. Influence of age on symptoms at presentation in patients with community-acquired pneumonia. Arch Intern Med 1997;157(13):1453–1459.

85. Niederman MS, Mandell LA, Anzueto A, Bass JB, Broughton WA, Campbell GD et al. Guidelines for the management of adults with community-acquired pneumonia. Diagnosis, assessment of severity, antimicrobial therapy, and prevention. Am J Respir Crit Care Med 2001;163(7):1730–1754.

86. Fine MJ, Auble TE, Yealy DM, Hanusa BH, Weissfeld LA, Singer DE et al. A prediction rule to identify low-risk patients with community-acquired pneumonia. N Engl J Med 1997;336 (4):243–250.

87. Meehan TP, Fine MJ, Krumholz HM, Scinto JD, Galusha DH, Mockalis JT et al. Quality of care, process, and outcomes in elderly patients with pneumonia. JAMA 1997;278(23): 2080–2084.

88. Falsey AR, Walsh EE. Viral pneumonia in older adults. Clin Infect Dis 2006;42(4):518–524.

89. Thompson WW, Shay DK, Weintraub E, Brammer I, Bridges CB, Cox NJ et al. Influenza-associated hospitalizations in the United States. JAMA 2004;292(11):1333–1340.

90. Bradley SF. Prevention of influenza in long-term-care facilities. Infect Control Hosp Epidemiol 1999;20(9):629–637.

91. Falsey AR, Hennessey PA, Formica MA, Cox C, Walsh EE. Respiratory syncytial virus infection in elderly and high-risk adults. N Engl J Med 2005;352(17):1749–1759.

92. Looney RJ, Falsey AR, Walsh E, Campbell D. Effect of aging on cytokine production in response to respiratory syncytial virus infection. J Infect Dis 2002;185(5):682–685.

93. Hicks LA, Shepard CW, Britz PH, Erdman DD, Fischer M, Flannery BL et al. Two outbreaks of severe respiratory disease in nursing homes associated with rhinovirus. J Am Geriatr Soc 2006;54(2):284–289.

94. Louie JK, Yagi S, Nelson FA, Kiang D, Glaser CA, Rosenberg J et al. Rhinovirus outbreak in a long term care facility for elderly persons associated with unusually high mortality. Clin Infect Dis 2005;41(2):262–265.

95. Mosser AG, Vrtis R, Burchell L, Lee WM, Dick CR, Weisshaar E et al. Quantitative and qualitative analysis of rhinovirus infection in bronchial tissues. Am J Respir Crit Care Med 2005;171(6):645–651.
96. Bartlett JG, Mundy LM. Community-acquired pneumonia. N Engl J Med 1995;333 (24):1618–1624.
97. Doern GV, Pfaller MA, Kugler K, Freeman J, Jones RN. Prevalence of antimicrobial resistance among respiratory tract isolates of Streptococcus pneumoniae in North America: 1997 results from the SENTRY antimicrobial surveillance program. Clin Infect Dis 1998;27 (4):764–770.
98. Whitney CG, Farley MM, Hadler J, Harrison LH, Lexau C, Reingold A et al. Increasing prevalence of multidrug-resistant Streptococcus pneumoniae in the United States. N Engl J Med 2000;343(26):1917–1924.
99. Metlay JP, Hofmann J, Cetron MS, Fine MJ, Farley MM, Whitney C et al. Impact of penicillin susceptibility on medical outcomes for adult patients with bacteremic pneumococcal pneumonia. Clin Infect Dis 2000;30(3):520–528.
100. Nicolau D. Clinical and economic implications of antimicrobial resistance for the management of community-acquired respiratory tract infections. J Antimicrob Chemother 2002;50 (Suppl S1):61–70.
101. Bonomo RA. Resistant pathogens in respiratory tract infections in older people. J Am Geriatr Soc 2002;50(7 Suppl):S236–S241.
102. Gillissen A, Hoffken G. Early therapy with the neuraminidase inhibitor oseltamivir maximizes its efficacy in influenza treatment. Med Microbiol Immunol 2002;191(3–4):165–168.
103. Fagiolo U, Amadori A, Cozzi E, Bendo R, Lama M, Douglas A et al. Humoral and cellular immune response to influenza virus vaccination in aged humans. Aging (Milano) 1993;5 (6):451–458.
104. Artz AS, Ershler WB, Longo DL. Pneumococcal vaccination and revaccination of older adults. Clin Microbiol Rev 2003;16(2):308–318.
105. Gross PA, Hermogenes AW, Sacks HS, Lau J, Levandowski RA. The efficacy of influenza vaccine in elderly persons. A meta-analysis and review of the literature. Ann Intern Med 1995;123(7):518–527.
106. Sisk JE, Moskowitz AJ, Whang W, Lin JD, Fedson DS, McBean AM et al. Cost-effectiveness of vaccination against pneumococcal bacteremia among elderly people. JAMA 1997;278(16):1333–1339.
107. Butler JC, Breiman RF, Campbell JF, Lipman HB, Broome CV, Facklam RR. Pneumococcal polysaccharide vaccine efficacy. An evaluation of current recommendations. JAMA 1993;270(15):1826–1831.
108. Simberkoff MS, Cross AP, Al Ibrahim M, Baltch AL, Geiseler PJ, Nadler J et al. Efficacy of pneumococcal vaccine in high-risk patients. Results of a Veterans Administration Cooperative Study. N Engl J Med 1986;315(21):1318–1327.
109. Ortqvist A. Pneumococcal vaccination: current and future issues. Eur Respir J 2001;18 (1):184–195.
110. Dear K, Holden J, Andrews R, Tatham D. Vaccines for preventing pneumococcal infection in adults. Cochrane Database Syst Rev 2003;(4):CD000422.
111. Nichol KL, Margolis KL, Wuorenma J, Von Sternberg T. The efficacy and cost effectiveness of vaccination against influenza among elderly persons living in the community. N Engl J Med 1994;331(12):778–784.
112. Ghendon YZ, Kaira AN, Elshina GA. The effect of mass influenza immunization in children on the morbidity of the unvaccinated elderly. Epidemiol Infect 2006;134(1):71–78.
113. Reichert TA, Sugaya N, Fedson DS, Glezen WP, Simonsen L, Tashiro M. The Japanese experience with vaccinating schoolchildren against influenza. N Engl J Med 2001;344 (12):889–896.

Chapter 6
Influenza in the Elderly

Caterina Hatzifoti and Andrew William Heath

Introduction

Influenza is a highly contagious upper respiratory tract disease caused by the influenza (flu) viruses types A, B, and C. Worldwide, 20% of children and 5% of adults develop symptomatic infections due to influenza A or B viruses each year.[1] The virus causes asymptomatic disease as well as lung, brain, heart, kidney, and muscle disorders and predisposes patients of all age groups to bacterial pneumonia. Illness development depends on the patient's age, pre-existing immunity, immune competence, virus properties, smoking, and pregnancy. Rates of serious infection and death are highest among people aged >65 years and people with serious medical conditions. The virus is most commonly spread among humans by respiratory droplets containing virus via coughing and sneezing but can sometimes also be transmitted directly to humans by avian or swine species.

Virology and Epidemiology

Flu virus is a member of the family Orthomyxoviridae and there are three types of the virus A, B, and C, but only the first two cause widespread outbreaks. All types of influenza viruses have segmented genomes (eight single-stranded segments of RNA) enclosed within a lipid envelope derived from the host cell membrane (Fig. 6.1) and show great antigenic diversity, mainly resulting from single but accumulating nucleotide changes, known as *antigenic drift*. Mutation rates in RNA viruses such as influenza viruses and HIV are much higher than in eukaryotes or DNA viruses owing to the lack of repair mechanisms for RNA that exist for DNA replication.

Changes that replace entire genes through reassortment of RNA fragments in a cell infected with two or more virus strains, a process called *antigenic shift*, are less common, but can have a dramatic effect in enabling complete viral evasion of the immune system (Fig. 6.2). Antigenic shift often results in worldwide epidemics, or pandemics such as those that occurred in 1957 and 1968. Detailed molecular

C. Hatzifoti and A.W. Heath
University of Sheffield Medical School, Beech Hill Road, Sheffield, UK

S.L. Percival (ed.), *Microbiology and Aging*.
DOI: 10.1007/978-1-59745-327-1_6, © Springer Science + Business Media, LLC 2009

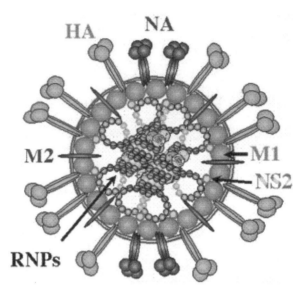

Fig. 6.1 Schematic structure presentation of an Influenza virus particle. (Courtesy of Dr. Paul Digard, Pathology Department, University of Cambridge.) The outer surface consists of a lipid envelope consisting of glycoprotein spikes of two types, hemagglutinin (HA) and neuraminidase (NA). The inner side of the envelope is lined by the matrix protein and the genome segments are packaged into the ribonucleoprotein (RNP) core (See Color Plates)

analysis of different flu strains is important for comprehending the evolution of influenza pandemic viruses.

The two surface glycoprotein antigens, hemagglutinin and neuraminidase (Fig. 6.1), are involved in flu virus attachment and pathogenesis, and it is largely changes in these surface antigens through antigenic drift or shift that allow a new viral strain to evade pre-existing immunity. Influenza B viruses have only 1 subtype of hemagglutinin and 1 type of neuraminidase and therefore do not undergo antigenic shift, whereas influenza A viruses have 15 different possible subtypes of hemagglutinin (H1–H15) and 9 potential neuraminidase subtypes (N1–N9). Birds can be infected by influenza A viruses with any combination of the 15 HA and 9 NA genes forming a global reservoir of virus. While human and swine pandemic influenza viruses have so far been largely restricted to a few surface antigens (H1, H2, H3, N1, N2; at least as far as can be ascertained, which is going back only a century or so!), there are potentially a large number of possible new surface antigen combinations that could arise and infect humans. It is thought that close association of birds, such as ducks, with mammals, such as pigs, in agriculture allows coinfection with avian and mammalian influenza virus strains, which occasionally leads to the production of a virus with different surface glycopoteins which is still able to infect humans[2] (Fig. 6.2).

In recent years, there have been a number of outbreaks of variously shifted strains that have so far, luckily, failed to transmit from human to human. For instance, between May 1997 and early 1998, there were 18 confirmed human cases of an H5N1 virus (similar to an avian strain that killed many thousands of chickens) and 6 of those 18 cases were fatal.[3] Overall, H5N1 virus has since this

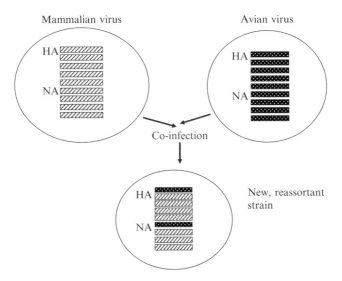

Fig. 6.2 Cartoon illustrating reassortment of influenza genes to produce a novel virus. Coinfection with a mammalian strain and an avian virus strain with different genes, including HA and NA, results in a virus with many internal proteins encoded by the original mammalian genes, but with new HA and NA derived from the avian strain. The new virus is able to replicate well in mammalian cells and is able to evade immune responses generated against earlier circulating strains. The rectangular blocks represent viral genes

chapter was prepared caused 79 human infections in Vietnam, Cambodia, and Thailand, of which 46 were fatal.[4] The danger posed to the world should these strains become capable of human to human transmission is obvious. During the production of the final draft of this manuscript, news has emerged from WHO indicating that the pattern of avian flu infections in northern Vietnam is now consistent with human-to-human spread.

In nonpandemic years (that is, most of the time), epidemics of influenza mainly occur during the winter months in temperate regions and are caused by drifted strains of virus related to those that had circulated in previous years. These epidemics are, on average, responsible for approximately 36,000 excess deaths annually in the United States alone. An estimated 90% of these deaths occur in persons aged >65 years.[5]

The timing and magnitude of influenza virus activity is unpredictable, but using efficient surveillance data, and assessing levels of activity in a timely manner using defined "threshold values," epidemiologists can indicate when sufficient flu activity is occurring in a population to warrant the use of interventions such as the prophylactic use of antiviral drugs.[6] Antiviral chemotherapy is discussed in the section "Antiviral Treatment."

Symptoms and Related Illnesses

The incubation period for influenza is 1–4 days with an average of 2 days,[7] although cough and malaise can persist for more than 2 weeks. Adults typically are infectious from the day before symptoms occur through approximately 5 days after illness.

Uncomplicated influenza illness is characterized by the abrupt onset of constitutional and respiratory signs and symptoms such as fever, myalgia, headache, nonproductive cough, sore throat, and rhinitis.[8] These symptoms are of course common to many viral infections, and respiratory viruses other than influenza are known to contribute to lower respiratory tract complications and deaths in elderly people during the winter months while producing symptoms very similar to those of influenza virus infection. In 1997, Nicholson and colleagues[9] studied the causes of respiratory infections in elderly people living at home in Leicestershire, UK, and concluded that 52% of the diseases were caused by rhinoviruses, 26% by coronaviruses, 9.5% by influenza, and 7% by respiratory syncytial virus (RSV).

Complications in the lower respiratory tract can occur following influenza virus infection in the elderly. The most common serious complication of influenza is pneumonia, which may occur at the same time as the influenza-like illness or up to 2 weeks afterwards. Viral pneumonia accompanied by toxemia can develop within 24 h following the onset of influenza, usually influenza Type A infection. The pneumonia is an interstitial pneumonitis with severe hyperemia and broadening of the alveolar walls together with a mononuclear cell infiltration, capillary dilatation, and thrombosis.[10] The symptoms include tachypneoa, tachycardia, high fever, and hypotension. Hypoxemia and death may follow between 1 and 4 days later. Initial improvement in those who survive occurs 5–16 days after onset of the pneumonia. Generally, there are no lasting complications after severe influenza infection, although a few patients develop a diffuse interstitial fibrosis accompanied by impaired lung function.[10]

Pneumonia and secondary infections, which commence after apparent recovery from the influenza infection, are usually caused by a bacterial superinfection with organisms such as *Streptococcus pneumoniae*, *Staphylococcus aureus* or *Hemophilus influenzae*. Infection with *S. aureus* affects the lung by causing oedema, hyperemia, hemorrhaging, consolidation, and formation of pus. When secondary bacterial infections are associated with type A influenza viruses they can be particularly harmful. During influenza A infections, there is apoptosis of leukocytes recruited into the airways, resulting in reduced efficiency of bacterial phagocytosis and destruction.[11] Many other immune functions may be compromised during influenza virus infection, and influenza virus infection of epithelial cells has been shown to directly enhance bacterial adherence to the cells.[12]

Antivirals and Influenza Vaccines for the Elderly

Flu hemagglutinin is the major component of current influenza vaccines and neuraminidase is the primary target for antiviral drug activity. The receptor for hemagglutinin is the terminal sialic acid residue on host cell surface sialyloligosaccharides, while the viral enzyme neuraminidase (sialidase) catalyzes the hydrolysis of sialic acid residues from sialyloligosaccharides. Most of the recently developed anti-influenza drugs inhibit sialidase of influenza viruses A and B.

Antiviral Treatment

Well-defined and validated antiviral drugs have proven to be curative in many cases and have a critical advantage over vaccine therapy. Flu vaccines need to be redesigned annually to immunize against particular strains or group of strains, a process that can take several months. Chemoprophylaxis should be considered for people at high risk during the time from vaccination until immunity has developed, since antibody responses in adults develop approximately 2-weeks post vaccination.[13] Prophylactic use of antiviral agents is also an option for preventing influenza among persons with anaphylactic hypersensitivity to eggs or other components of the influenza vaccine, or in "at-risk" individuals (including those aged over 65) recently exposed to a person with an influenza like illness, or for those same individuals during an epidemic. Indeed, the U.K. National Institute for Clinical and Health Excellence (NICE) recently published guidelines indicating that prophylactic postexposure use of ostelamivir (see below) is recommended for use in at-risk groups in residential care during periods when the virus is known to be circulating, or in unprotected at-risk people exposed to someone with an influenza-like illness. Unprotected people in the cases above means people not vaccinated since the previous flu season, or when the vaccine strain does not closely match the circulating strains of virus, or during the period before the vaccination takes effect.

Many experts consider that the best way of preparing for a flu pandemic (which would likely occur in the absence of any appropriate vaccine) is to prepare a stock of sufficient of doses of antiviral drugs, in order reduce the symptoms and possibly to slow transmission of the pandemic strain for long enough to allow the development and production of strain-specific vaccines. This policy has been adopted by a number of countries; however, only a fraction of the approximately 30 million doses needed in the UK are so far available. The most practical influenza medication is considered to be Tamiflu (ostelamivir-phosphate) produced by Roche. Although Tamiflu is available on the National Health Service (NHS) for treating high-risk groups, supply may be limited.

Zanamivir and ostelamivir belong to the neuraminidase inhibitor group of antiviral compounds and they are up to 84% (zanamivir) and 87% (ostelamivir) effective in preventing laboratory confirmed influenza illness.[14,15] Ostelamivir prophylaxis in particular led to a 92% reduction in influenza illness among nursing home residents during a 6-week study.[16] Zanamavir is not recommended for treatment for patients with underlying airway disease, since cases of respiratory dysfunction have been reported after inhalation together with allergic reactions such as oropharyngeal or facial edema.[17] Administration of ostelamivir has presented with fewer side effects such as nausea and/or vomiting[18,19] and these can be controlled if the drug is taken with food.[15]

Amantadine and rimantadine belong to another group of antiviral agents, which prevent the symptoms of influenza A illness by blocking of the M2 ion channel and altering optimal pH conditions to inhibit virus uncoating and replication. They are not effective against influenza B infection, since influenza B viruses lack the M2 protein. When used as prophylactic agent, amantadine can prevent illness while permitting subclinical infection and development of a protective antibody response, which does not interfere with the antibody response to the vaccine.[20]

Side effects related to amantadine and rimantadine are usually mild and stop immediately after treatment, but serious side effects have been reported such as central nervous system (CNS) symptoms, behavioral changes, hallucinations, agitation, and seizures.[21,22] These more severe side effects have been observed among older persons who have been taking amantadine as prophylaxis at a dosage of 200 mg per day[23] and can be reduced by lowering the dosage of the drug.

A novel antiviral agent, NA cyclopentane inhibitor RWJ-270201 was shown to have potent inhibitory activity against NAs of influenza A and B viruses and a unique pattern of activity against resistant variants. It proved to be approximately threefold more potent than zanamavir in inhibiting NA activity of A/H1N1 clinical isolates, approximately fourfold more potent than zanamavir in inhibiting NA activity of A/H3N2 clinical isolates, and approximately sixfold more potent than ostelamivir carboxylate in inhibiting NA activity of influenza B virus clinical isolates.[24] To test the commercial prospects of the drug, phase III trials commenced in North America and Europe in February 2000. RWJ-270201 significantly reduced viral titers in infected patients during phase II studies, without causing any side effects. Under a worldwide influenza collaboration formed in September 1998, Johnson & Johnson has received exclusive worldwide rights to RWJ-270201.[25]

Antiviral chemotherapy (choice of drug, dosage, and duration of therapy) depends on patient's age, weight, renal function, health problems, and related medication and should be taken only during the period of peak influenza activity in a community, in order to be more cost effective and reduce the risk of the appearance of resistant viral strains.[26] In a laboratory (ferret) model of infection, resistance of influenza virus A/LosAngeles/1/87 (H3N2) to amantadine was generated within 6 days, during a single course of treatment, similar to the situation in humans.[27]

Influenza surveillance information and diagnostic testing can guide treatment decisions. Early diagnosis of influenza could theoretically reduce the inappropriate use of antibiotics and exclude possible bacterial infections, which can produce symptoms similar to influenza as mentioned in the previous section. Diagnostic tests available for influenza include viral culture, serology, rapid antigen testing, polymerase chain reaction (PCR), and immunofluorescence-based assays.[28]

Current Influenza Vaccines

Flu vaccination has been a valuable means in protecting vulnerable groups such as children, the elderly, and people with chronic respiratory, heart, renal diseases, diabetes, and immunosuppression.

Current flu vaccines are generally produced from virus grown in fertile hens' eggs and then inactivated by formaldehyde or β-propiolactone (whole-killed vaccine). Other variations consist of detergent split virus, in which the viral envelope has been disrupted using detergents (split vaccine), and purified hemagglutin and neuraminidase antigens (subunit vaccine).[29,30]

The Trivalent Inactivated Influenza (TIV) vaccine currently consists of two influenza A strains (one H3N2, one H1N1) and an influenza B strain. It provides some protection against influenza complications in the elderly including pneumonia and death when given shortly before the beginning of flu season. Each year, the vaccine is reformulated, based on assessment of which viruses have been circulating globally. Not surprisingly, protection appears to vary depending upon how closely the challenge viruses are matched with the vaccine strains. A reduction of 61% in influenza-related deaths was seen when the vaccine and circulatory strains were well matched and only 35% when they were not well matched.[31]

Inactivated influenza vaccine administered to the elderly and other high-risk groups for the year 2004–2005 contained the formaldehyde inactivated strains: A/New Caledonia/20/99 (H3N2), A/Wyoming/3/2003 (H1N1), and B/Jiangsu/10/2003 (0.5 ml intramuscular dose). Common side effects of the vaccine found in less than one in ten persons are redness, bruising around the injection site, sweating, fever, headache, tiredness, or joint and muscular pain, but these symptoms usually disappear within 1–2 days without treatment. In general, healthy people in the age group of 65–74 years present minimal systemic side effects and only a low incidence of local side effects after influenza vaccination.[32] Subvirion and purified surface antigen preparations of the inactivated vaccine, as described above, are also available.

The vaccine can prevent hospitalizations, which constitute the principal direct cost of influenza, and studies from a number of countries with differing healthcare systems have shown vaccination of older and high-risk populations to be cost effective.[33] Vaccination of healthcare workers in nursing homes and hospitals is also associated with a substantial decline in mortality among patients.[34] The Institute of Medicine recently produced a report on future vaccines,[35] which ranked potential vaccines and vaccination strategies into four groups depending upon the projected cost of the program per quality adjusted life year (QALY) saved. Influenza vaccination for one-fifth of the population per year (or once every 5 years per individual) was put into the top group with the most favorable vaccines, those for which a vaccination strategy would save money as well as QALYs.

While the trivalent influenza vaccine is approximately 70–90% effective in preventing illness in healthy younger people, in older populations protection can be as low as 30%,[36] with the average from a number of studies being around 50%.[37–40] This low efficacy of influenza vaccination in the elderly is of great importance, as this group is among the most susceptible to the serious consequences of the infection.

Immune Responses in the Elderly

The reduced efficacy of influenza vaccines in the elderly mentioned in the section "Current Influenza Vaccines" is attributed to immunosenescence, the deterioration of immune responses to immunization, or infection associated with aging. Some ways in which immune responses are impaired in the elderly are summarized in Table 6.1.

Table 6.1 Summary of impaired immune responses in the elderly

Immunity component	Impact of aging	Reference
Macrophages	Decreased number, inefficient presentation of Ags to T cells, reduced phagocytosis, reduced generation of nitrous oxide and superoxide, delayed wound healing, decline in TLRs, cytokine and chemokine expression	41
NK cells	Decreased proliferation, cytokine secretion, and CD69 expression	42
Neutrophils	Impaired chemotaxis, degranulation, and phagocytosis	43, 44
Ag-specific T and B cells	Altered clonal expansion, diminished ability to generate high antibody titer	41
Naïve, mature T cells	Decreased number, reduced expression of MHC II	45
APC function (DCs, LCs)	Poor hypersensitivity to allergens	46
TLRs	Decline in the secretion of antimicrobial peptides and pro-inflammatory cytokines	47

Abbreviations: Ag antigen; *TLR* Toll-like receptor; *NK* natural killer; *MHC II* major histocompatibility complex class II; *APC* antigen presenting cell; *DCs* dendritic cells; *LC* Langerhans' cells

Innate Immune Responses

The initial site of influenza virus replication is thought to be the tracheobronchial ciliated epithelium, but the whole respiratory tract may be involved. Pulmonary infection is strongly related with mortality associated with influenza virus infection either because of viral pneumonia or because of bacterial superinfection. Aging is associated with a progressive decline in lung performance due to alterations in lung parenchyma and elastic recoil[48] and a decrease in tracheal mucus development[49] important for pathogen clearance. Lower sensitivity of the respiratory system to acute disease and infection delays important clinical symptoms such as dyspnoea and tachypnoea, which are important for diagnosis of influenza-associated diseases.

The first line of defense against pathogens, the innate immune functions of macrophages, natural killer (NK) cells, and neutrophils, are impaired with aging leading to lack of early protective immunity to influenza and bacterial infection, thus making the elderly susceptible to viral and bacterial pneumonia and skin and gastrointestinal tract infections.

Macrophages are present in the lungs as well as in other parts of the body and function as pathogen scavengers by initiating inflammatory responses and phagocytosis to eliminate pathogens. Their adherence, opsonization, and phagocytic ability have shown an age-related decline in several murine models.[50,51] Expression of the adhesion molecules VCAM-1 and ICAM-1 was delayed in the elderly[52] and the wound healing process was found to be delayed in older humans and rodents[53] because of delayed re-epithelialization, angiogenesis, collagen deposition, wound strength, and delayed infiltration of macrophages.

Table 6.2 Mammalian Toll-like receptor activity

Receptor	Ligand PAMP	Known activation cascades
TLR 1	Triacetylated lipoproteins	Unknown
TLR 2	Lipoproteins, peptidoglycan (Gram-positive bacteria), lipoteichoid acids, fungal structures	MyD88-dependent TIRAP
TLR 3	Double-stranded RNA	MyD88-independent TRIF
TLR 4	Lipopolysaccharide membrane (Gram-negative bacteria), HSP60, mBD2, fungal structures	MyD88-dependent TIRAP MyD88 independent TRIF/TICAM/TRAM
TLR 5	Flagellin	MyD88-dependent IRAK
TLR 6	Diacetylated lipoproteins	Unknown
TLR 7	Small synthetic compounds, immiquinod, imidazoquinoline, ss RNA	MyD88-dependent IRAK
TLR 8	ssRNA	MyD88-dependent IRAK
TLR 9	Unmethylated CpG DNA	MyD88-dependent IRAK
TLR 10	None defined	Unknown
TLR 11	Uropathogenic bacteria	MyD88-dependent IRAK

Abbreviations: PAMP pathogen associated molecular patterns; *TLR* Toll-like receptor; *MyD88* adaptor protein in the Toll IL-1 receptor family signaling; *TIRAP* Toll-IL-1 receptor domain-containing adaptor protein; *TRIF* TIR domain containing adaptor inducing IFN-β; *HSP 60* 60-kDa heat shock chaperonin protein; *mBD2* mouse β defensin 2; *TRAM* thyroid hormone receptor activator molecule; *IRAK* IL-1 receptor-associated kinase; *CpG* cytosine preceding a guanosine pattern

Innate immune responses are frequently initiated via Toll-like-receptors (TLRs), a set of conserved molecules that recognize pathogen-associated molecular patterns (PAMPs) and endogenous proteins associated with danger and stress signals. Upon TLR stimulation, a variety of antimicrobial peptides and proinflammatory cytokines (IL-6, TNF-α, etc.) are synthesized to assist in the clearance of the invading pathogen. The 11 TLRs recognized to date and their ligands, as well as their signaling activation pathways that may be altered during aging, are summarized in Table 6.2. Clearly, responses to viral infection are influenced by TLRs, such as TLR-3. This receptor is constitutively expressed in human alveolar and bronchial epithelial cells. Its ligand is double-stranded RNA, which is produced during influenza and other viral infections, and its expression was found to be positively regulated by the influenza A virus via the secretion of the cytokines IL-8, IL-6, RANTES, and interferon-beta, and the upregulation of the major adhesion molecule ICAM-1.[54] In a recent study, Renshaw and colleagues[47] assessed TLR expression on splenic and peritoneal macrophages of aged mice and concluded that decreased expression and function of TLRs resulting from aging may partially contribute to the increased susceptibility of the elderly population to bacterial, viral, and yeast infections.

The secretion of cytokines such as IL-6, TNF-α, and chemokines such as MIP-1a, CCL5 is also dysregulated in the aged population[47] (Table 6.1). Increased levels of prostaglandin E(2) have been linked to suppression of IL-12 and class II MHC expression on antigen presenting cells (APCs), an effect that can be reversed by vitamin E supplementation.[55] Both cytokine and chemokine molecules are involved in immune responses to inflammation such as fever. Thus the poor inflammatory response and the lack of presentation of clinical signs in the elderly may delay diagnosis and may contribute to the higher mortality rates seen in older people.

Adaptive Immunity

In relation to the impaired innate immune functions mentioned above, humoral and mainly cellular immune responses decline with age because of the limited generation of high-affinity, protective antibodies against pathogens and of thymus atrophy, respectively. The latter limits the quantity of naïve T cells against infectious agents and new antigens. Inefficient aged T-cell cooperation and limited production of cytokines may lead to the decline in specific antibody responses. Frail, elderly subjects exhibit a blunted and somewhat delayed type 1 T-cell response to influenza vaccination, which is correlated positively with the reduced IgG 1 subclass and the total antibody response.[56] On the other hand, an imbalance in the production of pro- and anti-inflammatory cytokines and the accumulation of $CD8^+$ $CD28^-$ IFN-γ producing T cells in the aging immune system could diminish the likelihood of elderly persons producing specific Abs of sufficient titer following influenza vaccination.[57] Also, an increase in self-reactive antibodies has been observed in older vaccinated patients.[58]

Influenza Vaccine Research and Future Prospects

Newer Methods of Inactivated Vaccine Production

The components of inactivated influenza virus vaccines are produced in embryonated hen's eggs and this presents some practical difficulties. First, the egg supply is often limited, and eggs must be ordered a long time in advance. Secondly, many people are allergic to egg proteins and therefore cannot receive the vaccine, and thirdly, not all strains grow well in eggs, and therefore sometimes the virus strain chosen for use in the vaccine is a compromise based upon antigenic similarity to circulating strains and ability to grow in eggs. Because of these problems with egg growth of the virus, there is interest in producing vaccine virus in tissue culture cells.

Madin Darby Canine Kidney (MDCK) cells are widely used for the isolation of the virus, and Vero cells derived from African green monkey kidney have been recently authorized by the WHO for vaccine production.[59] The safety and immunogenicity of an MDCK-cell-grown influenza vaccine was confirmed in a phase II clinical trial.[60]

Another potential means of avoiding production in eggs would be to use a recombinant subunit vaccine wherein components such as hemagglutinin and neuraminidase are produced in a heterologous system from cDNA introduced into the expression vector. To this end, Baculovirus-based production of intact hemagglutinin in insect cells has been demonstrated, and its immunogenicity has been proven.[61]

Generating Broadly Cross-Reactive Responses

The selection of stable antigenic targets is critical in the design of an influenza vaccine. To date, this area is somewhat under-researched, with the majority of studies focusing on the HA and NA antigens. A universal influenza virus vaccine that does not require frequent updates and/or annual immunizations would offer significant advantages over current seasonal flu vaccines, including, of course, protection against pandemic strains.

Influenza matrix protein, which lines the inside of the lipoprotein envelope enclosing the virus RNA (Fig. 6.1), is a promising antigenic target. It is a multifunctional protein that plays an important role in virus replication by regulating the bidirectional transport of ribonucleoprotein (RNP) into and out of the nucleus, inhibiting viral RNA polymerase activity by binding to RNP and mediating the association of RNP with viral envelope glycoproteins on the inner surface of the cytoplasmic membrane for virion formation and budding. Influenza-matrix-protein-derived peptide GILGFVFTL was found to be 100–1,000 times more effective than commonly used peptides in sensitizing HLA-A2$^+$ target cells to lysis by influenza-virus-specific cytotoxic T lymphocytes.[62]

The highly conserved M2 integral membrane protein encoded by influenza A viruses has also been suggested as a potential antigen for a universal vaccine. M2 protein possesses an ion channel activity that is required for efficient virus entry into host cells. The M2 cytoplasmic tail, in particular, plays a role in infectious virus production by coordinating the efficient packaging of genome segments into influenza virus particles.[63]

Synthetic peptides of M2 extracellular domain conjugated to keyhole limpet hemocyanin or *Neisseria meningitidis* outer membrane protein complex were found to be highly immunogenic in mice, ferrets, and rhesus monkeys and were able to confer protection against lethal challenge with either H1N1 or H3N2 virus in mice.[64,65] Disappointingly, antibody induced by the M2 vaccine did not cross-react with the H5N1 virus, which could be related to the next pandemic strain.[65]

Another conserved influenza protein, the nucleoprotein (NP), may be a potentially valuable vaccine because of its cross-reactivity against even distantly related virus subtypes. This antigen in combination with small amounts of IL-2 was shown to induce strong proliferation of resting CD4$^+$ and CD8$^+$ T cells from young and elderly donors.[66]

Antigen delivery systems can influence the immune response quantitatively as well as qualitatively and the route of administration might drastically affect the success of a vaccine. In the case of influenza, antigen delivery can be critically important, as it might be necessary to stimulate substantial levels of mucosal immunity, which is considered helpful in protection against mucosal infections, in the absence of side effects. New improved intervention strategies through immunization and/or vaccine delivery are therefore needed to reduce morbidity and mortality in the elderly due to influenza and related complications and provide adequate protection during influenza virus epidemics.[10]

Live Attenuated Vaccines

The intranasal vaccine FluMist, a cold-adapted, live-attenuated, trivalent influenza virus vaccine (LAIV) developed by MedImmune was approved by the U.S. Food and Drug Administration on June 17, 2003 only for administration to healthy persons aged 5–49 years.[32] The "cold adaptation" process encourages replication in the nasal passages to induce immunity but restricts replication in the increased temperatures of the lower respiratory tract and lungs.[67] Live attenuated virus vaccine has perceived advantages over killed vaccines in that administration is by the intranasal route. This may be considered preferable to injection by vaccines, and these vaccines may generate stronger mucosal-cell-mediated immune responses than conventional killed vaccines. FluMist's role in the general prevention of influenza is yet to become clear, and there have been some problems associated with distribution, as the vaccine had to remain frozen. In order to circumvent this problem, a next-generation live vaccine was recently produced by MedImmune named CAIV-T, assessed in clinical trials and shown to be immunogenic and safe in healthy and at-risk populations.[67]

Preclinical Vaccine Research and Development

Other methods of mucosal vaccine delivery have been investigated including the use of heterologous viral systems. In a recent report, Abe and colleagues[68] demonstrated protection against lethal influenza virus infection in mice immunized intranasally with a recombinant baculovirus expressing the hemagglutinin gene of the A/PR/8/34 (H1N1) flu virus. Protection was later linked to activation of immune cells by bAcNPV via the Toll-like receptor 9 (TLR9)/MyD88-dependent signaling pathway.[69] Similar to these findings, vaccination with influenza virosomes has shown to elicit high titer of influenza-specific antibodies and T-helper cell and cytotoxic T-cell responses against encapsulated antigens due to the intrinsic adjuvant activity of virosomal formulations.[70]

   Improved cell-mediated immune responses have long been considered a desirable attribute of influenza vaccines. Novel pH-triggered microparticles encapsulating a model MHC class I-restricted peptide Ag from the influenza A matrix protein were efficiently phagocytosed by human monocytes and dendritic cells, and led to increased antigen presentation and primed CTL responses with minimal cellular toxicity and no functional impairment.[71]

As described above, TLR stimulation may be important in immune responses to vaccines and is certainly important in the action of adjuvants designed to enhance vaccine responses. TLR expression and function may also decline in older people.[47] Binding of the cell surface protein CD154 on activated T cells to CD40 on B cells, dendritic cells, macrophages, and other cell types leads to B-cell activation, proliferation, and antibody production independently of Toll receptor recognition and signaling. We have described work showing that conjugates of anti-CD40 mAbs with antigens are very potent immunogens[72,73] and we have recently observed that CD40 adjuvant conjugates with influenza virus antigens were successful in inducing specific anti-influenza antibody and cellular responses.[74]

Similar approaches have been employed with anti-CD40 mAb and liposomally encapsulated nuclear protein peptide NP366-374, corresponding to a CTL epitope on NP. Intranasal immunization of this formulation effectively induced mucosal immunity to reduce virus replication in the lung, suggesting that anti-CD40 mAb also functioned as a mucosal adjuvant through MHC class I- and class II-dependent pathways.[75]

Another interesting approach compared the immunogenicity and safety of a novel, interleukin-2 (IL-2)-supplemented trivalent liposomal influenza vaccine (INFLU-SOME-VAC) with that of a commercial trivalent split virion vaccine in community-residing elderly volunteers of a mean age 81 years. At 1-month post vaccination, hemagglutination inhibition for the A/New Caledonia (H1N1) and A/Moscow (H3N2) strains was significantly higher in the INFLUSOME-VAC group. INFLUSOME-VAC also induced a greater anti-neuraminidase (NA–N2) response without the detection of IL-2 antibodies and no increase in anti-phospholipid IgG antibodies, while the adverse reactions were similar in both the liposomal and split virion vaccine.[30]

Similar delivery systems developed for mucosal immunization include immune-stimulating complexes (ISCOM), cage-like structures about 30–40 nm in diameter composed of glycosides, cholesterol, immunizing protein antigen, and phospholipids. ISCOM influenza vaccines have been shown to be more immunogenic than conventional vaccines in humans[76] but failed to protect monkeys against distant drift variants of influenza A (H3N2) viruses.[77]

Conclusion

The combination of vaccination with new antiviral agents in high-risk groups can be powerful tools in the fight against influenza. However, emphasis must be given to improvement in the efficiency of use of these tools. Influenza vaccination levels should hopefully continue to increase owing to greater acceptance of preventive medicine by physicians, increased administration of the vaccine by healthcare providers other than practitioners, and new information regarding vaccine effectiveness, cost effectiveness, and safety.[78] The Advisory Committee on Immunization Practices (ACIP) in the US recommends using strategies to improve vaccination levels in the elderly, including using reminder/recall systems and standing order programs.[79] They recommend that inpatient influenza immunization programs are practiced to target high-risk, hospitalized individuals >65 years who might otherwise have not received influenza vaccination.[80] Additional strategies are also needed to achieve the Healthy People 2010 objectives among all racial and ethnic groups, since vaccination levels among blacks and Hispanics lag behind those among whites.[81]

References

1. Turner D, Wailoo A, Nicholson K, Cooper N, Sutton A, Abrams K. Systematic review and economic decision modelling for the prevention and treatment of influenza A and B. Health Technol Assess 2003;7:1–170.
2. Wuethrich B. Infectious disease. An avian flu jumps to people. Science 2003;299:1504.
3. Hatta M, Neumann G, et al. Reverse genetics approach towards understanding pathogenesis of H5N1 Hong Kong influenza A virus infection. Philos Trans R Soc Lond B Biol Sci 2001;356:1841–3.
4. Bulletin of the WHO. May 1, 2005.
5. Bridges CB, Fukuda K, Uyeki TM, Cox NJ, Singleton JA; Centers for Disease Control and Prevention, Advisory Committee on Immunization Practices. Prevention and control of influenza. Recommendations of the Advisory Committee on Immunization Practices (ACIP). MMWR Recomm Rep 2002;51:1–31.
6. Goddard NL, Kyncl J, Watson JM. Appropriateness of thresholds currently used to describe influenza activity in England. Commun Dis Public Health 2003;6:238–45.
7. Clements ML, Betts RF, Tierney EL, Murphy BR. Serum and nasal wash antibodies associated with resistance to experimental challenge with influenza A wild-type virus. J Clin Microbiol 1986;24:157–60.
8. Nicholson KG, Baker DJ, Chakraverty P, Farquhar A, Hurd D, Kent J, Litton PA, Smith SH. Immunogenicity of inactivated influenza vaccine in residential homes for elderly people. Age Ageing 1992;21:182–8.
9. Nicholson KG, Kent J, Hammersley V, Cancio E. Acute viral infections of upper respiratory tract in elderly people living in the community: comparative, prospective, population based study of disease burden. BMJ 1997;315:1060–4.
10. Jennings R, Read R. Clinical Assessment. Influenza in Practice. The Royal Society of Medicine, London, 2005, pp. 19–27.
11. Colamussi ML, White MR, Crouch E, Hartshorn KL. Influenza A virus accelerates neutrophil apoptosis and markedly potentiates apoptotic effects of bacteria. Blood 1999;93:2395–403.
12. Okamoto S, Kawabata S, Nakagawa I, Okuno Y, Goto T, Sano K, Hamada S. Influenza A virus-infected hosts boost an invasive type of *Streptococcus pyogenes* infection in mice. J Virol 2003;77:4104–12.
13. Gross PA, Russo C, Dran S, Cataruozolo P, Munk G, Lancey SC. Time to earliest peak serum antibody response to influenza vaccine in the elderly. Clin Diagn Lab Immunol 1997;4:491–2.
14. Monto AS, Robinson DP, Herlocher ML, Hinson JM Jr, Elliott MJ, Crisp A. Zanamivir in the prevention of influenza among healthy adults: a randomized controlled trial. JAMA 1999;282:31–5.

15. Hayden FG, Atmar RL, Schilling M, Johnson C, Poretz D, Paar D, Huson L, Ward P, Mills RG. Use of the selective oral neuraminidase inhibitor ostelamivir to prevent influenza. N Engl J Med 1999;341:1336–43.
16. Peters PH Jr, Gravenstein S, Norwood P, De Bock V, Van Couter A, Gibbens M, von Planta TA, Ward P. Long-term use of ostelamivir for the prophylaxis of influenza in a vaccinated frail older population. J Am Geriatr Soc 2001;49:1025–31.
17. Gravenstein S, Johnston SL, Loeschel E, Webster A. Zanamivir: a review of clinical safety in individuals at high risk of developing influenza-related complications. Drug Saf 2001;24:1113–25.
18. Nicholson KG, Aoki FY, Osterhaus AD, Trottier S, Carewicz O, Mercier CH, Rode A, Kinnersley N, Ward P. Efficacy and safety of the oral neuraminidase inhibitor ostelamivir in treating acute influenza: a randomized controlled trial. US Oral Neuraminidase Study Group. JAMA 2000;283:1016–24.
19. Nicholson KG, Aoki FY, Osterhaus AD, Trottier S, Carewicz O, Mercier CH, Rode A, Kinnersley N, Ward P. Efficacy and safety of ostelamivir in treatment of acute influenza: a randomised controlled trial. Neuraminidase Inhibitor Flu Treatment Investigator Group. Lancet 2000;355:1845–50.
20. Tominack RL, Hayden FG. Rimantadine hydrochloride and amantadine hydrochloride use in influenza A virus infections. Infect Dis Clin North Am 1987;1:459–78.
21. Dayton N. Symmetrel Package Insert. Endo Pharmaceuticals, Inc., Chadds Ford, PA, 2000.
22. Atkinson WL, Arden NH, Patriarca PA, Leslie N, Lui KJ, Gohd R. Amantadine prophylaxis during an institutional outbreak of type A (H1N1) influenza. Arch Intern Med 1986;146:1751–6.
23. Guay DR. Amantadine and rimantadine prophylaxis of influenza A in nursing homes. A tolerability perspective. Drugs Aging 1994;5:8–19.
24. Gubareva LV, Webster RG, Hayden FG. Comparison of the activities of zanamivir, ostelamivir, and RWJ-270201 against clinical isolates of influenza virus and neuraminidase inhibitor-resistant variants. Antimicrob Agents Chemother 2001;45:3403–8.
25. Barnard DL. RWJ-270201 BioCryst Pharmaceuticals/Johnson & Johnson. Curr Opin Investig Drugs 2000;1:421–4.
26. Patriarca PA, Arden NH, Koplan JP, Goodman RA. Prevention and control of type A influenza infections in nursing homes. Benefits and costs of four approaches using vaccination and amantadine. Ann Intern Med 1987;107:732–40.
27. Herlocher ML, Truscon R, Fenton R, Klimov A, Elias S, Ohmit SE, Monto AS. Assessment of development of resistance to antivirals in the ferret model of influenza virus infection. J Infect Dis 2003;188:1355–61.
28. Cox NJ, Subbarao K. Influenza. Lancet 1999;354:1277–82.
29. Boyce TG, Hsu HH, Sannella EC, Coleman-Dockery SD, Baylis E, Zhu Y, Barchfeld G, DiFrancesco A, Paranandi M, Culley B, Neuzil KM, Wright PF. Safety and immunogenicity of adjuvanted and unadjuvanted subunit influenza vaccines administered intranasally to healthy adults. Vaccine 2000;19:217–26.
30. Ben-Yehuda A, Joseph A, Barenholz Y, Zeira E, Even-Chen S, Louria-Hayon I, Babai I, Zakay-Rones Z, Greenbaum E, Galprin I, Glück R, Zurbriggen R, Kedar E. Immunogenicity and safety of a novel IL-2-supplemented liposomal influenza vaccine (INFLUSOME-VAC) in nursing-home residents. Vaccine 2003;21:3169–78.
31. Nordin J, Mullooly J, Poblete S, Strikas R, Petrucci R, Wei F, Rush B, Safirstein B, Wheeler D, Nichol KL. Influenza vaccine effectiveness in preventing hospitalizations and deaths in persons 65 years or older in Minnesota, New York, and Oregon: data from 3 health plans. J Infect Dis 2001;184:665–70.
32. Harper SA, Fukuda K, Uyeki TM, Cox NJ, Bridges CB; Advisory Committee on Immunization Practices (ACIP), Centers for Disease Control and Prevention (CDC). Prevention and control of influenza: recommendations of the Advisory Committee on Immunization Practices (ACIP). MMWR Recomm Rep 2004;53:1–40.
33. Office of Technology Assessment. Cost Effectiveness if Influenza Vaccination. Washington, DC, 1981.

34. Carman WF, Elder AG, Wallace LA, McAulay K, Walker A, Murray GD, Stott DJ. Effects of influenza vaccination of health-care workers on mortality of elderly people in long-term care: a randomised controlled trial. Lancet 2000;355:93–7.
35. Stratton KR, Durch JS, Lawrence RS. Vaccines for the 21st Century; A Tool for Decision Making. Editors Institute of Medicine of the National Academies, Washington, DC, 1999.
36. Ginaldi L, Loreto MF, Corsi MP, Modesti M, De Martinis M. Immunosenescence and infectious diseases. Microbes Infect 2001;3:851–7.
37. Powers DC, Hanscome PJ, Pietrobon PJ. In previously immunized elderly adults inactivated influenza A (H1N1) virus vaccines induce poor antibody responses that are not enhanced by liposome adjuvant. Vaccine 1995;13:1330–5.
38. Beyer WE, Palache AM, Sprenger MJ, Hendriksen E, Tukker JJ, Darioli R, van der Water GL, Masurel N, Osterhaus AD. Effects of repeated annual influenza vaccination on vaccine sero-response in young and elderly adults. Vaccine 1996;14:1331–9.
39. Gluck R, Wegmann A. Influenza vaccination in the elderly. Dev Comp Immunol 1997; 21:501–7.
40. Crocetti E, Arniani S, Bordoni F, Maciocco G, Zappa M, Buiatti E. Effectiveness of influenza vaccination in the elderly in a community in Italy. Eur J Epidemiol 2001;17:163–8.
41. Plowden J, Renshaw-Hoelscher M, Engleman C, Katz J, Sambhara S. Innate immunity in aging: impact on macrophage function. Aging Cell 2004;3:161–7.
42. Solana R, Mariani E. NK and NK/T cells in human senescence. Vaccine 2000;18:1613–20.
43. Butcher SK, Chahal H, Nayak L, Sinclair A, Henriquez NV, Sapey E, O'Mahony D, Lord JM. Senescence in innate immune responses: reduced neutrophil phagocytic capacity and CD16 expression in elderly humans. J Leukoc Biol 2001;70:881–6.
44. Mancuso P, McNish RW, Peters-Golden M, Brock TG. Evaluation of phagocytosis and arachidonate metabolism by alveolar macrophages and recruited neutrophils from F344xBN rats of different ages. Mech Ageing Dev 2001;122:1899–913.
45. Herrero C, Sebastián C, Marqués L, Comalada M, Xaus J, Valledor AF, Lloberas J, Celada A. Immunosenescence of macrophages: reduced MHC class II gene expression. Exp Gerontol 2002;37:389–94.
46. Bhushan M, Cumberbatch M, Dearman RJ, Andrew SM, Kimber I, Griffiths CE. Tumour necrosis factor-alpha-induced migration of human Langerhans cells: the influence of ageing. Br J Dermatol 2002;146:32–40.
47. Renshaw M, Rockwell J, Engleman C, Gewirtz A, Katz J, Sambhara S. Cutting edge: impaired Toll-like receptor expression and function in aging. J Immunol 2002;169:4697–701.
48. Janssens JP, Krause KH. Pneumonia in the very old. Lancet Infect Dis 2004;4:112–24.
49. Ho PL, Yam WC, Cheung TK, Ng WW, Que TL, Tsang DN, Ng TK, Seto WH. Fluoroquino-lone resistance among Streptococcus pneumoniae in Hong Kong linked to the Spanish 23F clone. Emerg Infect Dis 2001;7:906–8.
50. Khare V, Sodhi A, Singh SM. Effect of aging on the tumoricidal functions of murine peritoneal macrophages. Nat Immun 1996;15:285–94.
51. De la Fuente M, Medina S, Del Rio M, Ferrández MD, Hernanz A. Effect of aging on the modulation of macrophage functions by neuropeptides. Life Sci 2000;67:2125–35.
52. Ashcroft GS, Horan MA, Ferguson MW. Aging alters the inflammatory and endothelial cell adhesion molecule profiles during human cutaneous wound healing. Lab Invest 1998; 78:47–58.
53. Gosain A, DiPietro LA. Aging and wound healing. World J Surg 2004;28:321–6.
54. Guillot L, Le Goffic R, Bloch S, Escriou N, Akira S, Chignard M, Si-Tahar M. Involvement of Toll-like receptor 3 in the immune response of lung epithelial cells to double-stranded RNA and influenza A virus. J Biol Chem 2005;280:5571–80.
55. Wu D, Mura C, Beharka AA, Han SN, Paulson KE, Hwang D, Meydani SN. Age-associated increase in PGE2 synthesis and COX activity in murine macrophages is reversed by vitamin E. Am J Physiol 1998;275:C661–8.

56. Deng Y, Jing Y, Campbell AE, Gravenstein S. Age-related impaired type 1 T cell responses to influenza: reduced activation *ex vivo*, decreased expansion in CTL culture in vitro, and blunted response to influenza vaccination *in vivo* in the elderly. J Immunol 2004;172:3437–46.

57. Saurwein-Teissl M, Schönitzer D, Grubeck-Loebenstein B. Dendritic cell responsiveness to stimulation with influenza vaccine is unimpaired in old age. Exp Gerontol 1998;33:625–31.

58. Huang YP, Gauthey L, Michel M, Loreto M, Paccaud M, Pechere JC, Michel JP. The relationship between influenza vaccine-induced specific antibody responses and vaccine-induced nonspecific autoantibody responses in healthy older women. J Gerontol 1992;47: M50–5.

59. Kistner O, Barrett PN, Mundt W, Reiter M, Schober-Bendixen S, Dorner F. Development of a mammalian cell (Vero) derived candidate influenza virus vaccine. Vaccine 1998;16:960–8.

60. Halperin SA, Nestruck AC, Eastwood BJ. Safety and immunogenicity of a new influenza vaccine grown in mammalian cell culture. Vaccine 1998;16:1331–5.

61. Treanor JJ, Wilkinson BE, Masseoud F, Hu-Primmer J, Battaglia R, O'Brien D, Wolff M, Rabinovich G, Blackwelder W, Katz JM. Safety and immunogenicity of a recombinant hemagglutinin vaccine for H5 influenza in humans. Vaccine 2001;19:1732–7.

62. Trojan A, Urosevic M, Hummerjohann J, Giger R, Schanz U, Stahel RA. Immune reactivity against a novel HLA-A3-restricted influenza virus peptide identified by predictive algorithms and interferon-gamma quantitative PCR. J Immunother 2003;26:41–6.

63. McCown MF, Pekosz A. The influenza A virus M2 cytoplasmic tail is required for infectious virus production and efficient genome packaging. J Virol 2005;79:3595–605.

64. Neirynck S, Deroo T, Saelens X, Vanlandschoot P, Jou WM, Fiers W. A universal influenza A vaccine based on the extracellular domain of the M2 protein. Nat Med 1999;5:1157–63

65. Fan J, Liang X, et al. Preclinical study of influenza virus A M2 peptide conjugate vaccines in mice, ferrets, and rhesus monkeys. Vaccine 2004;22:2993–3003.

66. Gschoesser C, Almanzar G, Hainz U, Ortin J, Schonitzer D, Schild H, Saurwein-Teissl M, Grubeck-Loebenstein B. CD4⁺ and CD8⁺ mediated cellular immune response to recombinant influenza nucleoprotein. Vaccine 2002;20:3731–8.

67. Filmore D. Flu trials. Mod Drug Discov 2004;7:44–48.

68. Abe T, Takahashi H, Hamazaki H, Miyano-Kurosaki N, Matsuura Y, Takaku H. Baculovirus induces an innate immune response and confers protection from lethal influenza virus infection in mice. J Immunol 2003;171:1133–9.

69. Abe T, Hemmi H, Miyamoto H, Moriishi K, Tamura S, Takaku H, Akira S, Matsuura Y. Involvement of the Toll-like receptor 9 signaling pathway in the induction of innate immunity by baculovirus. J Virol 2005;79:2847–58.

70. Huckriede A, Bungener L, Daemen T, Wilschut J. Influenza virosomes in vaccine development. Methods Enzymol 2003;373:74–91.

71. Haining WN, Anderson DG, Little SR, von Bergwelt-Baildon MS, Cardoso AA, Alves P, Kosmatopoulos K, Nadler LM, Langer R, Kohane DS. pH-triggered microparticles for peptide vaccination. J Immunol 2004;173:2578–85.

72. Barr TA, McCormick AL, et al. A potent adjuvant effect of CD40 antibody attached to antigen. Immunology 2003;109:87–92.

73. Barr TA, Carlring J, et al. Antibodies against cell surface antigens as very potent immunological adjuvants. Vaccine 2006;24S2:S20–21.

74. Hatzifoti C, Heath AW. CD40-mediated enhancement of immune responses against three forms of influenza vaccine. Immunology 2007;122:98–106.

75. Ninomiya A, Ogasawara K. Intranasal administration of a synthetic peptide vaccine encapsulated in liposome together with an anti-CD40 antibody induces protective immunity against influenza A virus in mice. Vaccine 2002;20:3123–9.

76. Ennis FA, Cruz J, Jameson J, Klein M, Burt D, Thipphawong J. Augmentation of human influenza A virus-specific cytotoxic T lymphocyte memory by influenza vaccine and adjuvanted carriers (ISCOMS). Virology 1999;259:256–61.

77. Rimmelzwaan GF, Baars M, van Beek R, van Amerongen G, Lövgren-Bengtsson K, Claas EC, Osterhaus AD. Induction of protective immunity against influenza virus in a macaque model: comparison of conventional and iscom vaccines. J Gen Virol 1997;78:757–65.
78. Singleton JA, Greby SM, Wooten KG, Walker FJ, Strikas R. Influenza, pneumococcal, and tetanus toxoid vaccination of adults – United States, 1993–7. MMWR CDC Surveill Summ 2000;49:39–62.
79. McKibben LJ, Stange PV, Sneller VP, Strikas RA, Rodewald LE; Advisory Committee on Immunization Practices. Use of standing orders programs to increase adult vaccination rates. MMWR Recomm Rep 2000;49:15–6.
80. Lawson F, Baker V, Au D, McElhaney JE. Standing orders for influenza vaccination increased vaccination rates in inpatient settings compared with community rates. J Gerontol A Biol Sci Med Sci 2000;55:M522–6.
81. CDC. Racial/ethnic disparities in influenza and pneumococcal vaccination levels among persons aged >65 years. United States 1989–2001. MMWR Morb Mortal Wkly Rep 2003;52:958–62.

Chapter 7
Changes in Oral Microflora and Host Defences with Advanced Age

Rimondia S. Percival

Introduction

It is now well established that the demographic structure of the ageing population in industrialized countries is changing with increasing numbers and proportions of elderly people aged 60 years and over. For example, in Europe 20% of the population is aged more than 60 years and this is predicted to increase to 25% by 2020.[1] In China, the most populous country on earth, numbers of individuals of 60 years of age and over will increase from 17 million estimated in 1982 to nearly 300 million by the year 2025.[2]

Infectious diseases are an increasingly important problem as the elderly population increases. Understanding their aetiology should assist in reducing prevalence of these diseases in the elderly and contribute to better treatment. Research efforts must therefore be focused on the effects of ageing on the relationship between infection and physiological changes in the host and on natural resistance to infection. This also includes determining the effect of the ageing process on the oral environment.

In addition to the increased number of elderly, it is evident that the proportion of dentate elderly individuals is increasing. The adult dental health survey of 1998[3] showed that 44% of English adults over 75 years retained some of their natural dentition and around 10% of this age group had more than 20 natural teeth. With increased retention of teeth into old age, the risk of diseases of the mouth and teeth is also enhanced. The association of poor oral health and systemic disease requires better understanding, and a more concerted research effort is required into the ageing process in relation to oral biology in order to identify risk factors that are associated with various disease states. Potentially, such research could reduce the number of aged individuals acquiring such diseases.

However, there are various problems associated with studies attempting to correlate the effect of the ageing process on the stability of the oral microflora. Many characteristics of the ageing population have to be taken into consideration,

R.S. Percival
Department of Oral Biology, Leeds Dental Institute, Clarendon way, Leeds, LS2 9LU, UK

S.L. Percival (ed.), *Microbiology and Aging.*
DOI: 10.1007/978-1-59745-327-1_7, © Springer Science + Business Media, LLC 2009

for instance, it is known that chronological age does not necessarily correlate with physiological age.[4] Furthermore, genuine age-related changes may be obscured by complicating factors such as disease and the use of medication, which increase in the elderly.[5] Other factors such as dental status, e.g. denture wearing, dietary habit, and salivation, can also influence age-related changes.

The aim of this chapter is to describe age-related effects on the oral environment and the consequent impact on the resident oral microflora along with a brief discussion of associated salivary host defence factors.

Overview of the Oral Environment

The oral cavity comprises a series of different environments such as the teeth, mucosal surfaces, and gingival crevice. The presence of soft shedding (mucosa) and hard non-shedding (tooth) surfaces is a distinctive feature of the mouth. Microorganisms flourish in the oral cavity and display remarkable tropism for different environments. The hard tooth surface provides sites colonized by microorganisms below (sub-gingival) and above (supra-gingival) the gingival margin whereas the mucosal surface is an environment characterized by continual desquamation of epithelial cells with rapid turnover of microorganisms.

The oral surfaces are also constantly bathed by two important physiological fluids, saliva and gingival crevicular fluid, both essential for the maintenance of oral ecosystems by providing water, nutrients, adherence, and antimicrobial factors.[6] The epithelial surfaces of the lips, cheeks, palate, and tongue are bathed in saliva, are intermittently exposed to dietary nutrients, and provide relatively aerobic environments.[7] *Streptococcus* spp. (*S. salivarius* and *S. mitis*) and *Veillonella* spp. are the predominant species of the tongue; other major members of the tongue also include the Gram-positive filamentous bacteria *Actinomyces* spp.[8,9] Obligately, anaerobic bacteria can also be recovered, including periodontal pathogens species such as *Porphyromonas gingivalis*, *Treponema denticola*, *Actinobacillus actinomycetemcomitans*, and *Prevotella intermedia*.[10-13] Similarities between the microflora composition of the saliva and the dorsum and the lateral surfaces of the tongue have been reported.[14]

The supragingival and subgingival environments on teeth differ in that the former is bathed in saliva, is essentially aerobic, and predominantly colonized by Gram-positive facultative anaerobic bacteria, for example, *Actinomyces* spp. and streptococci,[15] whereas the latter is bathed in crevicular fluid, is essentially anaerobic, and is mainly inhabited by Gram-negative bacteria including *Fusobacterium* spp., *Treponema* spp., small numbers of *A. actinomycetumcomitans* and black-pigmented rods.[16-18]

The teeth in the oral cavity provide several different surfaces which enable colonization by distinct microbial communities and the development of hard-tissue biofilms. In the fissures and at the margins of fillings, where mechanical entrapment of bacteria and food remnants occur, colonization by aciduric (acid-tolerating) bacteria is favoured and mutans streptococci are prevalent.[19,20] The areas between adjacent teeth (approximal) and the gingival crevice afford protection from adverse conditions in the mouth and support anaerobic microbial populations. Smooth surfaces of the teeth are more exposed to environmental factors and are only colonized by a limited number of bacterial species that are more adapted to such extreme conditions.[20]

Changes in Oral Microflora with Age

Microflora in the Young

At birth, the human mouth is predominantly edentulous and sterile, but about 8 h after birth there is a rapid increase in the number of detectable organisms.[21,22] Microorganisms from the infant's surroundings, which establish a more or less permanent residence in the oral cavity, are known as the *normal* or *indigenous flora*.[9] The composition of the microflora varies considerably for the first few days of life. However, certain species can be detected during this period such as streptococci, lactobacilli, and staphylococci, but in lower numbers than in adults. The most commonly detected species present from 8 h after birth is *S. salivarius*, which is normally resident on the tongue and constitutes about 25% of the total cultivable streptococci.[21,23] These studies have also reported the absence of *Candida* and some anaerobic species, such as *Veillonella*, *Prevotella*, and spirochaetes, from edentulous infants.

A longitudinal study[24] has shown the increased prevalence of *Veillonella* species and *Prevotella melaninogenica* within the first 2 months of life, whereas *Fusobacterium nucleatum*, *Porphyromonas catoniae*, non-pigmented *Prevotella* species, and *Leptotrichia* spp. were more frequently detected after 1 year. *Veillonella* and *A. odontolyticus* were also more frequently detected in the oral cavity of 1- and 3-month-old neonates.[25]

With the application of advanced methods, such as Checkerboard DNA–DNA hybridization,[26] polymerase chain reaction (PCR), and PCR-based denaturing gradient gel electrophoresis (PCR-DGGE techniques),[27–29] microorganisms present in low numbers or those difficult to culture have been detected. As a result, it has been possible to detect periodontal pathogens and other species, including *Streptococcus mutans*, *S. sobrinus*, *Actinomyces* species, *Campylobacter rectus*, *Fusobacterium nucleatum*, *P. intermedia* and *P. gingivalis*, at a very early age in both pre-dentate and dentate children aged 6–36 months.[30,31] *Tannerella forsythensis* (formerly *Bacteroides forsythus*) was also detected in children aged 18–48 months.[32]

One of the major changes in the oral environment that occurs around the age of 6 months is the eruption of teeth. The presence of teeth provides hard surfaces for attachment and colonization by microorganisms adapted to this niche, such as *S. sanguinis*, *S. mutans*, and *Actinomyces naeslundii* genospecies 2 (formerly *A.*

viscosus), which become regular inhabitants of the dentate mouth.[8,21,22] As the infant grows, continual exposure to microorganisms normally indigenous to the adult oral cavity and the presence of erupting teeth facilitate the accumulation of dental plaque with increasingly complex oral microflora. The increased frequency of isolation of species such as *Fusobacterium* and *Actinomyces* has also been reported after tooth eruption.[28,33] Throughout childhood, the bacterial population continues to increase, and further development is dependent on the frequency of introduction of organisms and the conditions present in the oral cavity.

The isolation frequency of strictly anaerobic bacteria such as *Prevotella* species increases with age from between 18 and 40% at the age of 5 to over 90% by 13–16 years of age.[21] An increased isolation frequency with age was also observed for spirochaetes. Similar studies have also reported an increased isolation of *Prevotella* and spirochaetes in children between the ages of 11 and 14 years[34] and in children aged 14 and 15 years.[35]

The increased prevalence of *Prevotella* species may be associated with elevated hormone levels, as was observed in puberty[36,37] and in pregnant women[38,39] A direct relationship between increased prevalence of *P. intermedia* in pregnant women and increased levels of oestrogens and progesterone in plasma has been demonstrated and attributed to hormones supplementing the menadione requirement of the bacteria.[40] Other studies, however, were unable to detect any relationship between hormone levels during puberty and pregnancy and the prevalence of black pigmented anaerobes.[41,42]

Microflora in the Elderly

The established resident microflora of the oral cavity remains relatively stable over time (microbial homeostasis) and lives in harmony with the host throughout life by means of the influences of specific and innate host defences.[43] The resident microflora supports the immune system in providing resistance to colonization by exogenous pathogenic microorganisms. However, the microflora can also act as a reservoir of potentially pathogenic bacteria, which may then express their pathogenicity when there is a perturbation of this stable relationship. The disruption of the stable relationship between the adult and its indigenous microflora can be due to changes in the host resulting in the breakdown of homeostasis,[43] and as the adult ages several physiological changes take place that can cause variability in the oral microflora.

Various studies have attempted to correlate changes in the composition of the oral microflora with age; however, there are several difficulties associated with the design of such studies. There is difficulty in distinguishing sub-groups: for example, the definition of elderly, the healthy, the sick, the housebound, or institutionalized. Ideally, for assessment of genuine age-related effects, individuals in a population group have to satisfy certain minimum requirements, such as number of teeth, absence of dentures and active disease, and no recent history of medication. Such requirements can be easily satisfied in a young study population, but are disproportionately represented in elderly individuals.

Age-Related Direct and Indirect Effects on the Oral Microflora

As the individual ages, a variety of related changes occur in the oral cavity. In the following sections, some of these changes, with direct or indirect impact on the composition of the resident oral microflora, will be discussed and reviewed in detail. Discrepancies reported often reflect differences in status and characteristics of the elderly population included in the study.

Tooth Loss and Denture Wearing

With increased age, increased loss of teeth can dramatically change the oral ecology and lead to the elimination of some types of oral bacteria due to the lack of a suitable habitat, such as tooth surfaces and subgingival sites.[21] The loss of teeth results in a marked reduction, or total elimination, of spirochaetes, as well as in a reduction of lactobacilli, *S. mutans* and *S. sanguinis*, due to lack of surfaces for colonization.[22] The importance of tooth surfaces for colonization by mutans streptococci has been reported, and it has been shown that their levels in saliva were significantly related to the numbers of teeth.[44] In an early study,[21] complete loss of teeth resulted in a reduction of black-pigmented obligate anaerobes (of the genera *Porphyromonas* and *Prevotella*) that are generally found in periodontal pockets. More recent studies have detected the presence of obligate anaerobes in saliva of geriatric edentulous subjects in the age ranges 61–71, 44–91, and 52–75 years.[45–48] However, in some of these studies the enhanced prevalence of black-pigmented obligate anaerobes in the elderly may have been primarily due to either the presence of dentures or oral implants,[45,48] or elderly subjects with periodontitis.[49]

In industrialized countries with improved oral health, there are increasing numbers of elderly individuals retaining some of their natural teeth. Consequently, one of the major dental problems facing this population is root caries. Various studies have indicated the increased prevalence of root caries among the elderly.[5,50,51] The increased incidence of root caries was directly related to either high salivary mutans streptococci and yeast counts[50] or *S. sobrinus* counts,[52] while in an elderly Chinese population *Actinomyces* spp., *Lactobacillus* spp., *Streptococcus* spp., and *Candida dubliniensis* counts[53,54] were related to the increased incidence of root caries.

The prevalence of denture wearing also increases significantly with age.[55] Placement of dentures will not only influence the total numbers of oral microorganisms but also influence the prevalence of particular species.[22] The presence of dentures restores the solid retention surfaces required for colonization and growth of microorganisms, and bacteria such as *S. mutans* and lactobacilli can re-establish growth in the oral cavity up to the levels found in dentate mouths.[44,56] Insertion of dentures also increased the regular recovery of *Staphylococcus aureus* both in healthy subjects[57] and in institutionalized elderly subjects.[58] Gram-negative bacteria, for example, enterobacteria, were also more frequently isolated from the mouth when dentures were present.[57,59]

Denture plaque can also act as a reservoir of potential respiratory pathogens and facilitate colonization of the oropharynx and subsequent aspiration pneumonia in dependent elderly subjects. An approximate 68% similarity between microbial flora colonizing dentures and the pharyngeal mucosa has been reported,[60,61] which suggests that the elderly may have a high level risk of contracting an opportunistic infection. However, the insertion of dentures has a more noticeable effect on the prevalence of some species than others; for example, the presence of dentures in the elderly significantly enhanced the growth of yeasts, with *Candida albicans* being the most prevalent species.[57,59,62–66] This increased prevalence was attributed to the tendency of *Candida* to adhere to denture material.[67] In a recent study, the first isolation of other *Candida* species such as *Candida pararugosa* from the oral cavity of systemically healthy denture wearers was reported.[68] In contrast to these studies, very low numbers of *Candida* were detected in a limited study group consisting of five geriatric (age range 66–71 years) denture wearers.[46]

The increased prevalence of *Candida* in the mouth of elderly people may be due to changes in local environmental conditions, such as the restriction of salivary flow underneath dentures. In particular, full upper dentures reduce the mechanical washing action of saliva and diminish the inhibitory effect of salivary antimicrobial factors on yeast colonization under dentures.[63] The increased presence of higher numbers of mutans streptococci and lactobacilli in elderly denture wearers has also been reported.[44,57,65,69] The presence of dentures may result in a decreased pH[62] and slow down oral sugar clearance[70] in the elderly, both of which will generate a more cariogenic environment. Prolonged conditions of low pH in plaque favour selection of aciduric microorganisms.[71] Overall, there is some agreement that in healthy, independent elderly individuals, irrespective of tooth loss or denture wearing, the carriage of aciduric microorganisms and yeast may indeed be a function of a genuine ageing process.[72–74]

Salivary Flow Rates

Numerous findings on the properties and secretion of saliva and histological studies of salivary glands have revealed age-related changes in the structure of these glands and a diminished secretory reserve capacity.[75–77] The effect of ageing on saliva flow still remains unclear since conflicting observations exist in the literature (Table 7.1).

Age-related reductions in secretion of both resting[78–81] and stimulated[5,79,82] whole saliva have been reported. A decrease in salivary secretion rates with age has also been observed in stimulated parotid,[78] resting and stimulated submandibular[83] and resting[84,85] and stimulated[86,87] minor glands. On the other hand, an age-related

Table 7.1 Summary of reported age-related changes in human salivary flow rates

Saliva secretion type	Effect of increased age on flow rate	Age range (years) and reference
Whole		
Resting	Decrease	20–83,[78] 18–83,[79] 20 to >80,[80] 18–90[81]
Stimulated	Decrease	18–83,[79] 18–90 only women,[82] 55 to >85[5]
Resting	No effect	21–93[87]
Stimulated	No effect	35–74[88]
Parotid		
Stimulated	Decrease	20–83[78]
Resting	No effect	23–81[89]
Stimulated	No effect	23–81,[89] 20 to >80,[80] 27–97,[83] 26–90[90]
Submandibular		
Resting and stimulated	Decrease	27–97[83]
Resting and stimulated	No effect	26–90[90]
Minor glands		
Resting	Decrease	17–81,[84] 18–74[85]
Stimulated	Decrease	17–76,[86] 21–93[87]
Resting and stimulated	No effect	20–55,[91]

decline was not observed in other studies of resting[87] and stimulated[88] whole salivary flow rate. Age effects were also not observed in other studies on resting[89] and stimulated[80,83,89,90] parotid salivary flow and in resting and stimulated submandibular saliva flow[90] and from minor salivary glands flow.[91] The controversy regarding the effect of ageing on salivary flow rates may have resulted partly from differences in experimental design, for example, selection of institutionalized or non-institutionalized population, or even inclusion in some studies subjects on systemic medication.

Sometimes, functional disturbances of the salivary glands can cause a reduction in salivary flow rate, such as the prevalence of xerostomia, which increasingly occurs (up to 30%) in aged populations of 65 years and over.[92] Insertion of dentures also may have an effect on whole and palatal salivary flow rates.[93] Hormonal levels in women of post-menopausal age[94,95] and gender differences (females generally have smaller salivary glands than males) can all cause variations in salivary flow rates.[96] Moreover, there is wide variation in salivary flow between individuals,[97] and the ageing process may also have variable effects on different glands; for example, it has been suggested that the parotid gland is less sensitive to ageing compared to submandibular glands.[81]

Nevertheless, it may be concluded that, although many factors can influence salivary flow in the elderly, increased age generally correlates with reduced flow from most salivary glands. This will inevitably have an effect on the resident oral microflora. A number of studies have reported that diminished salivary flow rates result in reduction of buffering capacity and access of antimicrobial substances. This creates an oral environment favouring the increased colonization of opportunistic pathogens, such as yeasts, and a microflora associated with the progression of caries, e.g. mutans streptococci and lactobacilli.[5,63,69,98–101] Such effects are therefore likely to increase in an ageing population.

Oral Hygiene, Medication, and Systemic Disease

Oral hygiene habits in elderly populations are regarded as important for the maintenance of oral health and of a microflora that is compatible with a healthy mouth. Since the mouth is a major entrance to internal organs, this will consequently also contribute to overall health and well-being, particularly in the elderly.[102] In an elderly population oral hygiene standards are low and regarded as a major caries predisposing factor that can lead to higher ratios of decayed tooth surfaces and the development of low-pH niches that favour the growth of yeasts and higher numbers of mutans streptococci.[69,103–106] Poor denture cleanliness has also been reported to correlate with high levels of yeasts and denture stomatitis.[104,107] Increased carriage of Gram-negative bacilli in the hospitalized elderly has also been demonstrated.[108] Elderly hospitalized patients with dentures and reliant on nursing assistance often have poor oral hygiene,[109] and increased isolation of methicillin-resistant *S. aureus* (MRSA) and coagulase-negative *S. aureus*, *Pseudomonas aeruginosa*, *E. coli*, and *Veillonella* spp. has been reported from those patients compared with independently living individuals.[110,111]

There is increased use of medication by elderly people; for example, mean numbers of drugs taken per day were shown to increase from 0.9 to 2.4 in 85-year-old subjects.[5] Dry mouth is often a side-effect of many of the estimated 430 pharmaceutical products used by the elderly population. Some of these drugs will decrease salivary flow rates and/or alter salivary composition.[65,101,112] Combined medication and psychological effects resulting in hyposalivation and subjective oral dryness have also been reported.[113] Lower salivary secretion rates of major and minor salivary glands in the elderly resulting from the use of medication has been shown to affect the oral microflora, with increased counts of yeasts, lactobacilli, and mutans streptococci.[5,59,95,114–116] It has also been reported that medication containing sucrose can increase numbers of mutans streptococci, lactobacilli, and yeasts in elderly subjects.[117]

Systemic disease can influence the composition of oral microflora in elderly subjects; for example, primary Sjögren's syndrome, which affects both salivary and lachrymal gland functions,[118] results in a marked reduction in both unstimulated and stimulated parotid and submandibular salivary flow rates. With increased age, the risk of cancer rises and the combined effect of irradiation and cytotoxic therapy and xerostomia induced by cytotoxic treatment have all been found to affect the composition of oral microflora. A reduction (66%) in salivary flow rate has been reported in a bone-marrow-transplant patient leading to increased prevalence of cariogenic bacteria.[119] Cytotoxic therapy has also resulted in increased carriage of yeasts.[120] Hyposalivation due to partial or total destruction of major and minor salivary glands[100,121] (caused by radiotherapy of head and neck regions of cancer patients) resulted in a marked increase in the prevalence of *S. mutans*, *Lactobacillus* spp., and *C. albicans*.[122,123] Various studies have also reported the increased isolation of yeasts, enterobacteria (e.g. *Klebsiella* spp., *Escherichia coli*, *Pseudomonas aeruginosa*), coagulase-positive staphylococci, *Prevotella*, *Porphyromonas*, *Veillonella*, and *Fusobacterium* spp. from debilitated and hospitalized elderly patients with oral carcinomas, advanced cancer, and bone marrow transplant.[108,124–127]

Overall, the data suggest that in the elderly oral health, disease, hospitalization, and medication can all have a profound influence on the oral environment and lead to changes in the oral microflora, particularly with increased isolation of Gram-negative bacilli. However, these effects were generally not apparent in un-medicated healthy ageing populations.[57,72]

Dietary Habits and Malnutrition

The maintenance of microbial homeostasis in the oral cavity is dependent upon diet, which can be modified with advancing age. While masticatory performance is usually not affected by the ageing process,[128] other changes such as loss of teeth, presence of dentures, reduced salivary flow rates, chewing ability, and medication will all lead to difficulty of eating various types of food. Consequently, this will lead to adaptation of dietary intake. It has been shown that the intake of some nutrient-rich foods declined in edentulous and denture-wearing elderly subjects and the ease of eating various types of food was dependent on the number of teeth present.[129,130]

This dietary adaptation will mean avoidance of hard and coarse foods, such as fruits, vegetables and meats, which are good sources of vitamins and minerals,[131,132] and will lead to a preference for softer and easy-to-swallow food.[133] Such a restricted diet will result in increased prevalence of nutrient and mineral deficiencies among the elderly and also a reduction in serum albumin levels, regarded as an indicator of good health.[131,134] It has been reported that the lack of minerals such as selenium and zinc can contribute to immunodeficiency in the elderly.[135] Poor nutrient intake and malnutrition have been shown to impair the immune responses and make the elderly more vulnerable to common and opportunistic infectious diseases.[136,137]

Dry mouth-associated eating and swallowing problems among elderly individuals can inhibit intake of fibre-rich foods, restricting the elderly to a soft and carbohydrate-rich diet.[138] Sugary drinks and sweets used to ease the discomfort of a dry mouth are another source of carbohydrate substrate which will also sustain the growth of yeasts.[139] In the elderly, the frequency of daily carbohydrate intake increased with age, from five events in those aged 55 years to six or more times a day in those aged 85 years.[5,73]

Table 7.2 Summary of age-related effects on oral microflora

Factors	Effect on oral microflora						Reference
	Y	MS	LB	ST	G-AB	ANs	
Loss of teeth	↓	↓	↓	–	–	V	21, 22, 44–48
Denture wearing	↑	↑	↑	↑	↑	–	44, 56–59, 62–66
Salivary flow rates	↑	↑	↑	–	–	–	5, 63, 69, 98–101
Oral hygiene	↑	↑	↑	↑	↑	–	69, 103–106, 110, 111
Medication	↑	↑	↑	–	↑	↑	5, 59, 95, 114–116
Systemic disease	↑	↑	↑	↑	↑	↑	108, 119, 120, 122–127
Dietary habits and malnutrition	↑	↑	↑	–	↑	–	5, 16, 52, 59, 69, 73, 103, 117, 139, 140

Y yeasts; *MS* mutans streptococci; *LB* lactobacilli; *ST* staphylococci; *G-AB* Gram-negative aerobic bacilli; *ANs* anaerobes; ↑ increase observed; *V* variable effect observed; ↓ decrease observed; – no effect observed

As discussed earlier, numerous studies have demonstrated that the frequent consumption of high-sucrose diet enhances the development of more cariogenic microorganisms, including mutans streptococci and lactobacilli.[5,16,52,69,73,103,117,140] A positive correlation between salivary levels of mutans streptococci, lactobacilli, and yeasts and the number of snacks per day in dental patients of 55 years and over has also been reported.[141] In contrast, an increased prevalence of aerobic and facultatively anaerobic Gram-negative rods and yeasts was recorded in ageing vegetarian Buddhist monks 27–96 years old.[59]

These studies highlight the influence of the ageing process on the relationship between dental status, diet, and nutritional status in the elderly and emphasize the need to implement a well-balanced diet to reduce the risk of diet-related oral problems. A summary of all age-related effects on oral microflora is presented in Table 7.2.

Host Defences in the Oral Cavity

The mucosal surfaces constitute an enormous surface area; they include the entire gastrointestinal and respiratory tracts, salivary and lachrymal glands, and portions of the genito-urinary system. It is at mucosa that microbial pathogens and toxic agents frequently make their first contact with the host and potentially cause systemic or local disease.[142] The oral cavity, being a part of the gastrointestinal tract, with increased time becomes progressively infected with microorganisms via ingested food or inspired air. Gradually, these microorganisms establish themselves as indigenous microflora. The oral microflora, like the indigenous flora of other sites in the body, has the potential to be pathogenic. This potential can be manifested when, for example, physical injury or nutritional change upsets the balance in the host–microbial relationship or causes these microorganisms to reach sites in the body not normally accessible to them.[43]

Since the oral cavity is exposed to the external environment, internal defence mechanisms are required for the protection of oral tissues and maintenance of oral health. Salivary gland secretions have the most important influence on the aqueous portion of the oral milieu. The mixed oral fluids are usually referred to as *whole saliva*, which consists of the secretions from the major salivary glands, namely, parotid, submandibular, and sublingual glands, as well as from numerous minor salivary glands that are found in the lower lip, tongue, cheeks, and palate.[22]

Whole saliva also contains a number of constituents of non-salivary origin and among these is gingival crevicular fluid (GCF) which continually flows from blood across the gingival epithelium and eventually reaches saliva via the gingival crevice around the roots of teeth.[143] This fluid can contain all the elements of a functioning immune system, including high levels of IgG (the principal immunoglobulin of GCF and serum) and also lower levels of IgA and IgM.[16,17] Antibody activity in GCF to both supragingival and subgingival bacteria has also been detected in both IgG and IgA isotypes.[144] GCF also contains neutrophils and complement, and defects in neutrophils can predispose to disease, such as increased risk of periodontitis. Analysis of salivary components is also frequently used for the diagnosis and assessment of systemic diseases, since saliva is easy to collect and it contains serum constituents. Diseases of salivary glands can often be diagnosed from secretions obtained directly from the glands.[145] However, whole saliva is not the best liquid for assessment of salivary gland performance; for this purpose collection of saliva from various individual glands is more useful.[146] Both salivary flow and salivary constituents also play a role in the maintenance of oral and general health. It has been suggested that a low flow rate can contribute to either dental caries or periodontal disease and consequently to subsequent tooth loss.[147,148] Reduced flow rates may also lead to increased risk of mucosal infections not only in the mouth but also in the gastrointestinal tract.[149]

Saliva contains a variety of specific and non-specific factors with antimicrobial activity, which often work together synergistically to either limit the growth of bacteria or kill them directly. The principal specific defence factor in the oral cavity is secretory IgA (S-IgA). Most S-IgA is locally produced and the cells responsible are plasma cells that predominate the area (lamina propria) just below the mucous membranes.[150] Most (60%) of IgA secreted into the oral cavity from major and minor salivary glands belongs to the S-IgA1 subclass and the remaining to S-IgA2.[151] S-IgA is the major immunoglobulin isotype of external secretions in humans and many mammalian species, and plays a role in protection against microbial invasion and is considered to be the first line of defence of the host against invading pathogens. Several protective mechanisms have been proposed for S-IgA including neutralization of viruses, inhibition of adherence, and modulation of enzyme activity. The major functions of S-IgA are summarized in Table 7.3.

Although S-IgA is the predominant immunoglobulin in salivary secretions, other immunoglobulin classes, primarily IgG and IgM, are also present but at lower levels. Most salivary IgG reaches the oral cavity through the gingival crevice and is mainly derived from serum, whereas monomeric serum IgA and IgM make a lesser contribution.[150] The second most abundant immunoglobulin in secretions is S-IgM, which is locally produced at mucosal sites and can compensate when there is a deficiency of S-IgA.[152]

Table 7.3 Functions of secretory IgA at mucosal surfaces

Neutralization of
Viruses
Exotoxin
Bacterial enzymes important in virulence
Prevention of
Antigen penetration across the mucosa
Adherence
Colonization
Motility (antiflagellar antibodies)
Interaction with
Lysozyme, lactoferrin, peroxidase, mucin
Summarized from Refs. [6, 150, 154]

Table 7.4 Salivary functions in relation to oral health

Function	Salivary components involved	Reference
Mechanical cleansing	Physical flow of saliva enabling removal of food and bacterial cells for elimination via the alimentary tract	[43, 147]
Buffering action	Bicarbonate, phosphate	[143, 145, 155]
Anti-bacterial, antifungal, antiviral activity	S-IgA, lysozyme, lactoferrin, lactoperoxidase, histatins, cystatins, SLPI, micelles, β-defensins	[150, 153, 155–158]
Lubrication and protection of mucous membrane	Basic proline-rich glycoproteins, mucins	[145, 150, 155, 159]

Other non-specific salivary components with antimicrobial activities include lysozyme, which can hydrolyse the bacterial cell wall of Gram-positive bacteria; lactoferrin, which has a high affinity for iron (consequently depriving microorganisms of this essential mineral); and lactoperoxidase, which protects host proteins and cells from hydrogen peroxide. Other protective agents include hisatins, cystatins, SLPI (secretory leukocyte protease inhibitors), and β-defensins, and recently many of these protective components, along with IgA, have been detected associated with micelles (macromolecular complexes) in saliva.[153] A summary of salivary protective mechanisms and antimicrobial agents are listed in Table 7.4.

Changes in Oral Host Defences with Age

Infectious diseases are major causes of morbidity and mortality in the elderly population,[160] and a variety of factors contribute to the increased susceptibility to infection in the elderly. For example, prevalence of infections may result from an underlying dysfunction of an aged immune system[161] or may be due to physiological and biological changes that normally occur with ageing, which result in structural and functional changes of many organs. In the oral cavity, various changes also take place with the ageing process, as was discussed in previous sections, and all these changes will have an impact on saliva and its protective components (S-IgA immunoglobulin and antimicrobial factors) that continuously bathe all the mucosal surfaces of the mouth and inhibit colonization. With advanced age, there is a reduction in salivary flow rates, sometimes resulting from disease of salivary glands, medication, or treatment (e.g. cytotoxic and radiation therapy). These will have an impact on the levels of salivary immunoglobulins and antimicrobial factors secreted into the oral cavity, leading to reduced protection of the oral surfaces. With increased microbial colonization, risk of oral diseases, such as caries and periodontitis, is enhanced.

Studies on age-related effects on oral host defence factors and the subsequent impact on the resident oral microflora have reported variable findings. Some indicated an increase in host defence components, while others reported a decrease or no change with respect to age. In an early study, an age-related decline in IgA levels in nasal secretions of hospitalized patients with respiratory disease was described.[162] However, many subsequent investigations, which included healthier and older subjects, reported that total salivary IgA concentrations did not decline[86] or, more commonly, increased with age.[81,163,164] Other studies have demonstrated that salivary IgA secretion rates, regarded as a more accurate measurement of mucosal function,[165] declined with increased age in whole saliva of healthy individuals.[166,167]

Age-related differences in salivary IgA subclasses (IgA1 and IgA2) have also been investigated; studies generally report no changes in IgA subclass levels when elderly and young subjects are compared.[164,168,169] However, the ability to produce secretory antibodies to various antigens has been shown by some investigators to be affected by the ageing process. For instance, parotid saliva IgA antibody levels to glucosyltransferase (GTF) from *S. mutans* and killed polio virus were shown to decline in old subjects compared with the young.[170] Others have reported that both levels and secretion rates of S-IgA antibodies to *S. mutans* and *A. naeslundii* genospecies 2[171] and S-IgA antibodies to influenza virus[172] were not impaired with increased age.

Although variable total immunoglobulin and specific antibody levels are observed in the elderly, it has been suggested that antibody activity and responses may have physiological significance and hence could be regarded as more important parameters to consider when relating secretory antibody levels to protection of mucosal surfaces.[173] For example, it has been demonstrated that the opsonic activity of saliva towards *C. albicans* was markedly diminished in individuals of about 70 years of age compared to young adults, despite both groups having similar IgA levels.[174] It was also reported that aberrations in immunoglobulin synthesis and appearance of ineffective fragments of S-IgA can also occur with increased age.[175]

Variable observations regarding the ageing effects on salivary antimicrobial factors have also been reported. Both lysozyme and lactoferrin levels have been shown to increase with advanced age.[176] However, diminished levels of SLPI and lysozyme have also been seen in healthy, elderly individuals.[177] Loss of teeth and insertion of complete dentures in elderly subjects also affect the levels of salivary antimicrobial factors,[178] and denture wearers had significantly lower concentrations of lactoferrin and myeloperoxidase compared with dentate subjects. In subjects with radiation-induced hyposalivation, increased levels of lactoferrin were also detected, which negatively correlated with the numbers of *F. nucleatum* and *P. intermedia/P. nigrescens.*[179]

The concentration and secretion rate of histatin have been reported to decrease with increased age in healthy unmedicated elderly subjects.[180] Both histatin and human β-defensin have antifungal activity against *C. albicans* and inhibit adherence to mucosal surfaces.[157,158,181] Hence, any reduction in their levels may contribute to the increased susceptibility of the elderly to *Candida* infection. Salivary mucins MUC5B (formally MG1) and MUC7 (formally MG2)[179] have also been reported to decrease with age.[79] Mucins are salivary-protective components that prevent overgrowth of the oral microflora and assist in the maintenance of a stable oral environment. Thus a decrease in mucin level may enhance the colonization of oral surfaces with harmful species.

Although much of the evidence in the literature suggests that age-related changes do occur in the secretory immune system, data on the nature and specificity of age-related changes in the oral defence system is limited, variable, and sometimes contradictory. Variable findings may be due to a number of factors, such as differences in study populations, disease status, and methodology employed, e.g. type of saliva and assays used. However, there would appear to be some consensus in that there is an age-related negative correlation between salivary flow rates and levels of S-IgA and antimicrobial factors.

Conclusion

From all the factors discussed in this chapter, it is evident that genuine age-related changes in healthy elderly are different to those seen in people who are on medication and hospitalized. Studies investigating genuine age-related changes in oral biology, such as composition of oral microflora, are essential to identify and confirm consistent changes with age. Such studies are valuable to determine the treatment needs for this increasing proportion of elderly population and may identify individuals at risk of certain infections.

Studies attempting to correlate changes in oral microflora with age are faced with various problems, such as the lack of universally accepted definition of any age group, and it is known that chronological age does not necessarily correlate with physiological age. Genuine age-related effects in the elderly may also be obscured by other factors that also change with increased age, such as dental status, e. g. presence of dentures, impaired salivary flow, changes in dietary habits, disease, and the use of medication. Overall, it is evident that in the healthy elderly population genuine age-related changes in the oral microflora have resulted in the increased carriage of aciduric microorganisms and yeasts, whereas in medicated and hospitalized elderly subjects Gram-negative bacilli increase in prevalence. With respect to salivary flow rates, most studies are in agreement that secretory ability does not diminish with age for the parotid gland. A negative correlation also exists between salivary flow rates and levels of both S-IgA and antimicrobial factors, which consequently will have an impact on the resident oral microflora and maintenance of oral health in elderly. Further research is required to fully elucidate the effect of age on such responses.

References

1. WHO (World Health Organisation). Keeping fit for life: meeting the nutritional needs of older persons. WHO, Geneva, 2002.
2. Steel K, Maggi S. Ageing as a global issue. Age Ageing 1993;22:237–239.
3. Steele JG, Sheiham A, Marcenes W, Walls AWG. National Diet and Nutritional Survey: People Aged 65 Years and Over. Report of the Oral Health Survey, vol 2, London: HMSO, 1998.
4. Gardner ID. The effect of aging on susceptibility to infection. Rev Infect Dis 1980;2:801–810.
5. Fure S. Ten-year cross-sectional and incidence study of coronal and root caries and some related factors in elderly Swedish individuals. Gerodontology 2004;21:130–140.
6. Marcotte H, Lavoie MC. Oral microbial ecology and the role of salivary immunoglobulin A. Microbiol Mol Biol Rev 1998;62:71–109.
7. Roth GI, Calmes R. Oral microbiology. In: Oral Biology. St. Louis, MO: C.V. Mosby, 1981, pp. 307–339.
8. Smith DJ, Anderson JM, King WF, van Houte J, Taubman MA. Oral streptococci colonization in infants. Oral Microbiol Immunol 1993;8:1–4.
9. Theilade E. Factors controlling the microflora of the healthy mouth. In: Hill MJ, Marsh PD eds. Human Microbial Ecology, West Palm Beach, FL: CRC Press, 1990:1–56.
10. Asikainen S, Alaluusua S, Saxen L. Recovery of A. actinomycetemcomitans from teeth, tongue and saliva. J Periodontol 1991;62:203–206.
11. Dahlen G, Manji F, Baelum V, Fejerskov O. Putative periodontopathogens in "diseased" and "non-diseased" persons exhibiting poor oral hygiene. J Clin Periodontol 1992;19:35–42.
12. Bosy A, Kulkarni GV, Rosenberg M, McCullock CAG. Relationship of oral malodor to periodontitis: evidence of independence in discrete subpopulations. J Periodontol 1994;65:37–46.
13. De Boever EH, Loesche WJ. Assessing the contribution of anaerobic microflora of the tongue to oral malodor. J Am Dent Assoc 1995;126:1384–1393.
14. Mager DL, Ximenez-Fyvie LA, Haffajaee AD, Socransky SS. Distribution of selected bacterial species on intraoral surfaces. J Clin Periodontol 2003;30:644–654.
15. Nolte WA. Oral microbiology: with basic microbiology and immunology, 4th ed. St. Louis, MO: C.V. Mosby, 1982.
16. Schonfeld SE. Oral microbial ecology. In: Slots J, Taubman MA, eds. Contemporary and Microbiology and Immunology. St. Louis: Mosby Yearbook, 1992, pp. 267–274.
17. Loesche WJ. Ecology of the oral flora. In: Nisengard RJ, Newman MG eds. Oral Microbiology and Immunology. Canada: Saunders, 1994, pp. 307–319.
18. Lee KH, Tanner ACR, Maiden MFJ, Weber HP. Pre- and post-implantation microbiota of the tongue, teeth, and newly-placed implants. J Clin Periodontol 1999;26:822–832.

19. Krasse B. Oral microflora: establishment and preventive effects. Wenner-Gren Int Symp Ser 1989;52:253–262.
20. Marsh PD, Martin M. The mouth as a microbial habitat. In: Oral Microbiology. Chapman & Hall, London, 1992, pp. 6–26.
21. Socransky SS, Manganiello SD. The oral microbiota of man from birth to senility. J Periodontol 1971;42:485–496.
22. Miller CH. Microbial ecology of the oral cavity. In: Schuster GS, ed. Oral Microbiology and Infectious Disease, 3rd ed. Hamilton, ON: B.C. Decker, 1990, pp. 465–478.
23. Pearce C, Bowden GH, Evans M, Fitzsimmons SP, Johnson J, Sheridan MJ, Wientzen R, Cole MF. Identification of pioneer viridans streptococci in the oral cavity of human neonates. J Med Microbiol 1995;42:67–72.
24. Könönen E, Kanervo A, Takala A, Asikainen S, Jousimies-somer H. Establishment of oral anaerobes during the first year of life. J Dent Res 1999;78:1634–1639.
25. Zou J, Zhou XD, Li SM. Analysis of oral microflora early colonised in infants. Hua Xi Kou Qiang Yi Xue Za Zhi 2004;22:126–128.
26. Socransky SS, Smith C, Martin L. "Checkerboard" DNA–DNA hybridization. Biotechniques 1994;17:788–793.
27. Kimura S, Ooshima T, Takiguchi M, Sasaki Y, Amano A, Morisaki I, Hamada S. Periodontopathic bacterial infection in childhood. J Periodontol 2002;73:20–26.
28. Haraldsson G, Holbrook WP, Könönen E. Clonal persistence of oral *Fusobacterium nucleatum* in infancy. J Dent Res 2004;83:500–504.
29. Li Y, Ku CYS, Xu J, Saxena D, Caufield PW. Survey of oral microbial diversity using PCR-based denaturing gradient gel electrophoresis. J Dent Res 2005;84:559–564.
30. Tanner ACR, Milgrom PM, Kent R Jr, Mokeem SA, Page RC, Liao SIA, Riedy CA, Bruss J. Similarity of the oral microbiota of pre-school children with that of their caregivers in a population-based study. Oral Microbiol Immunol 2002;17:379–387.
31. Tanner ACR, Milgram PM, Kent R Jr, Mokeem SA, Page RC, Riedy CA, Weinstein P, Bruss J. The microbiota of young children from tooth and tongue samples. J Dent Res 2002;81:53–57.
32. Yang EY, Tanner ACR, Milgrom P, Mokeem SA, Riedy CA, Spadafora AT, Page RC, Bruss JON. Periodontal pathogen detection in gingival/tooth and tongue flora samples from 18- to 48-month-old children and periodontal status of their mothers. Oral Microbiol Immunol 2002;17:55–59.
33. Hardie JM, Bowden GH. The normal microbial flora of the mouth. In: Skinner FA, Carr JG, eds. The Normal Microbial Flora of Man. New York: Academic Press, 1974, pp. 47–83.
34. Gusberti FA, Mombelli A, Lang NP, Minder CE. Changes in subgingival microbiota during puberty: a 4-year longitudinal study. J Clin Periodontol 1990;17:685–692.
35. Ashley FP, Gallagher J, Wilson RF. The occurrence of *Actinobacillus actinomycetemcomitans, Bacteroides gingivalis, Bacteroides intermedius* and spirochaetes in the subgingival microflora of adolescents and their relationship with the amount of supragingival plaque and gingivitis. Oral Microbiol Immunol 1988;3:77–82.
36. Wojcicki CJ, Scott Harper D, Robinson PJ. Differences in periodontal disease-associated microorganisms of subgingival plaque in prepubertal, pubertal and postpubertal children. J Periodontol 1987;58:219–223.
37. Moore WEC, Burmeister JA, Brooks CN, Ranney RR, Hinkelmann KH. Investigation of the influences of puberty, genetics and environment on the composition of subgingival periodontal floras. Infect Immun 1993;61:2891–2898.
38. Kornman KS, Loesche WJ. The supragingival microbial flora during pregnancy. J Periodontal Res 1980;15:111–122.
39. Jensen J, Liljemark W, Bloomquist C. The effect of female sex hormones on subgingival plaque. J Periodontol 1981;52:599–602.
40. Kornman KS, Loesche WJ. Effects of estradiol and progesterone on *Bacteroides melaninogenicus* and *Bacteroides gingivalis*. Infect Immun 1982;35:256–263.

41. Yanover L, Ellen RP. A clinical and microbiologic examination of gingival disease in parapubescent females. J Periodontol 1986;57:562–567.
42. Jonsson R, Howland BE, Bowden GHW. Relationship between periodontal health, salivary steroids and *Bacteroides intermedia* in males, pregnant and non-pregnant women. J Dent Res 1988;67:1062–1069.
43. Marsh PD. Host defenses and microbial homeostasis: role of microbial interactions. J Dent Res 1989;68:1567–1575.
44. Loesche WJ, Schork A, Terpenning MT. Factors which influence levels of selected organisms in saliva of older individuals. J Clin Microbiol 1995;33:2550–2557.
45. Könönen E, Asikainen S, Alaluusua S, Könönen M, Summanen P, Kanervo A, Jousimies-Somer H. Are certain pathogens part of normal oral flora in denture-wearing edentulous subjects? Oral Microbiol Immunol 1991;6:119–122.
46. Sato M, Hoshino E, Nomura S, Ishioka K. Salivary microflora of geriatric edentulous persons wearing dentures. Microb Ecol Health Dis 1993;6:293–299.
47. Külekçi G, Bilgin T, Eğilmez S, Turfaner M, Anğ Ö. The presence of black-pigmented Gram-negative anaerobes in the oral cavity of edentulous subjects. FEMS Immunol Med Microbiol 1993;6:219–222.
48. Kalykakis GK, Mojon P, Nisengard R, Spiekermann H, Zafiropoulos GG. Clinical and microbial findings on osseo-integrated implants; comparisons between partially dentate and edentulous subjects. Eur J Prosthodont Restor Dent 1998;6:155–159.
49. Schlegel-Bregenzer B, Persson RE, Lukehart S, Braham P, Oswald T, Persson GR. Clinical and microbiological findings in elderly subjects with gingivitis or periodontitis. J Clin Periodontol 1998;25:897–907.
50. Närhi TO, Vehkalahti MM, Siukosaari P, Ainamo A. Salivary findings, daily medication and root caries in the old elderly. Caries Res 1998;32:5–9.
51. Hugoson A, Koch G, Slotte C, Bergendal T, Thorstensson B, Thorstensson H. Caries prevalence and distribution in 20–80-years-olds in Jönköping, Sweden, in 1973, 1983, and 1993. Community Dent Oral Epidemiol 2000;28:90–96.
52. Lundgren M, Emilson CG, Österberg T. Root caries and some related factors in 88-year-old carriers and non-carriers of *Streptococcus sobrinus* in saliva. Caries Res 1998;32:93–99.
53. Tingfa Z, Yuxing Z, Chunmei Z, Shenghui Y. Pathogen of root surface caries in the elderly. Chin Med J (Engl) 2001;114:767–768.
54. Shen S, Samaranayake LP, Yip HK, Dyson JE. Bacterial and yeast flora of root surface caries in elderly, ethnic Chinese. Oral Dis 2002;8:207–217.
55. Redford M, Drury TF, Kingman A, Brown LJ. Denture use and the technical quality of dental prostheses among persons 18–74 years of age: United States, 1988–1991. J Dent Res 1996;75:714–725.
56. Köhler B, Persson M. Salivary levels of mutans streptococci and lactobacilli in dentate 80- and 85-year-old Swedish men and women. Community Dent Oral Epidemiol 1991;19:352–356.
57. Marsh PD, Percival RS, Challacombe SJ. The influence of denture-wearing and age on the oral microflora. J Dent Res 1992;71:1374–1381.
58. Honda E. Oral microbial flora and oral malodour of the institutionalized elderly in Japan. Gerodontology 2001;18:65–72.
59. Sedgley CM, Chu CS, Lo ECM, Samaranayake LP. The oral prevalence of aerobic and facultatively anaerobic Gram-negative rods and yeasts in semi-recluse human vegetarians. Arch Oral Biol 1996;41:307–309.
60. Sumi Y, Miura H, Sunakawa M, Michiwaki Y, Sakagami N. Colonization of denture plaque by respiratory pathogens in dependent elderly. Gerodontology 2002;19:25–29.
61. Sumi Y, Kagami H, Ohtsuka Y, Kakinoki Y, Haruguchi Y, Miyamoto H. High correlation between the bacterial species in denture plaque and pharyngeal microflora. Gerodontology 2003;20:84–87.
62. Coulter WA, Strawbridge JL, Clifford T. Denture induced changes in palatal plaque microflora. Microb Ecol Health Dis 1990;3:77–85.

63. Närhi TO, Ainamo A, Meurman JH. Salivary yeasts, saliva, and oral mucosa in the elderly. J Dent Res 1993;72:1009–1014.
64. Pires FR, Santos EBD, Bonan PRF, De Almeida OP, Lopes MA. Denture stomatitis and salivary *Candida* in Brazilian edentulous patients. J Oral Rehabil 2002;29:1115–1119.
65. Närhi TO, Kurki N, Ainamo A. Saliva, salivary micro-organisms, and oral health in the home-dwelling old elderly-a five year longitudinal study. J Dent Res 1999;78:1640–1646.
66. Nikawa H, Hamada T, Yamamoto T. Denture plaque – past and recent concerns. J Dent 1998;26:299–304.
67. Radford DR, Challacombe SJ, Walter JD. Denture plaque and adherence of *Candida albicans* to denture-base materials in vivo and in vitro. Crit Rev Oral Biol Med 1999;10:99–116.
68. Giammanco GM, Melilli D, Pizzo G. *Candida pararugosa* isolation from the oral cavity of an Italian denture wearer. Res Microbiol 2004;155:571–574.
69. Närhi TO, Ainamo A, Meurman JH. Mutans streptococci and lactobacilli in the elderly. Scand J Dent Res 1994;102:97–102.
70. Hase JC, Birkhed D. Oral sugar clearance in elderly people with prosthodontic reconstructions. Scand J Dent Res 1991;99:333–339.
71. Bradshaw DJ, McKee AS, Marsh PD. Effect of carbohydrate pulses and pH on population shifts within oral microbial communities in vitro. J Dent Res 1989;68:1298–1303.
72. Percival RS, Challacombe SJ, Marsh PD. Age-related microbiological changes in the salivary and plaque microflora of healthy adults. J Med Microbiol 1991;35:5–11.
73. Fure S. Five-year incidence of caries, salivary and microbial conditions in 60-, 70- and 80-year-old Swedish individuals. Caries Res 1998;32:166–174.
74. Lockhart SR, Joly S, Vagras K, Swails-Wenger J, Enger L, Soll DR. Natural defenses against *Candida* colonization breakdown in the oral cavities of the elderly. J Dent Res 1999; 78:857–868.
75. Scott J. Structural age changes in the salivary glands. In: Ferguson DB, ed. The Ageing Mouth. Basel: Karger, 1987, pp. 40–62.
76. Vissink A, Spijkervet FK, Van Nieuw Amerongen A. Ageing and saliva: a review of the literature. Spec Care Dentist 1996;16:95–103.
77. Ghezzi EM, Ship JA. Ageing and secretory reserve capacity of major salivary glands. J Dent Res 2003;82:844–848.
78. Yaegaki K, Ogura R, Kameyama T, Sujaku C. Biochemical diagnosis of reduced salivary gland function. Int J Oral Surg 1985;14:47–49.
79. Navazesh M, Mulligan RA, Kipnis V, Denny PA, Denny PC. Comparison of whole saliva flow rates and mucin concentrations in healthy Caucasian young and aged adults. J Dent Res 1992;71:1275–1278.
80. Percival RS, Challacombe SJ, Marsh PD. Flow rates of resting whole and stimulated parotid saliva in relation to age and gender. J Dent Res 1994;73:1416–1420.
81. Nagler RM, Hershkovich O. Relationships between age, drugs, oral sensorial complaints and salivary profile. Arch Oral Biol 2005;50:7–16.
82. Streckfus C, Bigler L, O'Bryan T. Ageing and salivary cytokine concentrations as predictors of whole saliva flow rates among women: a preliminary study. Gerontology 2002; 48:282–288.
83. Wu AJ, Baum BJ, Ship JA. Extended stimulated parotid and submandibular secretion in a healthy young and old population. J Gerontol 1995;50A:M45–M48.
84. Sivarajasingam V, Drummond JR. Measurements of human minor salivary gland secretions from different oral sites. Arch Oral Biol 1995;40:723–729.
85. Lee SK, Lee SW, Chung SC, Kim YK, Kho HS. Analysis of residual saliva and minor salivary gland secretions in patients with dry mouth. Arch Oral Biol 2002;47:637–641.
86. Smith DJ, Joshipura K, Kent R, Taubman MA. Effect of age on immunoglobulin content and volume of human labial gland saliva. J Dent Res 1992;71:1891–1894.
87. Shern RJ, Fox PC, Li SH. Influence of age on the secretory rates of the human minor salivary glands and whole saliva. Arch Oral Biol 1993;38:755–761.

88. Mazengo MC, Söderling E, Alakuijala P, Tiesko J, Tenovuo J, Simell O, Hausen H. Flow rates and composition of whole saliva in rural and urban Tanzania with special reference to diet, age, and gender. Careis Res 1994;28:468–476.

89. Heft MW, Baum BJ. Unstimulated and stimulated parotid salivary flow rate in individuals of different ages. J Dent Res 1984;63:1182–1185.

90. Ship JA, Nolan NE, Puckett SA. Longitudinal analysis of parotid and submandibular salivary flow rates in healthy, different-aged adults. J Gerontol 1995;50:M285–M295.

91. Ferguson DB. The flow rate of unstimulated human labial gland saliva. J Dent Res 1996;75:980–985.

92. Ship JA, Pillemer SR, Baum BJ. Xerostomia and the geriatric patient. J Am Geriatr Soc 2002;50:535–543.

93. Márton K, Boros I, Fejérdy P, Madléna M. Evaluation of unstimulated flow rates of whole and palatal saliva in healthy patients wearing complete dentures and in patients with Sjogren's syndrome. J Prosthet Dent 2004;91:577–581.

94. Streckfus CF, Baur U, Brown LJ, Bacal C, Metter J, Nick T. Effects of estrogen status and ageing on salivary flow in healthy Caucasian women. Gerontology 1998;44:32–39.

95. Eliasson L, Carlěn A, Laine M, Birkhed D. Minor gland and whole saliva in postmenopausal women using a low potency oestrogen (oestriol). Arch Oral Biol 2003;48:511–517.

96. Dawes C, Cross HG, Baker CG, Chebib FS. The influence of gland size on the flow and composition of human parotid saliva. J Can Dent Assoc 1978;44:21–25.

97. Ghezzi EM, Lange LA, Ship JA. Determination of variation of stimulated salivary flow rates. J Dent Res 2000;79:1874–1878.

98. Simons D, Braisford SR, Kidd EAM, Beighton D. The effect of medicated chewing gums on oral health in frail older people: a 1-year clinical trial. J Am Geriatr Soc 2002;50:1348–1353.

99. Almståhl A, Wikström M. Oral microflora in subjects with reduced salivary secretion. J Dent Res 1999;78:1410–1416.

100. Ferguson DB. The flow rate and composition of human labial gland saliva. Arch Oral Biol 1999;44:S11–S14.

101. Bardow A, Nyvad B, Nauntofte B. Relationships between medication intake, complaints of dry mouth, salivary flow rate and composition, and the rate of tooth demineralization in situ. Arch Oral Biol 2001;46:413–423.

102. Peltola P, Vehkalahti MM, Simoila R. Oral health-related well-being of the long-term hospitalized elderly. Gerodontology 2005;22:17–23.

103. Wyatt CCL. Elderly Canadians residing in long-term care hospitals: part II. dental caries status. J Can Dent Assoc 2002;68:359–363.

104. Budtz-Jørgensen E, Mojon P, Banon-Clément JM, Baehni P. Oral candidosis in long-term hospital care: comparison of edentulous and dentate subjects. Oral Dis 1996;2:285–290.

105. Simons D, Brailsford S, Kidd EAM, Beighton D. Relationship between oral hygiene practices and oral status in dentate elderly people living in residential homes. Community Dent Oral Epidemiol 2001;29:464–470.

106. Ueda K, Toyosato A, Nomura S. A study on the effect of short-, medium- and long-term professional oral care in elderly persons requiring long-term nursing care at a chronic or maintenance stage of illness. Gerodontology 2003;20:50–56.

107. Kulak-Ozkan Y, Kazazoglu E, Arikan A. Oral hygiene habits, denture cleanliness, presence of yeast and stomatitis in elderly people. J Oral Rehabil 2002;29:300–304.

108. Preston AJ, Gosney MA, Noon S, Martin MV. Oral flora of elderly patients following acute medical admission. Gerontology 1999;45:49–52.

109. Peltola P, Vehkalahti MM, Wuolijoki-Saaristo K. Oral health and treatment needs of the long-term hospitalized elderly. Gerodontology 2004;21:93–99.

110. Imsand M, Janssens JP, Auckenthaler R, Mojon P, Budtz-Jørgensen E. Bronchopneumonia and oral health in hospitalized older patients. A pilot study. Gerodontology 2002;19:66–72.

111. Tada A, Watanabe T, Yokoe H, Hanada N, Tanzawa H. Oral bacteria influenced by the functional status of the elderly people and the type and quality of facilities for the bedridden. J Appl Microbiol 2002;93:487–491.

112. Sreebny LM, Schwartz SS. A reference guide to drugs and dry mouth – 2nd edition. Gerodontology 1997;14:33–47.
113. Bergdahl M, Bergdahl J. Low unstimulated salivary flow and subjective oral dryness: association with medication, anxiety, depression and stress. J Dent Res 2000;79:1652–1658.
114. Närhi TO, Meurman JH, Ainamo A, Nevalainen JM, Schmidt-Kaunisaho KG, Siukosaari P, Valvanne J, Erkinjuntti T, Tilvis R, Mäkilä E. Association between salivary flow rate and the use of systemic medication among 76-, 81-, and 86-year-old inhabitants in Helsinki, Finland. J Dent Res 1992;71:1875–1880.
115. Wu AJ, Ship JA. A characterization of major salivary gland flow rates in the presence of medications and systemic disease. Oral Surg Oral Med Oral Pathol 1993;76:301–306.
116. Meurman JH, Rantonen P. Salivary flow rate, buffering capacity, and yeast counts in 187 consecutive adult patients from Kuopio, Finland. Scand J Dent Res 1994;102:229–234.
117. Beighton D, Hellyer PH, Lynch EJR, Heath MR. Salivary levels of mutans streptococci, lactobacilli, yeasts and root caries prevalence in non-institutionalized elderly dental patients. Community Dent Oral Epidemiol 1991;19:302–307.
118. Baum BJ, Ship JA, Wu AJ. Salivary gland function and ageing: a model for studying the interaction of ageing and systemic disease. Crit Rev Oral Biol Med 1992;4:53–64.
119. Dens F, Boogaerts M, Boute P, Declereck D, Demuynck H, Vinckier F, Belgium B. Caries-related salivary microorganisms and salivary flow rate of bone marrow recipients. Oral Surg Oral Med Oral Pathol Oral Radiol Endod 1996;81:38–43.
120. Almståhl A, Wikström M. Oral microflora on the tongue and tooth surfaces in subjects with hyposalivation because of radiation therapy. Int J Dent Hygiene 2004;2:45–47.
121. Niedermeie W, Huber M, Fischer D, Beier K, Müller N, Schuler R, Brinninger A, Fartasch M, Diepgen Th, Matthaeus C, Meyer C, Hector MP. Significance of saliva for the denture-wearing population. Gerodontology 2000;17:104–118.
122. Schwarz E, Chiu GKC, Leung WK. Oral health status of southern Chinese following head and neck irradiation therapy for nasopharyngeal carcinoma. J Dent 1999;27:21–28.
123. Almståhl A, Wikström M, Stenberg I, Jakobsson A, Fagerberg-Mohlin B. Oral microbiota associated with hyposalivation of different origins. Oral Microbiol Immunol 2003;18:1–8.
124. Jobbins J, Bagg J, Parsons K, Finlay I, Addy M, Newcombe, RG. Oral carriage of yeasts, coliforms and staphylococci in patients with advanced malignant disease. J Oral Pathol Med 1992;21:305–308.
125. Sweeney MP, Bagg J, Baxter WP, Aitchison TC. Oral disease in terminally ill cancer patients with xerostomia. Oral Oncol 1998;34:123–126.
126. Nagy KN, Sonkodi I, Szöke I, Nagy E, Newman HN. The microflora associated with human oral carcinomas. Oral Oncol 1998;34:304–308.
127. Napeñas JJ, Brennan MT, Fox PC, Lockhart PB. Oral microflora changes in patients receiving chemotherapy: a systemic review. Oral Surg Oral Med Oral Pathol 2004;97:452–453.
128. Hatch JP, Shinkai RSA, Sakai S, Rugh JD, Paunovich ED. Determinants of masticatory performance in dentate adults. Arch Oral Biol 2000;46:641–648.
129. Nowjack–Raymer RE, Sheiham A. Association of edentulism and diet and nutrition in US adults. J Dent Res 2003;82:123–126.
130. Steele JG, Sheiham A, Marcenes W, Walls AWG. Diet and nutrition in Great Britain. Gerodontology 1998;15:100–106.
131. Morais JA, Heydecke G, Pawliuk J, Lund JP, Feine JS. The effects of mandibular two-implant overdentures on nutrition in elderly edentulous individuals. J Dent Res 2003;82:53–58.
132. Budtz-Jørgensen E, Chung JP, Rapin CH. Nutrition and health. Best Pract Res Clin Gastroenterol 2001;15:885–896.
133. Kwok T, Yu CNF, Hui HW, Kwan M, Chan V. Association between functional dental state and dietary intake of Chinese vegetarian old age home residents. Gerodontology 2004;21:161–166.
134. Pickering G. Frail elderly, nutritional status and drugs. Arch Gerontol Geriatr 2004;38;174–180.

135. Malaguarnera L, Ferlito L, Imbesi RM, Gulizia GS, Di Mauro S, Maugeri D, Malaguarnera M, Messina A. Immunosenescence: a review. Arch Gerontol Geriatr 2001;32:1–14.
136. Chandra RK. Impact of nutritional status and nutrient supplements on immune responses and incidence of infection in older individuals. Ageing Res Rev 2004;3:91–104.
137. Gavazzi G, Herrmann F, Krause KH. Ageing and infectious diseases in the developing world. Clin Infect Dis 2004;39:83–91.
138. Ship JA. Diagnosing, managing, and preventing salivary gland disorders. Oral Dis 2002;8:77–89.
139. MacEntee MI, Nolan A, Thomason JM. Oral mucosal and osseous disorders in frail elders. Gerodontology 2004;21:78–84.
140. Steele JG, Sheiham A, Marcenes W, Fay N, Walls AWG. Clinical and behavioural risk indicators for root caries in older people. Gerodontology 2001;18:95–101.
141. Beighton D, Hellyer PH, Heath MR. Association between salivary levels of mutans streptococci, lactobacilli, yeasts and black-pigmented *Bacteroides* spp. and dental variables in elderly dental patients. Arch Oral Biol 1990;35:173S–175S.
142. McNabb PC, Tomasi TB. Host defense mechanisms at mucosal surfaces. Ann Rev Microbiol 1981;35:477–496.
143. FDI Working Group 10, CORE. Saliva: its role in health and disease. Int Dent J 1992;42:291–304.
144. Smith DJ, van Houte J, Kent R, Taubman MA. Effect of antibody in gingival crevicular fluid on early colonization of exposed root surfaces by mutans streptococci. Oral Microbiol Immunol 1994;9:65–69.
145. Kaufman E, Lamster IB. The diagnostic applications of saliva – a review. Crit Rev Oral Biol Med 2002;13:197–212.
146. Nederfors T, Dahlöf C. A modified device for collection and flow rate measurement of submandibular – sublingual saliva. Scand J Dent Res 1993;101:210–214.
147. Lagerlöf F, Oliveby A. Caries–protective factors in saliva. Adv Dent Res 1994;8:229–238.
148. Lenander-Lumikari M, Loimaranta V. Saliva and dental caries. Adv Dent Res 2000;14:40–47.
149. Jamieson GG, Duranceau AC. The defense mechanisms of the esophagus. Surg Clin North Am 1983;63:787–799.
150. Van Nieuw Amerongen A, Bolscher JGM, Veerman ECI. Salivary proteins: protective and giagnostic value in cariology. Caries Res 2004;38:247–253.
151. Smith DJ, Taubman MA. Association of specific host immune factors with dental caries experience. In: Johnson NM, ed. Risk Markers for Oral Diseases Volume 1. Dental Caries, Cambridge: Cambridge University Press, 1991, pp. 340–357.
152. Underdown BJ, Mestecky J. Mucosal immunoglobulins. In: Ogra P, Lamm M, McGhee JR, Mestecky J, Strober W, Bienenstock J, eds. Handbook of Mucosal Immunology. New York: Academic Press, 1994, pp. 79–97.
153. Soares RV, Lin T, Siqueira CC, Bruno LS, Li X, Oppenheim FG, Offner G, Troxler RF. Salivary micelles: identification of complexes containing MG2, sIGA, lactoferrin, amylase, glycosylated praline-rich protein and lysozyme. Arch Oral Biol 2004;49:337–343.
154. Russell MW, Hajishengallis G, Childers NK, Michalek SM. Secretory immunity in defense against cariogenic mutans streptococci. Caries Res 1999;33:4–15.
155. Van Nieuw Amerongen A, Veerman ECI. Saliva – the defender of the oral cavity. Oral Dis 2002;8:12–22.
156. Tenovuo J. Clinical applications of antimicrobial host proteins lactoperoxidase, lysozyme and lactorerrin in xerostomia: efficacy and safety. Oral Dis 2002;8:23–29.
157. Feng Z, Jiang B, Chandra J, Ghannoum M, Nelson S. Human beta-defensins: differential activity against Candidal species and regulation by *Candida albicans*. J Dent Res 2005;84:445–450.
158. Joly S, Maze C, McCray PB Jr, Guthmiller JM. Human β-defensin 2 and 3 demonstrate strain–selective activity against oral microorganisms. J Clin Microbiol 2004;42:1024–1029.

159. Tabak LA. In defense of the oral cavity: structure, biosynthesis, and function of salivary mucins. Ann Rev Physiol 1995;57:547–564.
160. Yoshikawa TT. Epidemiology and unique aspects of ageing and infectious diseases. Clin Infect Dis 2000;30:931–933.
161. Ginaldi L, Loreto MF, Corsi MP, Modesti M, De Martinis M. Immunosenescence and infectious disease. Microb Infect 2001;3:851–857.
162. Alford RH. Effects of chronic bronchopulmonary disease and aging on human nasal secretion IgA concentrations. J Immunol 1968;101:984–988.
163. Ben–Aryeh H, Fisher M, Szargel R, Laufer D. Composition of whole unstimulated saliva of healthy children: changes with age. Arch Oral Biol 1990;35:929–931.
164. Childers NK, Greenleaf C, Li F, Dasanayake AP, Powell WD, Michalek SM. Effect of age on immunoglobulin A subclass distribution in human parotid saliva. Oral Microbiol Immunol 2003;18:298–301.
165. Chandler DC, Silverman MS, Lundblad RL, McFall WT. Human parotid IgA and periodontal disease. Arch Oral Biol 1974;19:733–735.
166. Challacombe SJ, Percival RS, Marsh PD. Age–related changes in immunoglobulin isotypes in whole and parotid saliva and serum in healthy individuals. Oral Microbiol Immunol 1995;10:202–207.
167. Miletic ID, Schiffman SS, Miletic VD, Sattely-Miller EA. Salivary IgA secretion rate in young and elderly persons. Physiol Behav 1996;60:243–248.
168. Greenleaf CR, Michalek SM, Dasanayake AP, Powell WD, Childers NK. Comparison of salivary IgA subclass distribution between children and adults. J Dent Res 2002;81:Abst No 0773.
169. Russell MW, Prince SJ, Ligthart GJ, Mestecky J, Radl J. Comparison of salivary and serum antibodies to common environmental antigens in elderly, edentulous and normal adult subjects. Aging: Immunol Infect Dis 1990;2:275–286.
170. Smith DJ, Taubman MA, Ebersole JL. Ontogeny and senescence of salivary immunity. J Dent Res 1987;66:451–456.
171. Percival RS, Marsh PD, Challacombe SJ. Age–related changes in salivary antibodies to commensal oral and gut biota. Oral Microbiol Immunol 1997;12:57–63.
172. Waldman RH, Bergmann K-C, Stone J, Howard S, Chiodo V, Jackowitz A, Waldman ER, Khakoo R. Age-dependent antibody response in mice and humans following oral influenza immunization. J Clin Immunol 1987;7:327–332.
173. Smith DJ, King WF, Taubman MA. Salivary IgA antibody to oral streptococcal antigens in predentate infants. Oral Microbiol Immunol 1990;5:57–62.
174. Ganguly R, Stablein J, Lockey RF, Shamblin P, Vargas L. Defective antimicrobial functions of oral secretions in the elderly. J Infect Dis 1986;153:163–164.
175. Arranz E, O'Mahony S, Ferguson A. Serum and salivary immunoglobulins and food antibodies in normal elderly subjects. In: MacDonald T, Challacombe SJ, Bland P, Stokes C, Heatley R, McInwat A, eds. Advances in Mucosal Immunology. The Netherlands: Kluwer, 1990, pp. 467–468.
176. Fox PC, Heft MW, Herrera M, Bowers MR, Mandel ID, Baum BJ. Secretion of antimicrobial proteins from the parotid glands of different aged healthy persons. J Gerontol 1987;42:466–469.
177. Shugars DC, Watkins CA, Cowen HJ. Salivary concentration of secretory leukocyte protease inhibitor, an antimicrobial protein, is decreased with advanced age. Gerontology 2001;47:246–253.
178. Närhi TO, Tenovuo J, Ainamo A, Vilja P. Antimicrobial factors, sialic acid, and protein concentration in whole saliva of the elderly. Scand J Dent Res 1994;102:120–125.
179. Almståhl A, Wikström M, Groenink J. Lactoferrin, amylase and mucin MUC5B and their relation to the oral microflora in hyposalivation of different origins. Oral Microbiol Immunol 2001;16345–16352.
180. Johnson DA, Yeh CK, Dodds MWJ. Effect of donor age on the concentrations of histatins in human parotid and submandibular/sublingual saliva. Arch Oral Biol 2000;45:731–740.
181. Ruissen ALA, Groenink J, Krijtenberg P, Walgreen-Weterings E, van't Hof W, Veerman ECI, Van Nieuw Amerongen A. Internalisation and degradation of histatin 5 by *Candida albicans*. Biol Chem 2003;384:183–190.

Chapter 8
Influence of the Gut Microbiota with Ageing

Eileen Murphy, Caroline Murphy, and Liam O'Mahony

Introduction

The mucosal surface of the human gastrointestinal tract is approximately 200–300 m^2 in area and is colonized by 10(13–14) bacteria of greater than 1,000 different species and subspecies. The number of bacterial cells within the gastrointestinal tract outnumbers the host cell populations by 10:1, highlighting the relative importance of microbiota composition and metabolic activity on host homeostasis.[1] This review will discuss some of the better described microbiota-related activities that influence host function and the relationship with host ageing. However, most of the bacterial species present within the gastrointestinal tract still remain to be characterized, and many of the mechanisms underpinning their activities remain unexplored.

Bacterial populations are not distributed evenly throughout the gastrointestinal tract. Bacterial numbers in different parts of the gastrointestinal tract appears to be influenced by multiple factors, including pH, peristalsis, redox potential, bacterial adhesion sites, bacterial cooperation/quorum signalling, mucin secretion, nutrient availability, diet, and bacterial antagonism. Because of the low pH of the stomach and the relatively swift peristalsis through the stomach and the small bowel, the stomach and the upper two-thirds of the small intestine (duodenum and jejunum) contain only low numbers of microorganisms, which range from 10^3 to 10^4 bacteria per millilitre of the gastric or intestinal contents. These are primarily acid-tolerant lactobacilli and streptococci. In the distal small intestine (ileum), the microbiota begins to resemble those of the colon, with numbers approaching 10^7–10^8 bacteria per millilitre of the intestinal contents. With decreased peristalsis, acidity, and lower oxidation–reduction potentials, the ileum maintains a more diverse microbiota and a higher bacterial population. The colon is the primary site of microbial colonization in humans, probably because of slow intestinal motility and the low oxidation–reduction potential. The colon harbours tremendous numbers and species of bacteria, most of which are obligate anaerobes.

E. Murphy, C. Murphy, and L. O'Mahony
Alimentary Pharmabiotic Centre, University College Cork, Cork, Ireland

S.L. Percival (ed.), *Microbiology and Aging.*
DOI: 10.1007/978-1-59745-327-1_8, © Springer Science + Business Media, LLC 2009

The gastrointestinal microbiota has been broadly classified into two types, autochthonous flora (indigenous flora) and allochthonous flora (transient flora). Autochthonous microorganisms colonize particular habitats, i.e. physical spaces in the gastrointestinal tract, whereas allochthonous microorganisms cannot colonize particular habitats except under abnormal conditions. Most pathogens are allochthonous microorganisms; nevertheless, some pathogens can be autochthonous to the ecosystem and normally live in harmony with the host, except when the system is disturbed. Historically, microbial research focused on the mechanisms by which enteric pathogens mediate tissue damage and disease. More recently, a circumstantial role of intestinal bacteria in the pathogenesis of various intestinal disorders has been recognized. For example, in genetically susceptible individuals, some components of commensal organisms can trigger aberrant immune responses that contribute to the pathogenesis of inflammatory bowel disease (IBD).[2]

Under normal circumstances, commensal bacteria are an essential health asset that exert a conditioning and protective influence on intestinal structure and homeostasis. Intestinal bacteria protect against infection, and actively exchange developmental and regulatory signals with the host that prime and instruct mucosal immunity.[1] Colonization of germ-free mice with a single species, *Bacteroides thetaiotaomicron*, has been shown to affect the expression of a variety of host genes. These include genes associated with nutrient uptake, metabolism, angiogenesis, mucosal barrier function, and the development of the enteric nervous system.[3] Interactions between gut-associated lymphoid tissues and colonizing bacteria early in life are crucial for appropriate development of functioning mucosal and systemic immunoregulatory systems.[4,5] Thus, individual variations in immunity may be influenced by the composition of the colonizing microbiota. Bacterial metabolism confers many benefits to gut physiology, and commensal bacteria represent a rich repository of metabolites that can be mined for therapeutic benefit.[1] Intestinal bacteria are not uniform in their ability to drive mucosal inflammatory responses. Some commensal species such as *B. vulgatus* are pro-inflammatory.[6] Conversely, other species lack inflammatory capacity, and certain bacteria including strains of bifidobacteria and lactobacilli can even attenuate inflammatory responses.[7–9] The composition of the gut microbiota is dramatically different between infants and the elderly and this relationship will be discussed in more detail below.

Activities of the Gut Microbiota

Nutrition

There is a longstanding belief that human health is linked to the activities of the resident microbial population. In particular, the gut microbiota plays a significant role in nutrition through the conversion of many dietary substances into nutrients that can be absorbed and utilized by the host and by altering the intrinsic metabolic machinery of host cells, leading to more efficient nutrient uptake and utilization. Most notably, the gut microbiota plays a significant role in the breakdown of non-digestible carbohydrates.

The gut microbiome, which may contain >100 times the number of genes in our genome, endows us with functional features that we have not had to evolve ourselves.[10] One such attribute is the ability to extract energy from non-digestible polysaccharides. The diet not only provides substrates for host metabolism but also supports the growth and metabolism of the bacteria in our gut. Mammals can readily absorb simple sugars, such as glucose and galactose, via active transport in the proximal regions of their small intestine which contains only a relatively small number of bacteria.[11] Mammals can, in addition, hydrolyse disaccharides such as sucrose, maltose, and lactose to their constituent monosaccharides and can degrade starch to glucose. However, they are limited in their intrinsic capacity to digest other dietary polysaccharides. As a consequence, a significant amount of undigested dietary carbohydrate reaches the distal portion of the gastrointestinal tract. This undigested carbohydrate includes polysaccharides such as cellulose, xylan, and pectin (mostly from plant cell walls) and undigested starch. Together with host-derived glycans (mucins and glycosphingolipids), they pass into the distal regions of the small intestine (ileum) and colon where they are degraded by resident microbes. The resulting monosaccharides are fermented by bacteria to yield short-chain fatty acids (SCFAs) which are absorbed and utilized by the host. The three major SCFAs produced in the gut are acetate, propionate, and butyrate, and these (not glucose) are the preferred energy substrate of the colonic epithelial cells.[12] It has been estimated that in humans 50–60 g of carbohydrate is typically fermented per day, yielding 0.5–0.6 mol of SCFA, with a total energy value of 140–180 kcal.[11] However, the amount and type of SCFA produced varies according to the dietary factors such as the fibre content. In addition to their nutritional value, SCFAs have important effects on gut physiology, with butyrate, in particular, affecting epithelial proliferation and differentiation.[13]

The ability to degrade and ferment a wide variety of polysaccharides is particularly evident among members of the genus *Bacteroides* which are very common in the human gut.[14] Molecular analysis of the polysaccharide utilizing machinery of these bacteria has provided useful insight into how microbes in the intestine sense and exploit nutrients in their environment. The best understood example of polysaccharide utilization is the starch utilization system (sus) of *Bacteroides thetaiotaomicron*.[15] This bacterium is a prominent member of the normal intestinal flora of both mice and humans and lends itself to genetic manipulation. Its proteome contains 172 glycosylhyrolases that are predicted to cleave most glycosidic linkages encountered in human diets.[16] The use of germ-free (GF) inbred strains of mice has proven valuable in the study of microorganisms in the gastrointestinal tract. These mice are raised without any resident microorganisms and they, therefore, represent a genetically defined, simplified in vivo assay system aimed at defining the impact of colonizing the gut with specific species. Interestingly, colonization of GF mice with *B. thetaiotamicron* has shown that its polysaccharide processing activity is associated with changes in the expression of a number of genes involved in the processing and absorption of carbohydrates (such as NA+/− glucose co-transporter, the principal mediator of glucose uptake in epithelial cells), as well as the breakdown and absorption of complex dietary lipids (e.g. pancreatic lipase-related protein 2, fasting-induced adipocyte factor (FIAF), apolipoprotein IV, and the liver-derived fatty acid binding protein).[17] *B. thetaiotamicron* has an extraordinary capacity for acquiring and degrading polysaccharides and also affects the metabolic machinery of host cells, leading to more efficient nutrient uptake and utilization.

The gut microbiota represents a key source of nutrients other than SCFAs. Unlike humans, many species of bacteria can synthesize folate[18,19] and their contribution to the folate content of the large intestine in human infants is sufficiently great to potentially affect the folate status of the host.[20] The gut bacteria are also a signifi-cant source of a range of vitamins, particularly those of the B group and vitamin K. It has been shown that germ-free mice require vitamin K and higher amounts of B vitamins (B_{12}, biotin, folic acid, and pantothetane) in their diets, in contrast to those that are colonized with a conventional microbiota.[21] In addition, the gut bacteria aid in the absorption of minerals such as calcium, magnesium, and iron.[1]

The use of GF mice or rats has provided additional insights into the mutually beneficial interactions that are manifest between the host and the intestinal micro-biota. A key observation, from studies using adult male GF Wistar rats, was that conventionally reared rats required 30% less caloric intake to maintain their body weight compared to germ-free animals. This indicates the importance of the microbiota in assisting the host to obtain the maximum nutritional value (i.e. energy) from the diet. Additional comparative studies involving GF and colonized animals have confirmed that the intestinal microbiota affects the host machinery and plays an important role in the control of energy storage in the host. Gordon and colleagues showed that GF mice have 40% less total body fat compared to conven-tionally raised animals even though the latter consume less per day.[22] One proposed mechanism for this phenomenon is that the microbiota promotes storage of calories harvested from the diet into fat, acting through the intestinally derived protein FIAF, which is involved in coordinating increased hepatic lipogenesis with increas-ing lipoprotein lipase (LPL) activity in adipocytes. Conventionalization of adult GF mice with the caecal contents harvested from conventional donors results in an increase in body fat to levels equivalent to those of conventionally raised animals. Therefore, the gut microbiota not only affects energy harvest from the diet but also influences energy storage in the host.

While the symbiotic relationship between the gut microbiota and the host is clearly crucial in salvaging energy from the diet, recent evidence from animal and human studies suggests that obesity alters the composition of the microbiota and this may be a factor involved in the development of obesity. The distal gut and faecal microbiota are numerically dominated by two bacteria divisions, the *Bacter-oides* and the *Firmicutes*. A comparative survey of 16S-rRNA-gene sequences of the distal gut microbiota of leptin-deficient obese mice and their lean littermates revealed a 50% reduction in the number of *Bacteroides* in the obese animals with a corresponding increase in the *Firmicutes*.[23] These differences are important be-cause *Firmicutes* seem to have biochemical pathways that can extract more energy from non-digestible carbohydrates and may explain the finding that the obese mice had more fermentation products and fewer calories remaining in their faeces than the lean mice. These observations have also been made in obese humans. An increased ratio of *Firmicutes* to *Bacteroides* was observed in the gut of obese compared to lean individuals, which suggests that the obese 'microbiome' is more efficient at extracting energy from the diet.[24] Interestingly, calorie restriction over a 1-year period resulted in the restoration of the balance between the *Firmicutes* and the *Bacteroides* in these obese individuals. A further study in obese mice showed that the altered ratio of *Firmicutes* to *Bacteroides* leads to an alteration of in body fat gain when the microbiota from obese mice was transferred to lean mice.[25] Over a 2-week period, the microbiota from mice give the obese microbiota gained more fat and extracted more calories from their food compared to the GF mice who received microbiota from lean mice. These studies suggest that obesity is associated with alterations in the composition of the gut microbiota and that these differences in the efficiency of caloric extraction from food may contribute to differential body weights.

These studies provide insights into the relatively recent and somewhat surprising revelations with regard to the role of the gut microbiota in relation of the energy balance of the host, fat deposition, and the risk of obesity. They provide further evidence that the human microbiota contributes positively towards nutrition and health and suggest that appropriate manipulation of the microbiota may represent a useful tool in strategies aimed at optimizing the health status of individuals.

Metabolism

The metabolic activities of the intestinal microbiota are very important to host health and well-being. Microbial metabolism can have a variety of effects, with the potential to influence areas outside of the colon. These can include lactose tolerance, decreased serum cholesterol levels and risk for cardiovascular disease, and detoxification of harmful substances.

Individuals with low levels of the enzyme lactase have limited ability to digest lactose, which can result in intestinal distress, or lactose intolerance. People with lactose intolerance suffer from bloating, flatulence, abdominal pain, and diarrhoea. Typically, they will restrict their intake of dairy products, which puts them at risk of deficiencies in several nutrients, most notably calcium.[26] *Streptococcus thermophilus*, a species belonging to the *S. salivarius* group of microorganisms, has been used as a probiotic because of its ability to ferment lactose. The contribution of lactase by bacterial cultures is thought to improve the digestion of lactose in lactose-intolerant individuals.[27] The inability of adults to digest lactose is widespread, although generally these patients tolerate lactose better from yogurt than from milk.[28] The yogurt starter cultures (*S. thermophilus* and *Lactobacillus delbrueckii* subspecies *bulgaricus*), present at levels normally seen in yogurt ($\geq 10^8$/g), effectively improve the digestion of lactose in lactose maldigesters.

Elevated levels of certain blood lipids are a risk factor for cardiovascular disease. The effect of bacterial cultures containing dairy products or probiotic bacteria on cholesterol levels has yielded equivocal results.[29] A proposed mechanism is based on the ability of certain probiotic lactobacilli and bifidobacteria to deconjugate bile acids enzymatically, increasing their rates of excretion.[30] Cholesterol is a precursor of bile acids, and the loss of bile acids through excretion is replaced by the conversion of cholesterol molecules to bile acids. Probiotic bacteria also ferment food-derived indigestible carbohydrates to produce short-chain fatty acids in the gut. This can cause a decrease in the systemic levels of blood lipids by inhibiting hepatic cholesterol synthesis and/or redistributing cholesterol from plasma to the liver.[31]

Approximately 80% of all kidney stones contain significant amounts of calcium oxalate, indicating that high dietary oxalate levels may be a risk factor contributing to the formation of renal stones.[32] Hyperoxaluria complicated by renal tract stones is an important clinical problem in humans, particularly those with enteric hyperoxaluria secondary to conditions such as Crohn's disease.[33] Oxalate degrading bacteria have the potential to reduce urinary excretion of oxalic acid, which is considered the most important risk factor in the formation of renal stones. Several studies have demonstrated the presence of oxalate-degrading bacteria in the human intestine.[34–36] Treatment of patients with an oral administration of freeze-dried lactic acid bacteria is associated with a reduced urinary oxalate excretion.[37] Additional studies have demonstrated oxalate degradation by *Oxalobacter formigenes*, a Gram-negative anaerobic bacterium that inhabits the gastrointestinal tracts of humans and mammals.[38–40] The presence of *O. formigenes* has been shown to reverse hyperoxaluria in a rat model and reduce urinary oxalate excretion in humans.[41]

A substantial number of published studies have investigated conjugated linoleic acid (CLA) because of its potential health-promoting properties and the proposed positive effects that CLA has on many aspects of human health, most notably the anti-carcinogenic, immune modulation, anti-atherosclerotic, and anti-obesity activities.[42–47] Production of the *cis*-9, *trans*-CLA isomer from dietary linoleic acid by the enteric microbiota may have an important influence on the evolving and interactive intestinal mucosal environment, thereby influencing long-term health. In addition to the increased interest in the possible physiological effects on humans following CLA consumption, there has been a concomitant increase in interest in the isolation of novel human-derived bacterial cultures with the ability to produce the bioactive fatty acid.[48–51] Some, but not all, human-derived bifidobacteria are capable of producing the fatty acid metabolite CLA.

Not all bacterial metabolites have beneficial effects on the host; indeed, negative influences may be observed associated with colonizing or invading microorganisms. Microbial metabolites may possess genotoxic, mutagenic, or carcinogenic activity and contribute substantially to the risk of developing cancer over a period of long-term exposure. It is likely that the appropriate balance between different microbial species, rather than one particular organism, is the primary putrefaction controlling feature. When adequate levels of beneficial anaerobic bacteria, such as *Bifidobacteria*, are present in the intestine, they ferment carbohydrates to produce acetic and lactic acid. This decrease in the luminal pH inhibits putrefaction.

However, in the absence of beneficial species or strains, certain groups such as *Clostridia* ferment proteins and release harmful nitrogenous metabolites into the lumen (e.g. biogenic amines, indoles, and ammonia). In the long term, this can lead to toxicity and inflammation and increases the risk of colon cancer.[52,53]

Immune System

The gastrointestinal tract is home to the largest accumulation of leukocytes in the body where they are constantly being exposed to a wide array of foreign antigens. Complex signalling networks between multiple cell types ensure that the appropriate balance is maintained between immune protection from infection and tolerance of harmless antigens, such as the resident bacterial flora.[54] Disturbance of this balance results in inappropriate immune activation as observed in patients with IBD. The small intestine is highly adapted to facilitate immunological sampling of intestinal contents. Specialized epithelial cells, M cells, actively transport antigen to underlying lymphoid follicles for immunological processing, while dendritic cells extend dendrites between epithelial cells in order to sample adherent bacterial species. Microbiota composition and metabolic activity impact the mechanisms by which the intestinal immune system samples luminal antigen and the controlling features that determine immunological tolerance. This phenomenon is still poorly described, and a significant portion of our understanding is derived from animal models and resected diseased tissue.

The single most important environmental factor that impacts intestinal immune signalling is the presence of microorganisms.[55] While most studies have focused on the immune response to pathogens, these are the exception in our coexistence with vast numbers of non-pathogenic microorganisms. Studies in GF mice have revealed dramatic alterations in the anatomy and function of both the mucosal and systemic immune compartments. GF mice have hypoplastic Peyer's patches that contain few germinal centres, as well as greatly reduced numbers of IgA-producing plasma cells and lamina propria CD4+ T cells. The lymph nodes and spleen are poorly organized and mice are hypogammaglobulinaemic. Acquisition of a bacterial flora results in the normalization of these abnormalities. Thus, the commensal bacteria drive and condition the mucosal immune system.

This observation has led investigators to further examine the therapeutic potential of specific bacterial species in driving regulatory immune responses within the mucosa. Murine studies have demonstrated that the deliberate administration of commensal, or probiotic, bacteria to susceptible colitis models results in reduced inflammatory activity associated with reduced pro-inflammatory cytokine production and maintained regulatory cytokine production.[56] This suggests that certain bacterial strains can drive immuno-regulatory responses via direct interaction with the mucosal immune system. In humans, dendritic cells isolated from mesenteric lymph nodes preferentially secrete the regulatory cytokines IL-10 and TGF-β when co-incubated with commensal bacteria, while the same dendritic cells preferentially secrete pro-inflammatory cytokines, but not regulatory cytokines, when exposed to the pathogenic organism *Salmonella typhimurium*.[57] This suggests that intestinal dendritic cells exposed to commensal organisms in vivo may drive the in vivo development of regulatory T cells, resulting in improved immunological tolerance.

The host response to infection is characterized by innate and acquired cellular and humoral immune reactions, designed to limit spread of the offending organism and to restore organ homeostasis. However, to limit the aggressiveness of collateral damage to host tissues, a range of regulatory constraints may be activated. Regulatory T cells (Treg) serve one such mechanism.[58] These are derived from the thymus but may also be induced in peripheral organs, including the gut mucosa.[59,60] For example, encounter with specific experimental microbes within the murine gut has been shown to drive the development of mucosal Tregs, which is associated with attenuation of inflammation in a murine model of colitis[61] and contributes to protection of the host from mucosal damage and systemic inflammation associated with infection by invasive pathogens.

These studies and others have led investigators to examine the potential anti-inflammatory properties of selected commensal species in human disease. Clinical studies assessing the impact of probiotic consumption on the symptoms of IBD are conflicting and are often confounded by small numbers.[62] However, the best evidence for probiotic efficacy in patients with IBD has been seen with a cocktail of eight different strains which effectively maintains remission in patients with pouchitis. Probiotic treatments have also been examined for the treatment of irritable bowel syndrome (IBS). While most of the bacterial strains examined have no demonstrable efficacy, consumption of one commensal bacterium, *Bifidobacterium infantis* 35,624, resulted in significant improvement of patient symptoms.[63, 64] Interestingly, an imbalance in cytokine signalling networks observed in IBS patients was normalized by *Bifidobacterium infantis* 35,624 consumption, suggesting an association between probiotic-induced immuno-regulation and clinical efficacy.

Influence of Ageing

Microbiota of the Infant

The importance of the relationship between the human gut and its microbiota has been highlighted already, and together they represent a dynamic biological system that has co-evolved from birth. It is well accepted that the ability of the gut to sustain a beneficial commensal microbiota, in contrast to harmful and opportunistic members, in a desirable community structure is essential for host health and reduction of disease risk. The acquisition and development of the desired gut microbiota, which begins at birth, is particularly important for infant health as well as having implications in later life. The establishment of the microbiota is a dynamic process consisting of a number of phases and leads to the emergence of a relatively stable microbiota that contributes to the development of a fully functional immune system.[65,66] Members of the Bifidobacterium species are thought to be among the most beneficial components of the gut microbiota and, therefore, have received considerable research attention with regard to their roles in optimizing the health status of both infants and adults.

At the outset, the foetal gut is sterile or germ free at birth, but colonization begins during birth or immediately afterwards. A number of factors including the microbial flora of the genital tract, sanitary condition, obstetric techniques, vaginal or caesarean mode of delivery, geographical distribution of bacterial species, and type of feeding influence the level and frequency at which various species of bacteria colonize the infant gut.[67] The choice of delivery (vaginal compared to caesarean section) has a significant impact on the types of bacteria to which the newborn is exposed. During vaginal delivery (i.e. natural birthing), the neonate is exposed to a wide diversity of microorganisms from the mother's microbiota and these can be cultivated from the faeces of the infant.[68] In the case of caesarean delivery, the infants are exposed to microorganism from the air, equipment, other infants, and the nursing staff, as well as the mother's microbiota.[69] Bacteria such as enterobacteria (including *E. coli*), streptococci and lactobacilli are among the first colonizers, and are followed by anaerobic species such as *Bacteriodes*, *Bifidobacterium*, and *Clostridium*. The ability of the anaerobes to colonize is facilitated by the reduction of the redox potential of the intestinal lumen caused by the initial growth of the facultative bacteria.

The next phase of microbiota acquisition and development involves the period in which milk is exclusively fed to the infant. The key factors that influence the bacterial flora of the microbiota at this stage are diet (in particular whether the infant consumes breast milk or infant formula), host genetics, and bacteria–bacteria interactions. Breast milk is a rich source of bacteria with counts of up to 10^9 microbes per litre in the case of healthy mothers.[69] Considerable attention has been devoted to the analyses of differences in the flora of breast-fed infants compared to those on infant formula. The prevalence of Bifidobacterium species has received particular emphasis because they are considered to have a number of beneficial properties including the reduction of gut pH which results in a concomitant reduction in potentially harmful species. In addition, bifidobacteria are able to exert directly antagonistic activities against gut pathogens and may promote the development of the mucosal immune system. The microbiota of breast-fed infants is considered to be dominated by populations of bifidobacteria, which make up 60–90% of the total faecal microbiota, with lactobacilli present in much smaller numbers. In the case of infant formula feeding, bifidobacteria are also present, but the microbiota is usually more complex with a higher frequency of facultative anaerobes such as bacteroides and clostridia compared to breast-fed infants.[70,71] Analysis of the composition of the gut microbiota of infants have been hindered by the limitations of conventional cultivation techniques. The emergence of modern molecular-based techniques is helping to provide more specific details of the numbers and types of bifidobacteria present in infant faeces. The most common species of Bifidobacterium encountered include *B. infantis*, *B. breve*, *B. longum*, and *B. bifidum*.

The predominance of Bifidobacterium within the microbiota of breast-fed infants has drawn attention to the fact that human milk contains a myriad of components that have significant bioactive and immuno-modulatory roles. Human milk oligosaccharides (HMOs) are considered the main components that influence the development of the intestinal flora.[72,73] The occurrence of these HMOs in human breast milk is considered to contribute to an evolutionary selection process for the growth of bifidobacteria in the gut. Over 100 different HMOs have been identified, and the presence of variable combinations of glucose, sialic acid, galactose, fucose and n-acetylglucosamine contributes to their complexity. Since the breast-milk HMOs are only partially digested in the intestine, they reach the colon and stimulate the bifidogenic microbiota. In addition, the HMOs have a protective effect against enteric pathogens.[74] This effect on the wider population, rather than just the stimulation of bifidobacteria, is in agreement with the expected effect of 'prebiotics' as defined elsewhere.[75]

In addition to HMOs, other factors in human milk influence the composition of the bacterial microbiota and contribute to the control of infections. These include proteins such as immunoglobulins, κ-caesin, lysozyme, lactoferrin, haptocorrin, α-lactalbulim, and lactoperoxidase, which possess anti-microbial activity and support the immune defence of breast-fed infants against pathogenic bacteria and viruses.[76,77] During milk feeding, the infant microbiota appears to stabilize at about 4 weeks of age and remains so until weaning, when the introduction of solid foods takes places place. After weaning, the infant gut becomes colonized by a diverse, but unstable, consortium of species belonging mainly to the genera Bifidobacterium, Bacteroides, Streptococcus, and Clostridium. The ecosystem becomes stable by 2 years of age and the composition continues to remain stable throughout most of the early adult life.[78]

Colonization of the infant intestine by a balanced microbiota results in the stimulation of a number of key functions such as intestinal maturation, the mucosal barrier and immune system, and nutrient absorption.[79] The gut microbiota plays an important role in the immuno-physiological regulation of the gastrointestinal tract by providing crucial signals for the development of the immune system in infancy and by actively influencing gut-associated immunologic homeostatic mechanisms later in life. Therefore, there is considerable interest in modulating the gut microbiota towards a more beneficial community, particularly early in life. Supplementation with prebiotics or probiotics may promote the optimum balance in the context of the normal microbiota, while also protecting against the detrimental effects on the microbiota caused by stress and certain disease situations. Some examples are provided herewith in the case of infant diseases, but the concepts are also applicable to adult populations.

The concept of prebiotic supplementation to the infant is supported by the recognition that HMOs nourish the developing microbiota. In addition, a review of studies involving over 400 pre-term and full-term infants showed that prebiotic mixtures containing short-chain galacto-oligosaccharides and long-chain fructo-oligosaccharides stimulated the growth of bifidobacteria and lactobacilli, decreased faecal pH, and normalized short-chain fatty acid patterns in infant stools.[80]

In addition, it is likely that certain types of oligosaccharides may act as soluble receptors in the mucosa for different pathogens, thereby increasing the resistance of breast-fed infants to these pathogens.

Probiotics (usually Bifidobacteria or Lactobacilli) have also been administered to infants to support a well-balanced microbiota. Probiotic supplementation in infant formulas has shown that strains may persist in the infant gut and lower stool pH.[81] A number of studies have shown that probiotics can be an effective treatment option in the case of viral- or antibiotic-associated diarrhoea in infants and children. In the case of the commonly occurring rotavirus gastroenteritis, the beneficial effects of probiotics have been observed as evidenced by shortening of the duration of the diarrhoea and reduced requirement for hydration.[82] A detailed review of the published randomized, placebo-controlled trials on the use of probiotics in acute diarrhoea has highlighted the benefits of the *Lactobacillus rhamnosus* GG strain. It is noteworthy that diarrhoeal disease is a serious problem in the developing world where the most common causes of infantile diarrhoea are rotaviruses which are responsible for greater that 10% of infectious episodes. There is also preliminary data available on the potential for selected probiotic strains to prevent necrotizing enterocolitis, which is a severe inflammatory reaction of the small and large intestine in pre-term infants.[83]

Clinical evidence to support the use of selected probiotics in the prevention of allergy in children is accumulating. According to the 'hygiene hypothesis', the increasing number of allergic diseases in the developed world is attributable to reduced exposure to microbial challenge in early infancy, improved hygiene standards, changes in diet, different delivery modes, and smaller family sizes.[84] The microbiota of children with atopic disease has been shown to be different in composition to the microbiota of non-atopic children. The allergic infants were colonized less frequently by bifidobacteria, enterococci, and bacteroides but displayed increased levels of clostridia and coliform species.[85] In addition to an overall reduction in the numbers of bifidobacteria, the species composition was also changed. Allergic infants displayed higher levels of *Bifidobacterium adolescentis* and fewer *Bifidobacterium bifidum*.[86]

These findings prompted investigators to examine the role for probiotics in influencing the risk of developing allergy. Although not all strains and combinations of strains were effective, selected probiotic strains were successful in the treatment of atopic eczema when used with an extensively hydrolysed formula.[87] In a further study by the same group, the administration of probiotics to pregnant mothers and, later, to their children, reduced the number of children that later developed allergy.[88] These studies highlight the beneficial effect of *Lb. Rhamnosus* GG but, as mentioned already, strain specificity is important and not all probiotics tested give positive results. While the precise roles of the normal gut microbiota in the development of allergy remain to be elucidated, accumulating evidence suggests that probiotics have a role in preventing allergy when administered early in life, which is consistent with the view that exposure to a wide diversity of microbial flora is desirable and promotes a well-regulated immune system.

In summary, the importance of the gut microbiota in the health status of the infant is clearly recognized. The flexibility of the developing microbiota in early childhood offers the potential to influence and modulate bacterial populations to achieve health benefits. Already there are defined applications in which probiotics have been shown to have therapeutic effects. However, despite the increasing number of well-defined studies indicating the benefits of probiotics, we still do not understand the mechanisms underpinning their biological activity. In addition, the influence of long-term administration of probiotics on allergy, autoimmune diseases, and infection control are not understood. These aspects, as well as the selection of the optimum probiotic strains or combinations for specific purposes, offer exciting research challenges for the near future.

Microbiota of the Elderly

Advances in medical science and improved living standards have increased the overall age expectancy of Western society. People over 60 represent 20% of the current population and this is estimated to increase to 33% by the year 2030.[89] Although the microbiota of adults and children has been significantly studied, little is known of the changes that occur in the microbiota during ageing.

The composition of the resident intestinal microbiota varies between individuals, but the dominant populations are relatively stable during adult life under normal conditions.[90–92] The total number of anaerobic bacteria seems to remain relatively constant in older people; however, the composition of the microbiota does change considerably with age. The gut microbiota of healthy adults is dominated by species such as the *Bacteriodes/Prevotella* group, *Clostridium coccoides* group, and *Clostridium leptum* subgroup. However, 22% of the elderly person's microbiota is represented by species that are outside the bacteria normally represented in the adult population. Most of the elderly species were within the lineages *Clostridium lituseburense* subgroup, *Clostridium ramosum* group, and the *Prosthecobacter* group of organisms.[93] Some studies have indicated that *Bifidobacteria* levels decrease in older people, while levels of the potential detrimental clostridia and enterobacteria groups increase.[94] A wide range of *Bifidobacteria* species are found in adults and children, but in the elderly the population is reduced to one or two dominant organisms, in particular *Bifidobacterium adolescentis* and *B. longum*.[95] The absence of *Bifidobacteria*, or their low numbers in the elderly, may have metabolic and health consequences for the host because they play a role in the immune responsiveness of the gut and in resistance to gastrointestinal infections.

In addition to the decreased levels of *Bifidobacteria*, *Bacteriodes* were also shown to be decreased in the elderly population.[96] *Bacteriodes* are nutritionally versatile and can utilize a wide variety of carbon sources. As discussed above, these bacteria are thought to be responsible for most of the polysaccharide digestion that occurs in the large intestine. A reduction in *Bacteriodes* numbers may affect the host through short chain fatty acid changes and may also impact other bacterial species that depend nutritionally on polysaccharide digestion. Interestingly, malnutrition is a common observation in elderly individuals. A number of different mechanisms contribute to this malnutrition including a decrease in the amount and type of food consumed by the elderly, due to a decline in taste and smell, and a decreased ability to masticate.[97] Furthermore, decreased intestinal motility, resulting in faecal impaction and constipation, is a major problem.[98,99] It is postulated that malnourishment leads to a damaged gut epithelium and reduced barrier function, resulting in decreased gut-mediated immunity, reduced absorption of essential dietary components, and loss of appetite which further compounds the nutrient deficit. The concomitant associated decrease in *Bacteroides* numbers during this time is intriguing and deserves further study to determine the relationship with the physiological changes in the gastrointestinal tract, as well as modifications in diet and host immune system activity.

The normal intestinal microbiota provides an important natural defence mechanism against invading pathogens and prevents the overgrowth of autochthonous opportunistic pathogens in a process known as *colonization resistance*. The large intestinal ecosystem provides colonization resistance by a variety of mechanisms such as occupying adhesion sites in the gut and the production of antimicrobial agents. Quorum sensing is an important mechanism of cell-to-cell communication that involves density-dependent recognition of signalling molecules, resulting in modulation of gene expression. The development and maintenance of our commensal intestinal microbial system and the virulence mechanisms of enteric pathogens are linked to each other by quorum sensing. These detrimental changes in gastrointestinal ecology and function can have major consequences for the elderly, and a higher incidence of gastrointestinal infections is observed in older individuals.

The elderly gut is disrupted by a number of mechanisms, such as a loss in beneficial intestinal microbes, overgrowth of pathogenic bacteria, and possibly the most dramatic alteration of the microbiota that occurs during the administration of antibiotics. The alteration of the normal gastrointestinal microbiota by antibiotics can lead to significant changes in the colonic micro-environment, especially with regard to the concentration and distribution of organic compounds such as carbohydrates, short-chain fatty acids, and bile acids.[100] The elderly are hospitalized more frequently than younger people, their length of stay is longer, and they receive many more medications including antibiotics. This increased use of antibiotics has a profound impact on the microbiota, and several studies have examined alterations in gut microbiota post-broad-spectrum antibiotic treatment. The disruption of the normal microbiota by clindamycin, a broad-spectrum antibiotic, depletes *Bifidobacteria* and *Bacteriodes*, but other components of the gut microbiota (total facultative anaerobes, lactose fermentors, enterococci, and Gram-positive cocci) increase in numbers.[101] A study to compare the faecal microbiotas of young, healthy adults, non-antibiotic-treated elderly subjects, and antibiotic-treated elderly subjects demonstrated that antibiotic-treated and non-antibiotic-treated elderly subjects had decreased *Bifidobacterium* and *Bacteriodes* when compared to healthy, young adults. Additionally, antibiotic-treated elderly subjects had increased levels of clostridia.

These alterations of the gut microbiota in the elderly population post-antibiotic treatment may result in putrification of the colon and a greater susceptibility to disease, such as gastroenteritis and *Clostridium difficile* infection. Indeed, the frequency with which *C. difficile* is isolated is greater in the elderly. Clostridia in general have been found to occur in significantly higher numbers in healthy, elderly volunteers compared to younger subjects.[102]

Changes in the composition of the intestinal microbiota have been implicated in the initiation or maintenance of various disease states. A well-known example of this is *C. difficile* infection resulting in *Clostridium difficile*-associated diarrhoea (CDAD), which occurs predominantly in patients whose colonic microbiotas have been disturbed by antibiotic therapy. First described in 1935, *C. difficile* was not recognized as the causative agent of nosocomial diarrhoea until the 1970s.[103,104] However, CDAD is the now the most common hospital-acquired diarrhoea and is a major problem of gastroenteritis infection and antibiotic-associated diarrhoea in nursing homes and care facilities for the elderly. Indeed, the health protection agency in the UK reported 42,625 cases of *C. difficile* infection in patients aged 65 and over in England for the first 9 months of 2006, which was a 5.5% increase in cases over the same period in 2005. The main predisposing factor for the acquisition of CDAD is antibiotic therapy. In the 1970s, the administration of clindamycin followed by ampicillin and amoxicillin was implicated as responsible for CDAD, and these were replaced by cephalosporins in the 1980s and by flouroquinolones more recently. There is also the added problem of the hyper-virulent strain of *C. difficile* PCR ribotype 027, the incidence of which is increasing in the US, Canada, and Europe. During normal human growth and development, bacterial competitors crowd this slow-growing anaerobe out of the gut. However, if the commensal bacterial strains decrease in numbers (when patients are given broad-spectrum antibiotics), *C. difficile* can germinate and grow, resulting in CDAD. The clinical presentation of CDAD may vary from mild diarrhoea to severe dehabilitating infection. Antibiotics such as third-generation cephalosporins are accepted as the main risk factors, and antibiotic restriction is the most effective control.[105] Older age, female gender, and a prolonged hospital stay were also identified as risk factors in hospitalized CDAD patients. In addition, more recent studies reported the association of the use of proton pump inhibitors within the preceding 8 weeks, the use of nasal feeding tubes, and exposure to anginoplastic agents with an increased risk of developing *C. difficile* diarrhoea.[106] When compared to a healthy elderly group, CDAD patients have higher enterobacterial and enterococcal counts, with a marked increase in the diversity of clostridia and lactobacilli. The higher numbers of clostridia, enterobacteria, and enterococci may lead to putrification of the colon due to the breakdown of proteins forming toxic end products that may harm host cells. The associated high numbers of lactobacilli suggests that *Bifido-bacteria* and *Bacteriodes* may have a more prominent role in colonization resistance against *C. difficile*.

Antibiotic therapy breaks down the defence mechanisms of the ageing gut, leaving individuals more susceptible to infection with opportunistic pathogens such as *C. difficile* (as discussed above). Consumption of probiotics, in particular those that produce antimicrobial components such as bacteriocins and organic acid, may protect the elderly gut from infection. For example, *Lactobacillus rhamnosus* produces a substance that is inhibitory to both Gram-positive and Gram-negative microorganisms. In addition, *L. rhamnosus* has been shown to interfere with the in vitro adherence of several human pathogens to intestinal cells.[107] Attempts to increase colonization resistance by using probiotics and faecal enemas have yielded favourable results in some clinical trials.[108,109] Using meta-analysis, three types of probiotics (*Sacchromyces boulardii*, *L. rhamnosus* GG, and probiotic mixtures) significantly reduced the development of antibiotic-associated diarrhoea.[110] Probiotics offer an attractive strategy to reduce unfavourable changes in the ageing gut and to maintain a more 'healthy' intestinal microbiota, to help maintain bowel function, and to reduce the susceptibility to infection in elderly persons. Intervention with a probiotic supplement may decrease the numbers of proteolytic bacteria, such as *Clostridia* in the gastrointestinal tract. Colonization resistance may also prevent the outgrowth of endogenous or newly acquired strains post-antibiotic treatment. Probiotics may also increase resistance to gut infections by directly improving host immunity. In addition to probiotics, prebiotic supplementation of the elderly may have beneficial effects. Carbohydrates such as lactulose and fructo-oligosaccharides (FOS) have been shown to affect the growth of *C. difficile* both in vitro and in vivo. Several prebiotics are known to stimulate the growth of *Bifido-bacteria*, which can in turn affect the growth and metabolism of other microorganisms in the bowel. Hopkins and Macfarlane in 2003 demonstrated that prebiotics stimulated *Bifidobacteria* growth, which results in concomitant reductions in *C. difficile* populations. In the presence of clindamycin, they also demonstrated further augmentation of *Bifidobacteria* in the presence of prebiotics, resulting in a further loss of *C. difficile* colonization. Modification of the large intestinal microbiota by combining probiotics and prebiotics (symbiotic) could beneficially affect the host and could be viewed as an attractive method of treatment or prophylaxis for CDAD.[111]

Concluding Remarks

In defining the microbial flora of the human gastrointestinal tract, a major deficiency immediately becomes apparent: there are substantially more cells present than are measured using conventional microbiological methods. In other words, the total number of bacteria that can be cultured is only of 10–20% of the total microbiota. A metagenomic approach enables the study of a microbial community as a single dynamic entity, and has been used to investigate complex environments such as soil and water. It may provide a more comprehensive method for providing information on of the effects of several factors, such as antibiotic therapy, ageing, and disease, on the intestinal microbial balance.

This chapter has documented the influence of the gut microbiota on host nutrition, metabolism, and immune function in both the infant and elderly populations.

It is clear that the microbiota have a profound influence on human health, in particular, resistance to infectious agents such as *C. difficile*. The mucosal immune system is especially vulnerable, since its function is closely linked to the luminal contents of the gut. It is certainly becoming clear that the enteric commensal bacteria can alter the effectiveness of the mucosal immune system, and there is promising research on the use of pre/pro/syn-biotics in maintaining a healthy gut. However, the probiotic mechanism of action is uncertain and is likely to depend on the individual strain itself and the clinical condition for which it is used.

References

1. O'Hara AM, Shanahan F. The gut flora as a forgotten organ. EMBO Rep 2006;7:688–693.
2. Shanahan F. Host-flora interactions in inflammatory bowel disease. Inflamm Bowel Dis 2004;10(Suppl 1):S16–S24
3. Hooper LV, Wong MH, Thelin A, Hansson L, Falk PG, Gordon JI. Molecular analysis of commensal host-microbial relationships in the intestine. Science 2001;291:881–884.
4. Cebra JJ. Influences of microbiota on intestinal immune system development. Am J Clin Nutr 1999;69:1046S–1051S.
5. Shanahan F. The host-microbe interface within the gut. Best Pract Res Clin Gastroenterol 2002;16:915–931.
6. Sartor RB. The influence of normal microbial flora on the development of chronic mucosal inflammation. Res Immunol 1997;148:567–576.
7. O'Hara AM, O'Regan P, Fanning A, O'Mahony C, MacSharry J, Lyons A, Bienenstock J, O'Mahony L, Shanahan F. Functional modulation of human intestinal epithelial cell responses by *Bifidobacterium infantis* and *Lactobacillus salivarius*. Immunology 2006;118:202–215.
8. Ma D, Forsythe P, Bienenstock J. Live *Lactobacillus reuteri* is essential for the inhibitory effect on tumor necrosis factor alpha-induced interleukin-8 expression. Infect Immun 2004;72:5308–5314.
9. Otte JM, Podolsky DK. Functional modulation of enterocytes by gram-positive and gram-negative microorganisms. Am J Physiol Gastrointest Liver Physiol 2004;286:G613–G626.
10. Backhed F, Ley RE, Sonnenburg JL, Peterson DA, Gordon JI. Host-bacterial mutualism in the human intestine. Science 2005;307:1915–1920.
11. Bergman EN. Energy contributions of volatile fatty acids from the gastrointestinal tract in various species. Physiol Rev 1990;70:567–590.
12. Roediger WE. Utilization of nutrients by isolated epithelial cells of the rat colon. Gastroenterology 1982;83:424–429.
13. O'Keefe SJ. Nutrition and colonic health: the critical role of the microbiota. Curr Opin Gastroenterol 2008;24:51–58.
14. Rajilic-Stojanovic M, Smidt H, de Vos WM. Diversity of the human gastrointestinal tract microbiota revisited. Environ Microbiol 2007;9:2125–2136.
15. Hooper LV, Midtvedt T, Gordon JI. How host-microbial interactions shape the nutrient environment of the mammalian intestine. Annu Rev Nutr 2002;22:283–307.
16. Xu J, Bjursell MK, Himrod J, Deng S, Carmichael LK, Chiang HC, Hooper LV, Gordon JI. A genomic view of the human-Bacteroides thetaiotaomicron symbiosis. Science 2003;299: 2074–2076.
17. Sonnenburg JL, Xu J, Leip DD, Chen CH, Westover BP, Weatherford J, Buhler JD, Gordon JI. Glycan foraging in vivo by an intestine-adapted bacterial symbiont. Science 2005;307: 1955–1959.

18. Crittenden RG, Martinez NR, Playne MJ. Synthesis and utilisation of folate by yoghurt starter cultures and probiotic bacteria. Int J Food Microbiol 2003;80:217–222.
19. Klipstein FA, Samloff IM. Folate synthesis by intestinal bacteria. Am J Clin Nutr 1966;19:237–246.
20. Kim TH, Yang J, Darling PB, O'Connor DL. A large pool of available folate exists in the large intestine of human infants and piglets. J Nutr 2004;134:1389–1394.
21. Wostmann BS. The germfree animal in nutritional studies. Annu Rev Nutr 1981;1:257–279.
22. Backhed F, Ding H, Wang T, Hooper LV, Koh GY, Nagy A, Semenkovich CF, Gordon JI. The gut microbiota as an environmental factor that regulates fat storage. Proc Natl Acad Sci USA 2004;101:15718–15723.
23. Ley RE, Backhed F, Turnbaugh P, Lozupone CA, Knight RD, Gordon JI. Obesity alters gut microbial ecology. Proc Natl Acad Sci USA 2005;102:11070–11075.
24. Ley RE, Turnbaugh PJ, Klein S, Gordon JI. Microbial ecology: human gut microbes associated with obesity. Nature 2006;444:1022–1023.
25. Turnbaugh PJ, Ley RE, Mahowald MA, Magrini V, Mardis ER, Gordon JI. An obesity-associated gut microbiome with increased capacity for energy harvest. Nature 2006; 444:1027–1031.
26. Montalto M, Curigliano V, Santoro L, Vastola M, Cammarota G, Manna R, Gasbarrini A, Gasbarrini G. Management and treatment of lactose malabsorption. World J Gastroenterol 2006;14:187–191.
27. Sanders ME. Consideration for use of probiotic bacteria to modulate human health. J Nutr 2000;130:384S–390S.
28. Suarez FL, Savaiano DA, Levitt MD. Review article: the treatment of lactose intolerance. Aliment Pharmacol Ther 1995;9:589–597.
29. Taylor GRJ, Williams CM. Effects of probiotics and prebiotics on blood lipids. Br J Nutr 1998;80:S225–S230.
30. De Smet I, Van Hoorde L, De Saeyer N, Vande Woestyne M, Verstraete W. *In vitro* study of bile salt hydrolase (BSH) activity of BSH isogenic *Lactobacillus plantarum* 80 strains and estimation of cholesterol lowering through enhanced BSH activity. Microb Health Dis 1994;7:315–329.
31. Wong JMW, de Souza R, Kendall CWC, Emam A, Jenkins DJA. Colonic health: fermentation and short chain fatty acids. J Clin Gasteroenterol 2006;40:235–243.
32. Coe FL, Parks JH, Asplin JR. The pathogenesis and treatment of kidney stones. N Engl J Med 1992;327:1141–1154.
33. Kumar R, Ghoshal UC, Singh G, Mittal RD. Infrequency of colonization with *Oxalobacter formigenes* in inflammatory bowel disease: possible role in renal stone formation. J Gastroenterol Hepatol 2004;19:1403–1409.
34. Allison MJ, Cook MH, Milne DB, Gallagher S, Calyman RV. Oxalate degradation by gastrointestinal bacteria from humans. J Nutr 1986;141:1–7.
35. Ito H, Kotake T, Masai M. *In vitro* degradation of oxalic acid by human faeces. Int J Urol 1996;3:207–211.
36. Hokama S, Honma Y, Toma C, Ogawa Y. Oxalate-degrading *Enterococcus faecalis*. Microbiol Immunol 2000;44:235–240.
37. Campieri C, Campieri M, Bertuzzi V, Swennen E, Matteuzzi D, Stefoni S, Pirovano F, Centi C, Ulisse S, Famularo G, De Simone C. Reduction of oxaluria after an oral course of lactic acid bacteria at high concentration. Kidney Intern 2001;60:1097–1105.
38. Allison MJ, Cook HM, Milne DB, Gallagher S, Clayman RV. Oxalate degradation by gastrointestinal bacteria from humans. J Nutr 1986;116:455–460.
39. Dawson KA, Allison MJ, Hartman PA. Isolation and some characteristics of anaerobic oxalate-degrading bacteria from the rumen. Appl Environ Microbiol 1980;40:833–839.
40. Duncan SH, Richardson AJ, Kaul P, Holmes RP, Allison MJ, Stewart CS. *Oxalobacter formigenes* and its potential role in human health. Appl Environ Microbiol 2002;68: 3841–3847.

41. Sidhu H, Allison MJ, Chow JM, Clark A, Peck AB. Rapid reversal of hyperoxaluria in a rat model after probiotic administration of *Oxalobacter formigenes*. J Urol 2001;166:1487–1491.
42. Belury MA. Inhibition of carcinogenesis by conjugated linoleic acid: potential mechanisms of action. J Nutr 2002;32:2995–2998.
43. Gaullier JM, Halse J, Hoye K, Kristiansen K, Fagertun H, Vik H, Gudmundsen O. Conjugated linoleic acid supplementation for 1 y reduces body fat mass in healthy overweight humans. Am J Clin Nutr 2004;79:1118–1125.
44. Ip MM, Masso-Welch PA, Ip C. Prevention of mammary cancer with conjugated linoleic acid: role of the stroma and the epithelium. J Mammary Gland Biol Neoplasia 2003;8:103–118.
45. Lee KN, Kritchevsky D, Pariza MW. Conjugated linoleic acid and atherosclerosis in rabbits. Atherosclerosis 1994;108:19–25.
46. Terpstra AH. Effect of conjugated linoleic acid on body composition and plasma lipids in humans: an overview of the literature. Am J Clin Nutr 2004;79:352–361.
47. Wahle KW, Heys SD, Rotondo D. Conjugated linoleic acids: are they beneficial or detrimental to health? Prog Lipid Res 2004;43:553–587.
48. Alonso L, Cuesta EP, Gilliland SE. Production of free conjugated linoleic acid by *Lactobacillus acidophilus* and *Lactobacillus casei* of human intestinal origin. J Dairy Sci 2003;86:1941–1946.
49. Coakley M, Ross RP, Nordgren M, Fitzgerald G, Devery R, Stanton C. Conjugated linoleic acid biosynthesis by human-derived *Bifidobacterium* species. J Appl Microbiol 2003;94:138–145.
50. Kishino S, Ogawa J, Omura Y, Matsumura K, Shimizu S. Conjugated linoleic acid production from linoleic acid by lactic acid bacteria. J Am Oil Chem Soc 2002;79:159–163.
51. Rosberg-Cody E, Ross RP, Hussey S, Ryan CA, Murphy BP, Fitzgerald GF, Devery R, Stanton C. Mining the microbiota of the neonatal gastrointestinal tract for conjugated linoleic acid-producing bifidobacteria. Appl Environ Microbiol 2004;70:4635–4641.
52. Smith EA, Macfarlane GT. Formation of phenolic and indolic compounds by ananerobic bacteria in the human large intestine. Microb Ecol 1997;33:180–188.
53. Cummings JH, Macfarlane GT. The control and consequences of bacterial fermentation in the human colon. J Appl Bacteriol 1991;70:443–459.
54. O'Mahony L. Immunology of the small intestine. In: Intestinal Failure: Diagnosis, Management and Transplantation. Blackwell, Oxford, 2008.
55. Macpherson AJ, Harris N. Interactions between commensal intestinal bacteria and the immune system. Nat Rev Immunol 2004;4:478–485.
56. McCarthy J, O'Mahony L, O'Callaghan L, Shiel B, Vaughan EE, Fitzsimons N, Fitzgibbon J, O'Sullivan GC, Kiely B, Collins JK, Shanahan F, Double blind, placebo controlled trial of two probiotic strains in interleukin 10 knockout mice and mechanistic link with cytokine balance. Gut 2003;52:975–980.
57. O'Mahony L, O'Callaghan L, McCarthy J, Shilling D, Scully P, Sibartie S, Kavanagh E, Kirwan WO, Redmond HP, Collins JK, Shanahan F. Differential cytokine response from dendritic cells to commensal and pathogenic bacteria in different lymphoid compartments in humans. Am J Physiol Gastrointest Liver Physiol 2006;290:839–845.
58. Belkaid Y, Rouse BT. Natural regulatory T cells in infectious disease. Nat Immunol 2005;6(4):353–360.
59. Karim M, Kingsley CI, Bushell AR, Sawitzki BS, Wood KJ. Alloantigen-induced CD25–CD4– regulatory T cells can develop *in vivo* from CD25–CD4– precursors in a thymus-independent process. J Immunol 2004;172:923.
60. Chen W, Jin W, Hardegen N, Lei KJ, Li L, Marinos N, McGrady G, Wahl SM. Conversion of peripheral CD4–CD25– naive T cells to CD4–CD25– regulatory T cells by TGF- induction of transcription factor Foxp3. J Exp Med 2003;198:1875.
61. Di Giacinto C, Marinaro M, Sanchez M, Strober W, Boirivant M. Probiotics ameliorate recurrent Th1-mediated murine colitis by inducing IL-10 and IL-10-dependent TGF-β bearing regulatory cells. J Immunol 2005;174:3237–3246.

62. Shanahan F. Probiotics in inflammatory bowel disease – therapeutic rationale and role. Adv Drug Deliv Rev 2004;56:809–818.
63. O'Mahony L, McCarthy J, Kelly P, Hurley G, Luo F, Chen K, O'Sullivan GC, Kiely B, Collins JK, Shanahan F, Quigley EM. *Lactobacillus* and *Bifidobacterium* in irritable bowel syndrome: symptom responses and relationship to cytokine profiles. Gastroenterology 2005;128:541–551.
64. Dinan TG, Quigley EM, Ahmed SM, Scully P, O'Brien S, O'Mahony L, O'Mahony S, Shanahan F, Keeling PW. Hypothalamic-pituitary-gut axis dysregulation in irritable bowel syndrome: plasma cytokines as a potential biomarker? Gastroenterology 2006;130(2): 304–311.
65. Duchmann R, Kaiser I, Hermann E, Mayet W, Ewe K, Meyer zum Buschenfelde KH. Tolerance exists towards resident intestinal flora but is broken in active inflammatory bowel disease (IBD). Clin Exp Immunol 1995;102:448–455.
66. Sudo N, Sawamura S, Tanaka K, Aiba Y, Kubo C, Koga Y. The requirement of intestinal bacterial flora for the development of an IgE production system fully susceptible to oral tolerance induction. J Immunol 1997;159:1739–1745.
67. Mountzouris KC, McCartney AL, Gibson GR. Intestinal microflora of human infants and current trends for its nutritional modulation. Br J Nutr 2002;87:405–420.
68. Fanaro S, Chierici R, Guerrini P, Vigi V. Intestinal microflora in early infancy: composition and development. Acta Paediatr Suppl 2003;91:48–55.
69. Mackie RI, Sghir A, Gaskins HR. Developmental microbial ecology of the neonatal gastrointestinal tract. Am J Clin Nutr 1999;69:1035S–1045S.
70. Vaughan EE, de Vries MC, Zoetendal EG, Ben-Amor K, Akkermans AD, de Vos WM. The intestinal LABs. Antonie Van Leeuwenhoek 2002;82:341–352.
71. Favier CF, Vaughan EE, De Vos WM, Akkermans AD. Molecular monitoring of succession of bacterial communities in human neonates. Appl Environ Microbiol 2002;68:219–226.
72. Boehm G, Stahl B, Jelinek J, Knol J, Miniello V, Moro GE. Prebiotic carbohydrates in human milk and formulas. Acta Paediatr Suppl 2005;94:18–21.
73. Coppa GV, Bruni S, Morelli L, Soldi S, Gabrielli O. The first prebiotics in humans: human milk oligosaccharides. J Clin Gastroenterol 2004;38:S80–S83.
74. Morrow AL, Ruiz-Palacios GM, Jiang X, Newburg DS. Human-milk glycans that inhibit pathogen binding protect breast-feeding infants against infectious diarrhea. J Nutr 2005;135:1304–1307.
75. Gibson GR, Roberfroid MB. Dietary modulation of the human colonic microbiota: introducing the concept of prebiotics. J Nutr 1995;125:1401–1412.
76. Andersson Y, Lindquist S, Lagerqvist C, Hernell O. Lactoferrin is responsible for the fungistatic effect of human milk. Early Hum Dev 2000;59:95–105.
77. Baldi A, Ioannis P, Chiara P, Eleonora F, Roubini C, Vittorio D. Biological effects of milk proteins and their peptides with emphasis on those related to the gastrointestinal ecosystem. J Dairy Res 2005;72:66–72.
78. Kimura K, McCartney AL, McConnell MA, Tannock GW. Analysis of fecal populations of bifidobacteria and lactobacilli and investigation of the immunological responses of their human hosts to the predominant strains. Appl Environ Microbiol 1997;63:3394–3398.
79. Hooper LV, Midtvedt T, Gordon JI. How host-microbial interactions shape the nutrient environment of the mammalian intestine. Annu Rev Nutr 2002;22:283–307.
80. Boehm G, Jelinek J, Stahl B, van Laere K, Knol J, Fanaro S, Moro G, Vigi V. Prebiotics in infant formulas. J Clin Gastroenterol 2004;38:S76–S79.
81. Bennet R, Nord CE, Zetterstrom R. Transient colonization of the gut of newborn infants by orally administered bifidobacteria and lactobacilli. Acta Paediatr 1992;81:784–787.
82. Allen SJ, Okoko B, Martinez E, Gregorio G, Dans LF. Probiotics for treating infectious diarrhoea. Cochrane Database Syst Rev 2004;CD003048.

83. Bin-Nun A, Bromiker R, Wilschanski M, Kaplan M, Rudensky B, Caplan M, Hammerman C. Oral probiotics prevent necrotizing enterocolitis in very low birth weight neonates. J Pediatr 2005;147:192–196.
84. Schaub B, Lauener R, von Mutius E. The many faces of the hygiene hypothesis. J Allergy Clin Immunol 2006;117:969–977; quiz 978.
85. Kirjavainen PV, Arvola T, Salminen SJ, Isolauri E. Aberrant composition of gut microbiota of allergic infants: a target of bifidobacterial therapy at weaning? Gut 2002;51:51–55.
86. Ouwehand AC, Isolauri E, He F, Hashimoto H, Benno Y, Salminen S. Differences in *Bifidobacterium* flora composition in allergic and healthy infants. J Allergy Clin Immunol 2001;108:144–145.
87. Viljanen M, Savilahti E, Haahtela T, Juntunen-Backman K, Korpela R, Poussa T, Tuure T, Kuitunen M. Probiotics in the treatment of atopic eczema/dermatitis syndrome in infants: a double-blind placebo-controlled trial. Allergy 2005;60:494–500.
88. Kalliomaki M, Salminen S, Poussa T, Isolauri E. Probiotics during the first 7 years of life: a cumulative risk reduction of eczema in a randomized, placebo-controlled trial. J Allergy Clin Immunol 2007;119:1019–1021.
89. McMurdo ME. A healthy old age: realistic or futile goal? Br Med J 2000;321:1149–1151.
90. Harmsen HJM, Raangs GC, Franks AH, Wilderboer-Veloo CM, Welling GW. The effect of prebiotic inulin and the probiotic *Bifidobacterium longum* in the faecal microflora of healthy volunteers measured by FISH and DGGE. Microbiol Ecol Health Dis 2002;14:211–219.
91. Vanhoutte T, Huys G, De Brandt E, Swings J. Temporal stability analysis of the microbiota in human faeces by denaturing gradient gel electrophoresis using universal and group-specific 16S rRNA gene primers. FEMS Microbiol Ecol 2004;48:437–446.
92. Zoetendal EG, Akkermans AD, De Vos WM. Temperature gradient gel electrophoresis analysis of 16S rRNA from human faecal samples reveals stable and host-specific communities of active bacteria. Appl Environ Microbiol 1998;64:3854–3859.
93. Blaut M, Collins MD, Welling GW, Dore J, van Loo J, de Vos W. Molecular biological methods for studying the gut microbiota: the EU human gut flora project. Br J Nutr 2002;87: S203–S211.
94. Gavini F, Cayuela C, Antoine JM, Lecoq C, Lefebvre B, Membre JM. Differences in the spatial distribution of bifidobacterial and enterobacterial species in human faecal microflora of three different (children, adults, elderly) age groups. Microb Ecol Health Dis 2001;13:40–45.
95. He FA, Ouwehand AC, Isolauri E, Hosoda M, Benno Y, Salminen S. Differences in composition and mucosal adhesion of *Bifidobacteria* isolated from healthy adults and healthy seniors. Curr Microbiol 2001;43:351–354.
96. Woodmansey EJ, McMurdo MET, Macfarlane GT, Macfarlane S. Comparison of compositions and metabolic activities of faecal microbiota in young adults and in antibiotic-treated and non-antibiotic treated elderly subjects. Appl Environ Microbiol 2004;70:6113–6122.
97. Walls AWG, Steele JG. The relationship between oral health and nutrition in older people. Mech Ageing Dev 2004;125:853–857.
98. Bitar KN, Patil SB. Aging and gastrointestinal smooth muscle. Mech Ageing Dev 2004; 125:907–910.
99. Saffrey MJ. Ageing of the enteric nervous system. Mech Ageing Dev 2004;125:899–906.
100. Hogenauer C, Hammer HF, Krejs GJ, Reisinger EC. Mechanisms and management of antibiotic-associated diarrhoea. Clin Infect Dis 1998;27:702–710.
101. Mylonakis E, Ryan ET, Claderwood SB. *Clostridium difficile*-associated diarrhoea. Arch Intern Med 2001;161:525–533.
102. Ljungberg B, Nilsson-Ehle I, Edlund C, Nord CE. Influence of ciprofloxacin on the colonic microflora in young and elderly volunteers: no impact of the altered drug absorption. Scand J Infect Dis 1990;22:205–208.

103. George RH, Symonds JM, Dimock F, Brown JD, Arabi Y, Shinagawa N, Keighley MR, Alexander-Williams J, Burdon DW. Identification of *Clostridium difficile* as a cause of pseudomembranous colitis. Br Med J 1978;1:695.
104. Hall IC, O'Toole E. Intestinal flora in new-born infants with a description of a new pathogenic anaerobe, *Bacillus difficilis*. Am J Dis Child 1935;49:390–402.
105. Al-Eidan FA, McElnay JC, Scott MG, Kearney MP. *Clostridium difficile*-associated diarrhoea in hospitalised patients. J Clin Pharm Ther 2000;25:101–109.
106. Cunningham R, Dale B, undy B, Gaunt N. Proton pump inhibitors as a risk factor for *Clostridium difficile* diarrhoea. J Hosp Infect 2003;54:243–245.
107. Forestier C, De Champs C, Vatoux C, Joly B. Probiotic activities of *Lactobacillus casei rhamnosus*: in vitro adherence to intestinal cells and antimicrobial properties. Res Microbiol 2001;152:167–173.
108. Roffe C. Biotherapy for antibiotic-associated and other diarrhoeas. J Infect 1996;32:1–10.
109. Tvede M, Rask-Madsen J. Bacteriotherapy for chronic relapsing *Clostridium difficile* diarrhoea in six patients. Lancet 1989;I:1156–1160.
110. McFarland LV. Meta-analysis of probiotics for the prevention of antibiotic associated diarrhoea and the treatment of *Clostridium difficile* disease. Am J Gastroenterol 2006;101:812–822.
111. Bartosch S, Woodmansey EJ, Paterson JCM, McMurdo MET, Macfarlane GT. Microbiological effects of consuming a symbiotic containing *Bifidobacterium bifidum*, *Bifidobacterium lactis*, and oligofructose in elderly persons, determined by real-time polymerase chain reaction and counting of viable bacteria. Clin Infect Dis 2005;40:28–37.

Chapter 9
A Gut Reaction: Aging Affects Gut-Associated Immunity

Joseph F. Albright and Julia W. Albright

The only way to keep your health is to eat what you don't want, drink what you don't like, and do what you'd druther not.

Mark Twain

Older people shouldn't eat health food, they need all the preservatives they can get

Robert Orben

Introduction

The digestive functions of the intestinal tract are familiar to everyone. The immuno-protective functions of the intestinal tract are not. Not long ago, when relatively little was known about the structure and function of the intestinal immune system, it was reasonable to conclude that aging affected gastrointestinal (GI) immunity to a minor extent, if at all. However, there were gerontologists who were not convinced because – given excessive functional potential beyond what is normally required – it was doubtful whether experiments involving whole animals or complex ex vivo systems were reliable. To illustrate the point, consider the following quotation[1]: "The multiorgan system that composes the gastrointestinal tract has a large reserve capacity, and thus there is little change in gastrointestinal function because of aging in the absence of disease." Although that quotation was directed at the digestive function of the GI system, it may reasonably be argued that it embraces the immunological function as well. We intend to develop that argument in this chapter. First, however, we will provide a review of current understanding and

J.F. Albright and J.W. Albright
Department of Microbiology, Immunology and Tropical Medicine, The George Washington
University School of Medicine, Washington, DC, USA

S.L. Percival (ed.), *Microbiology and Aging.*
DOI: 10.1007/978-1-59745-327-1_9, © Springer Science + Business Media, LLC 2009

175

thinking about the elements of the gut-associated immune system. After that, we will attempt a perception, with the aid of Minerva and a little help from Bacchus, of the aspects or features of gut-associated lymphoid tissue (GALT) that are most in need of investigation: most likely to yield new insight. Finally, we will argue that the gradual decline with advancing age in overall competence of GALT reaches a point at which the reserve potential is largely exhausted; and at that point, the elderly evince infections, autoimmune disorders, and neoplasias associated with resident microorganisms that had remained latent.

Architecture of Intestine and Distribution of GALT

The GALT is located primarily in the oral region (salivary glands, tonsils, adenoids) and in the small and large intestine. The gut may be pictured as a hollow tube closed at one end by the mouth and at the other by the anal sphincter. The lumen of the gut is external to the body. For that reason, the lumen is lined with an epithelium. The intestinal epithelium is a single-cell layer that extends all the way from the mouth to the anal opening. The epithelium serves as a barrier against injury and insult similar to the skin.

The wall of the gut, the "hollow tube," is a multilayered structure composed of four layers (tunics). The outer layer, the "serosa," is a membrane that surrounds the gut. On the dorsal/posterior aspect of the gut, the serosa forms a double-thickness, suspensory mesentery that is continuous with the lining of the peritoneal cavity. Beneath the serosa are the two strata of the "muscularis." In the outer stratum, the muscle fibers are aligned parallel to the longitudinal axis of the gut. The muscle fibers of the inner stratum are arranged in a circular orientation. The "submucosa" lies beneath the muscularis. It is a layer of connective tissue through which blood vessels, lymphatic vessels, and nerve fibers course. The GI tract is well endowed with both sensory and motor innervations. The innermost layer that surrounds the lumen is the "mucosa." The mucosa comprises several specialized layers and structures including those that constitute the gut-associated, mucosal immune system (the GALT).

Facing the lumen of the gut is the intestinal epithelium. This epithelium is the covering of the villi and crypts, i.e., evaginations and invaginations of the mucosa that are especially prominent in the jejunum and ileum of the human gut. The cells are polarized, their apical aspects face the lumen, and the basolateral aspects of adjacent cells are in close contact. As noted above, this is a monolayer of cells that creates a barrier against the penetration of pathogens and unsuitable gut contents. Although the epithelium is a monolayer, it is anything but monotonous. Many different, specialized cells lie in the epithelium. Enterocytes are specialized in absorbing digested nutrients from the lumen. Goblet cells secrete mucins that coat the outside of the epithelium and, among other properties, interfere with attachment of luminal microorganisms. Many lymphocytes, mostly T cells, referred to as intraepithelial lymphocytes (IEL), are interspersed among the other cells of the epithelium. The IEL are located in the basolateral spaces between the epithelial cells.

Inside the epithelium is a complex layer of the mucosa known as the lamina propria (LP). Fibroblasts and connective tissue cells are common in this layer. Capillaries, lymphatic vessels, and nerve fibers that supply the epithelium course through it. Most of the components of GALT are situated there. There are numerous

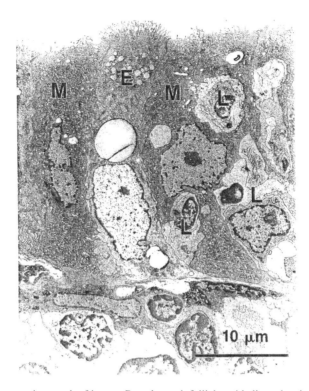

Fig. 9.1 Electron micrograph of human Peyer's patch follicle epithelium showing M cells with enfolded lymphocytes (L). Note the prominent microvilli on the surface of the enterocyte (E) and many fewer on the surface of the M cells (from T. Kato and R.L. Owen. Structure and Function of intestinal mucosal epithelium. Ch. 8 of *Mucosal Immunology*. With permission)

lymphoid follicles (LF), often with prominent germinal centers (GC). The latter are the organized foci of B lymphocytes, follicular dendritic cells (FDC), and occasional T cells. Most of the latter, however, are loosely organized, separate from the GC, in T-cell areas (interfollicular regions or IFR) where they are in association with dendritic cells (DC).

Dispersed within the mucosa of the small intestine, especially the ileum, are organized structures called Peyer's patches (PP). These resemble peripheral lymph nodes but have some unique features. Situated within the epithelium overlying PP are M (for microfold or multifenestrated) cells[2–4] (see Fig. 9.1). On the luminal aspect of these cells, the brush border (i.e., the vast number of microvilli that protrude into the lumen and create the enormous absorptive surface) is sparse, compared to that of enterocytes. That baldness favors the entrance into the M cells of antigenic material from the gut. Beneath the M cell lies an organized region called the subepithelial dome (SED). Many M cells are situated over the dome. Their membranes extend into the dome. The membranes are punctuated with infoldings called pockets. Within the pockets, lymphocytes and DC, occasionally macrophages, are situated, 2–8 cells enfolded within one pocket.

The SED is noted for its relatively high frequency of DC, of which three types have been distinguished.[5,6] In fresh preparations of tissues, the DC present in the SED are largely of the myeloid type (CD11b+). DC of the lymphoid type (CD8+) are concentrated in interfollicular regions (IFR). The third type lacks both CD11b and CD8a, is termed *double negative*, and is distributed both in the SED and IFR. In the process of characterizing the DC, it was demonstrated[6,7] that cells of the epithelium overlying the SED (the follicle-associated epithelium or FAE) express substantial amounts of two chemokines, CCL20 (MIP-3α) and CCL9 (MIP-1γ). The CD11b+ DC located in the SED were found to display receptors for both chemokines, viz., CCR6 for CCL20 and CCR1 for CCL9. On the other hand, the chemokine CCL19 (MIP-3β) was adduced to be present in the IFR where it attracts CD8α+ DC. It was reasoned that the CD11b+ DC undergo maturation in the SED and as they do, they express CCR7, the receptor for CCL19. They then "migrate" into the IFR.

The intestinal epithelium facing the lumen is not a smooth surface; rather it may be described as corrugated. It consists of alternating protrusions into the lumen, known as the *villi and pits* (crypts), which protrude into the lamina propria. The villi are lined with epithelial cells, most of them decorated with numerous, fingerlike protrusions of their apical membranes, collectively comprising the brush border.[8] The consequence of such corrugation is an enormous increase in surface area that is available for absorption of nutrients produced by digestion of foodstuffs. In addition, the number and variety of ecological habitats for commensal microbiota are vastly increased. The morphology of the villi varies considerably in different regions of the GI tract, reflecting the variety of functions dominating each region.

The Peyer's patches, as noted, are located within the lamina propria and may bulge into the submucosa. In addition to the T cells located in the IFR and to a limited extent in the SED, there are small congregations of T cells scattered along the lamina propria. Within the SED of the PPs, CD3+ and CD4+ T cells are present but not CD8+ T cells.[5] Both CD4+ and CD8+ cells are present in the IFR. B cells and macrophages are scarce in the SED, but B cells and FDC congregate in the lymphoid follicles and GC.

Closely associated with, but outside, the intestine are the mesenteric lymph nodes (MLN). Their organization and function appear to be typical of lymph nodes. However, unlike peripheral lymph nodes, the MLN receive the lymphatic drainage from the Peyer's patches. Any luminal microorganisms (commensal or potential pathogen) that traverse the FAE are collected in the MLN. The latter act "as a firewall to prevent live commensal intestinal bacteria from penetrating the systemic immune system."[9]

Intestinal Microbiota

The human gut is populated with as many as 100 trillion cells, whose collective genome, the microbiome, is a reflection of evolutionary selected pressures acting at the level of the host and at the level of the microbial cell. The ecological rules that govern the shape of microbial diversity in the gut apply to mutualists and pathogens alike.

RE Ley, DA Peterson, JI Gordon[10]

Table 9.1 The normal gastrointestinal flora of human

Total bacterial count	Stomach $0–10^3$	Jejunum $0–10^5$	Ileum $10^3–10^7$	Feces $10^{10}–10^{12}$
Aerobic or facultative				
Anaerobic bacteria				
Enterobacteria	$0–10^2$	$0–10^3$	$10^2–10^6$	$10^4–10^{10}$
Streptococci	$0–10^3$	$0–10^4$	$10^2–10^6$	$10^5–10^{10}$
Staphylococci	$0–10^2$	$0–10^3$	$10^2–10^5$	$10^4–10^7$
Lactobacilli	$0–10^3$	$0–10^4$	$10^2–10^5$	$10^6–10^{10}$
Fungi	$0–10^2$	$0–10^2$	$10^2–10^3$	$10^2–10^6$
Anaerobic bacteria				
Bacteroides	Rare	$0–10^2$	$10^3–10^7$	$10^{10}–10^{12}$
Bifidobacteria	Rare	$0–10^3$	$10^3–10^5$	$10^8–10^{12}$
Gram-positive cocci[a]	Rare	$0–10^3$	$10^2–10^5$	$10^8–10^{11}$
Clostridia	Rare	Rare	$10^2–10^4$	$10^6–10^{11}$
Eubacteria	Rare	Rare	Rare	$10^9–10^{12}$

From Ref. 11
[a]Includes Peptostreptococcus and Peptococcus

The distribution of bacteria in the major compartments of the gut is markedly uneven[11] (Table 9.1). The majority is present in the colon. In contrast to those in the stomach and small intestine, bacteria that thrive in the colon are anaerobes, generally Gram negative. The identification of the bacteria that colonize the gut is a difficult pursuit, partly because of the great variety, and partly because more than half of them cannot be cultured by conventional techniques. Nevertheless, it can be argued that given the vast variety of bacteria on earth, it is an exclusive group that inhabits the human intestine.[10] That exclusivity is taken to mean that microorganisms and mammals have co-evolved, reflecting the interdependence of microbes and humans for survival.[10]

The presence of endogenous, intestinal microbiota is of critical importance to the host (human or animals). The list of beneficial functions currently known includes processing of nutrients, facilitating intestinal angiogenesis, stimulating development of the GALT, participating in establishment of oral tolerance, preparing for gut mucosal immunity, and early (preimmune) diversification of the antibody specificity repertoire.

Prior to birth, the intestinal tract of the fetus is sterile. If it remains sterile in the neonate – as can be achieved experimentally – the GALT remains significantly underdeveloped.[12,13] Introduction of a single species of bacterium into the sterile ("germ-free" or GF) animal results in substantial improvement in the development of the GALT but still not equal to that of conventional (CVN) animals. The issue of the numbers and types of commensal microorganisms that are capable of provoking conventional development of GALT remains unresolved, and the index used to judge conventionalization may influence the conclusions drawn. Studies performed with GF mice are informative.[14] When judged by the number of IgA+ plasmablasts present in the duodenum of GF mice following infection, *Bacteroides* or *Escherichia* spp. were superior to a variety of other types of bacteria. Simultaneous exposure to four different types of gut bacteria produced within a few weeks a population of IgA plasma cells in the lamina propria close to the number in similar-aged CVN mice. Infections of GF mice with single commensals generally result in the slow, gradual development of IgA plasma cells in the lamina propria that attains only a fraction of the number present in CVN mice.

As noted above, it is assumed that the present condition of mutualism of a mammal and its commensal, intestinal microorganisms is an illustration of co-evolution. Which bacteria were the earliest to establish co-survival with humans? At present, there is little insight. That is not surprising given that there are more than 400 distinct species in the human gut and ways of culturing the majority of them remain to be discovered. However, there is one candidate type of bacterium that might have been an early commensal. The story is told in fascinating fashion by Cebra et al.[13] Joseph Leidy in 1849[15] described a dominant type of segmented filamentous bacterium that he found in the midgut of termites (Phylum Arthropoda, Class Insecta). Similar organisms have been found in chickens, rats, mice and are now described as Gram-positive, segmented, obligate anaerobes. Injection of segmented, filamentous bacteria into GF mice resulted in potent stimulation of the development of the state of intestinal IgA natural immunity.[13] A similar study produced results that led to the same conclusion.[16]

In the preceding section, emphasis was placed on the role of the intestinal epithelium as an essential barrier that separates the organism, including the GALT, from the microbiota of the intestinal lumen. However, there are events that involve penetration of the barrier: some beneficial, others detrimental. For example, in order for bacteria (introduced *per os* or intragastric) to stimulate development of the immature GALT in GF animals, presumably they must traverse the intestinal barrier. Similarly, luminal bacteria or their components probably traverse the barrier to stimulate the GALT in order to achieve physiological equilibrium (homeostasis) between the commensal population and the GALT. To generate protective immunity against pathogens that invade the gut, the pathogens or some immunogenic components must cross the barrier. Establishment of tolerance to antigenic materials introduced via the gut (see later) requires that the antigens reach the GALT by traversing the barrier. All the preceding events are beneficial. They involve the regulated transcytosis of bacteria, or foodstuff, or antigenic fragments/components across the intestinal epithelium via the M cells. The attachment of bacteria or antigenic materials to the apical aspect of the M cells may involve lectins or integrins. Recent evidence[17] has implicated Toll-like receptor (TLR) 4 along with platelet-activating factor receptor (PAF-R) and $\alpha_5\beta_1$ integrin in transcytosis of wild-type and several mutants of *Hemophilus influenzae*. The investigators concluded that their data and data from a small number of other studies "suggest that pathogen-associated molecular pattern (PAMP) interactions with pattern recognition receptors (PRRs) are key factors in M-cell recognition of intestinal antigens for mucosal immune priming."[17]

Once inside the M cell and presumably enclosed in vesicles, the organism or antigen is believed to be conducted to antigen processing cells (APC) (macrophages, DC) situated in the M-cell pocket(s). Individual pockets may have APC and

Color Plates

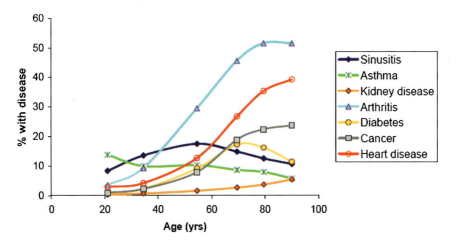

Chapter 1 Figure 1. Prevalence of selected chronic conditions, expressed in percentages, as a function of age for the US population (2002–2003 dataset). (Source: National Center for Health Statistics Data Warehouse on Trends in Health and Aging. Courtesy and permission from Dr João Pedro de Magalhães. http://www.senescence.info/definitions.html)[48]

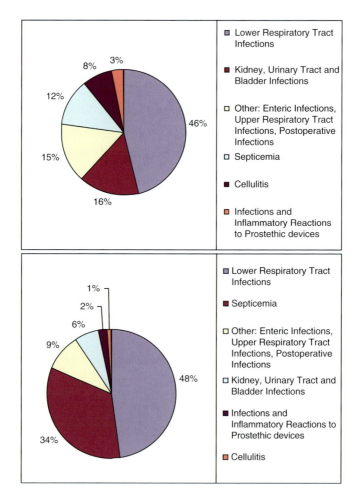

Chapter 1 Figure 2. Death by underlying or multiple cause, expressed in rates per 100,000 people, as a function of age for the 2001 US population aged 85 and older (Source: http://www.cdc.gov/nchs/nhcs.htm.National Center for Health Statistics Data Warehouse on Trends in Health and Aging. Courtesy and permission from Dr João Pedro de Magalhães. http://www.senescence.info/definitions.html)[48]

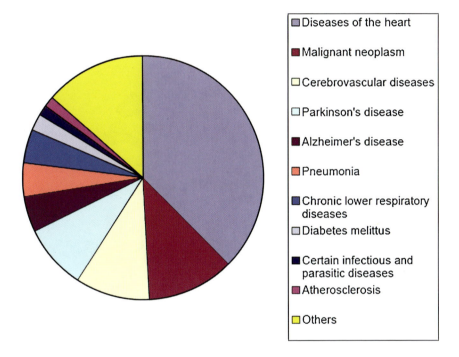

Chapter 3 Figure 1. Proportion of infectious disease hospitalizations (**a**) and infectious disease-related deaths (**b**) according to infectious disease group among patients 65 years or older in the United States from 2000 through 2002 (adapted from Ref. 1)

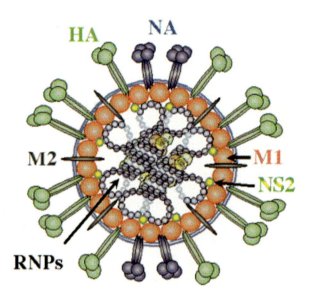

Chapter 6 Figure 1. Schematic structure presentation of an Influenza virus particle. (Courtesy of Dr. Paul Digard, Pathology Department, University of Cambridge.) The outer surface consists of a lipid envelope consisting of glycoprotein spikes of two types, hemagglutinin (HA) and neuraminidase (NA). The inner side of the envelope is lined by the matrix protein and the genome segments are packaged into the ribonucleoprotein (RNP) core

T cells together and (rarely) B cells that evince the memory phenotype.[18] However, as judged by events in the M cells following introduction of commensal bacteria into GF animals, immature DC predominate in the M-cell pockets, at least for a time, following uptake of immunogen.[19]

The M cells ingest bacteria and other particulate matter in a phagocytic fashion.[20,21] Viruses present in the lumen may be incorporated into M cells by endocytosis, involving clathrin-coated vesicles.[22] HIV-1 can be transcytosed via M cells located in tonsils and rectal epithelia.[23] Binding of the virus to the apical surface of the M cell is facilitated by the chemokine receptor, CCR5. Other small, nonadherent particulates enter by endocytosis.[24] Precisely what happens to these internalized substances is uncertain. They may be degraded in phagolysosomes or otherwise "processed" and delivered to professional APC situated in the M-cell pockets. Some investigators have suggested that M cells may be capable of processing and presenting antigenic material.[25,26]

Commensal microorganisms penetrate the intestinal epithelial barrier via the M cells with regularity in order to maintain the homeostatic truce between the microorganisms and the GALT. However, those transcytosed organisms or their constituents never get past the MLN and therefore never stimulate the systemic immune system. This is an element of the phenomenon of tolerance as discussed later. But what about potentially pathogenic organisms? There are numerous examples of pathogenic bacteria that penetrate the barrier via M cells. Infections with *Salmonella*,[26]*Shigella*,[27] and *Yersinia*[28] have been shown to target the M cells, resulting in a breach of the intestinal barrier. Studies with other organisms such as the R36a variant of *Streptococcus pneumoniae* have shown transcytosis of the microorganism without destruction of the barrier.[29] Indeed, the presence of *S. pneumoniae* R36a enhanced the transcytosis of microspheres employed as test material. The facilitated uptake stimulated by the bacterium appeared to result from increased activity per M cell as well as increased numbers of M cells in the FAE.[30,31] Thus, some bacteria may be able to amplify their own uptake. Whether or not an increase in numbers of M cells may be triggered by certain types of bacteria is an issue that requires further study. Pre-existing dormant or immature M cells may be stimulated to complete their maturation or morphogenesis. An alternative explanation, currently under debate, is whether or not enterocytes may convert to M cells under the influence of bacterial stimulation.

There are other, nondestructive pathways of transport of antigenic materials from lumen to GALT. For example, there are several reports of transport of peptides, even proteins, by enterocytes.[32] The latter might be able to function as APC although that is doubtful. They do express major histocompatibility complex (MHC) class I and class II surface molecules and class I-related CD1d molecules as well.

A second antigen-transport pathway that is attracting attention is the well-documented sampling of the intestinal lumen by subepithelial DC. A recent, trenchant report[33] revealed the nonuniform distribution of DC along the small intestine. DC displaying extensions into the lumen were found in the proximal jejunum of the conventional mouse but relatively few in the terminal ileum.

Following the introduction of *Salmonella* into the gut, the number of DC increased markedly in the terminal ileum, a response that was dependent on MyD88-TLR signaling. The extensions of the DC through the epithelial barrier and into the lumen frequently terminated in a balloonlike structure which was capable of engulfing bacteria.

The impenetrability of the intestinal epithelium is achieved by the force with which adjacent cells adhere to each other (see Ref. [34] for a review). Adherence of the epithelial cells is a function primarily of tight junctions (TJs) and adherens junctions (AJs). TJs are said to "seal neighboring cells together in an epithelial sheet to prevent leakage of molecules between them" and AJs are described as joining "an actin bundle in one cell to a similar bundle in a neighboring cell."[8] The following brief discussion will deal with TJs.

Knowledge about TJs has advanced rapidly in recent years.[35,36] In the case of intestinal epithelial cells, they form a continuous sheet covering the intestinal wall surrounding the lumen. Each villus and each crypt is lined with epithelial cells. The enterocytes, goblet cells, and others (but not the IEL, DC, or macrophages) in the epithelium of the villi and crypts are generated by pluripotent progenitors (stem cells) located near the bottom of the crypts. As the new progeny differentiate, they migrate upward to a site near the tip of the villus where they suffer apoptosis, are discharged, and die in the lumen. These migrating cells manage to form and maintain TJs and AJs. Each cell is surrounded by a band of TJs near its apical tip. The TJs form the barrier against entry of unsuitable materials between the cells. It is more of a selective barrier than an absolute barrier.

The TJs are formed by interaction of a number of constituent proteins: "occludins," "claudins," and "junction adhesion molecules" (JAMs) are the best known. Under high magnification, the TJ between contiguous cells appear as small foci or spots where the cells' membranes are conjoined.[8] The junctions are formed by the interactions between intermingled molecules of occludins and claudins contributed by each cell. JAM-1 contributed by apposed cells interact in a homophilic manner. Although they interact primarily with each other, JAM-1 are tethered to molecules of claudin, thereby providing additional strength to the junction. Both occludin and claudin molecules span the cell membrane four times and the carboxy and amino termini of both types of molecules are inside the cell membrane (cytosolic). This arrangement appears to be essential for their interaction with molecules of the ZO (zona occludens) proteins. There are three of the latter (ZO-1, ZO-2, ZO-3). They are members of a family of membrane-associated guanylate kinase homologs. ZO-1 and ZO-2, at any rate, behave like scaffolding proteins. Their amino-terminal regions can interact readily with occludins and claudins to form molecular clusters, while their carboxy-terminal regions interact with actin filaments thereby anchoring the TJ to the cytoskeleton.[36] The claudins are primarily responsible for recruiting ZO proteins to the forming TJs. Participation of occludin adds considerable additional strength to the junction.

As might be expected from the variety of ZO proteins (3 homologs), claudins of which there are at least 24, and JAMs (4 homologs), it appears that TJs might function as selective sites of entry into the extracellular spaces between the lateral surfaces of epithelial cells. It is known that the claudins are participants in the formation of various ion-selective pores.[36] Moreover, both occludin and claudins function in intracellular signaling.

There are several examples of viruses, bacteria, and even parasites that have adapted to use of TJ proteins to gain entry into gut tissue. Reovirus utilizes JAM-1, which results in a signal to the nucleus of the enterocyte and activation of NF-κB. The enterocyte dies by apoptosis but not before the virus has completed replication.[37] The bacterium *Clostridium perfringens* possesses an enterotoxin (CPE) that binds with high affinity to claudin-3 and claudin-4 but not to claudin-1 or claudin-2. Binding is accomplished via the carboxy-terminal half of the enterotoxin (C-CPE). When monolayers of cultured target cells (MDCK-I) were incubated with C-CPE, claudin-4 was selectively removed from TJ and degraded.[38] As a consequence, the TJ barrier of the monolayer of cells was degraded in proportion to the dose of C-CPE.

Disruption of the intestinal epithelial barrier is often observed following traumatic events such as systemic or local inflammation, surgery, physical injury, severe malnutrition, and others. When the barrier is breached, the microorganisms that escape may overwhelm the innate defenses, including GALT, and establish serious local or even systemic infections. As will be discussed later, an emerging "theory" of aging holds that the aging gut is in a perpetual state of subclinical inflammation (inflammaging) attributable to transcytosis of commensal organisms. Elevated transcytosis of luminal microorganisms is considered a pathognomonic feature of inflammatory bowel diseases (IBDs). At least some aspects of epithelial barrier disruption can be blamed on the cytokines IFN-γ and TNF-α and the effects they exert on TJs.[39–42] Studies performed in vitro with monolayers of epithelial cells (Caco-2, T84) revealed that IFN-γ treatment triggered disruption of TJs, internalization of some of the TJ components, and rearrangement of the actin cytoskeleton. The latter result involved disruption of actin interaction with myosin light chain.[40] Additional studies revealed a synergistic interaction of IFN-γ and TNF-α such that pretreatment with low, nondisruptive doses of IFN-γ primed the disruptive effects of subsequent low doses of TNF-α.[39] Similar results were obtained from studies performed in rats,[42] again suggesting that TJ disruption involves rearrangement of the enterocyte cytoskeleton. More details concerning the precise mechanisms of enterocyte ingestion of TJ components and cytoskeletal rearrangement are provided in Ref. [40]

Finally, to complete this section concerned with intestinal microorganisms, the presence in the gut of a variety of antimicrobial substances should be mentioned. This topic will be developed more fully in the section "oral Tolerance" which deals with innate immunity. Within the intestinal crypts of the duodenum, jejunum, and ileum, there are specialized epithelial cells known as *Paneth cells*. They are one of four principal derivatives of the pluripotential stem cells located at the bottom of the crypts. Various studies with mouse and/or human tissues have revealed that Paneth cells produce several antimicrobial proteins or peptides including several members of the α-defensin family (called "cryptdins" in the case of mice) (reviewed in Ref. 43). In the case of humans, six α-defensins have been discovered;

two are associated with Paneth cells and the other four are found in neutrophils. No leukocyte α-defensins have been identified in mice.

A second major family, the β-defensins, are not restricted to Paneth cells; rather, they are expressed by most epithelial cells of the small and large intestine. A relatively wide variety of β-defensins is known and they are widely expressed among mucosal epithelial surfaces. The expression of both α- and β-defensins at intestinal mucosal surfaces may be markedly enhanced by infection and inflammatory disorders.

Defensins are synthesized as prepropeptides and are then processed to yield the mature, active peptides. The latter are small, comprising 29–45 amino acid residues. Their lethal effects on bacteria are exerted on the surface membranes.

The production, characteristics, distribution, and actions of microbicidal proteins and peptides will be discussed in more detail in the section "oral Tolerance".

Oral Tolerance

When rodents are provided a protein antigen by the oral route (feeding or intragastric deposition) they are rendered unable to respond to the same antigen given by a parenteral route.[44] That unresponsive state is termed "oral tolerance" (OT). Also, antigen provided intranasally can induce systemic unresponsiveness to the same antigen.[45] OT has been demonstrated in several monogastric mammals as well as in humans.[46]

The gradual elucidation of OT has generated considerable interest and excitement, which is likely to continue for some time. There are at least three prominent reasons for the excitement. First, OT suggests an explanation for the fact that, in good health, humans live peacefully with their enteric microorganisms. Under abnormal conditions, those same microorganisms can induce severe, immune-mediated inflammation as occurs in inflammatory bowel disorders. Second, OT provides deep insight into the mechanisms that control autoimmune disorders and the prospects for successful clinical intervention in those disorders. Third, OT reveals how hypersensitivity (allergic) reactions to ingested food constituents are normally avoided. Experimental animal models in which OT has been prevented are extremely useful for studying mechanisms of allergic disorders.

Exposing the detailed mechanisms of OT has been the pursuit of a number of talented investigators. To understand some of the recent work, we should begin by recounting some of the established, accepted findings. It is important to emphasize that the precise anatomy of the GALT facilitates the establishment of OT. That has been explained clearly in a recent commentary[47] (see Fig. 9.2). The MLN occupy a pivotal position. Owing to the afferent lymphatic drainage of the intestinal epithelium and PP, nearly every prospective antigen is screened in the MLN. For example, DC carrying potentially antigenic components of commensal microbes are sequestered by the MLN and never reach systemic tissues where they might trigger immune responses. The situation appears to be similar for putative antigenic

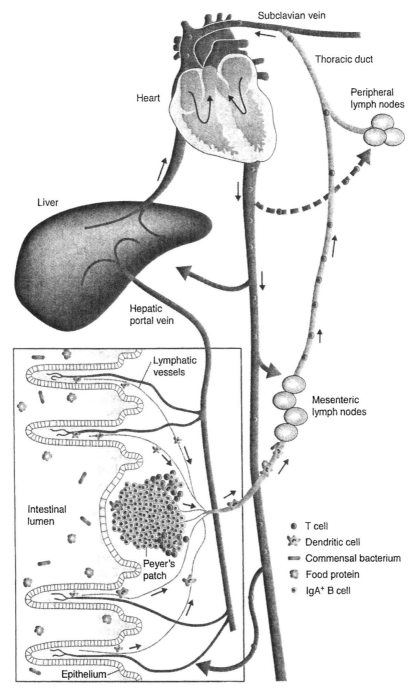

Fig. 9.2 Diagram of the lymphatic and blood vessels that serve the GALT with emphasis on the lymphatic connection between Peyer's patch and mesenteric lymph node (from Ref. 9 with permission)

components of food, although it is at least possible for such components to enter the bloodstream directly via venules of the hepatic portal vein. This pivotal function of the MLN is the reason they have been called a "firewall."[47]

Questions that have disturbed investigators for some time are concerned with routes of antigen administration, antigen dosage and distribution, quality of antigens, and the sites where tolerance originates and is manifested. Several of the established, accepted answers to questions regarding antigen and OT were discussed in a masterful review[48] and are simply summarized here. Feeding or intragastric administration of protein antigens severely restricts subsequent systemic or mucosal immune response even when subsequently the antigen is given with adjuvant (cholera toxin B subunit in the case of oral challenge or complete Freund's adjuvant in the case of parenteral challenge). However, in the absence of prior oral exposure, antigen given with adjuvant via the oral route elicits both mucosal and systemic immunity. Parenteral immunization with protein antigens elicits systemic but not mucosal immunity.[49] Orally administered antigen leads to significantly reduced cell-mediated immunity including delayed-type hypersensitivity.[48,50,51] The dose of oral antigen influences the characteristics of OT,[52,53] especially with repect to the mechanism that produces tolerance (see below).

Questions regarding the distribution of orally administered antigen relate to the sites of tolerance induction and persistence. Recent work[54] has resulted in partial clarification of the uncertainties. The results of several studies[55,56] led to the view that orally fed antigen induced tolerance concurrently both in the intestinal mucosa and peripheral sites. The reason was that antigen-activated, specific T cells could be demonstrated in various peripheral locations. Either antigens or antigen-bearing DC were reaching those peripheral sites, or T cells were migrating to peripheral locations after being primed in the GALT.

In order to determine whether or not the GALT is the locus of tolerance induction, a series of experiments were performed[54] in mice treated with the agent FTY720. The latter prevents the emergence of lymphocytes from lymphoid tissues into efferent lymphatics.[55] When those mice were provided oral antigen, there was no appearance of activated antigen-specific T cells in spleen or peripheral lymph nodes; and yet durable tolerance was established. Antigen-specific T-cell proliferation in the PP and MLN was unaffected by the FTY720. Clearly, GALT is the locus of OT induction. Additional experiments established that the MLN, rather than PP, are the key sites. The final set of experiments demonstrated that the proliferation of antigen-specific T cells in the MLN is effected by transport of the orally administered antigen (or antigen fragments) from the LP to the MLN. In mice lacking the chemokine receptor CCR7, giving antigen orally induced neither antigen-specific T-cell proliferation in the MLN or the induction of OT.

This recent demonstration that the MLN, not the PP, are the setting of OT confirms the findings of several other groups of investigators.[56–58] Moreover, the finding that CCR7 is required in the MLN, both for specific T-cell proliferation and OT, complements and extends previous work, all of which allows a view – although a clouded one – of what may underlie the emergence of OT. It has been established[59] that the SED of PP is an area populated by DC that appear to be immature.

When they mature after encountering antigen that has passed through the M cells, they express CCR7 and migrate to the IFR under the influence of CCL19 (MIP-3β). Although more evidence is required, it may be supposed that some of those DC, now activated and mature, continue the journey to the MLN. It is interesting to note that (a) estimates from studies in rats indicate that there are some 7–24 million DC in the small intestine of which approximately 8×10^5 normally migrate to the MLN every day[60] and (b) CCR7+ DC found in the MLN that had emigrated from the LP were characteristically vacuolated with vacuoles containing debris although the DC in the MLN are relatively inactive phagocytes.[61] There appears to be an active flow of DC charged with ingested immunogenic material from the PP to the MLN. It is important to mention that OT can be induced with much lower doses of antigen in mice that have been treated with flt3 ligand.[62] Treatment with the latter causes a substantial increase in the number of DC in the gut as well as in the spleen and elsewhere. The substantial increase in GALT DC allows OT to be induced with low doses of antigen that have no effect in normal animals.

The LP, PP, and MLN all contain typical T cells, both CD4+ and CD8+. In addition, there are substantial numbers of intraepithelial T cells, many of which are the γ/δ T cells that play an important role in establishing and maintaining the epithelial barrier.[62] Given the presence of diversified CD4+ T cells, antigen-laden DC, and a conducive microenvironment, conditions are suitable for development of regulatory T cells (Treg) that are instrumental in the creation of OT.

At least three types of T cell-mediated tolerance can be distinguished: central, peripheral, and oral. Treg play important roles in all three types. Each type has some unique aspects but there are aspects that are common to all. Central tolerance develops in the thymus, and pertains primarily to self-antigens and restriction of the potential for autoimmune disorders. It involves, in part, deletion of self-reactive clones of T cells when their receptors (TCR) react with cognate peptide-class II MHC complexes with high affinity. Most of the T cells involved (CD4+ or CD8+, double-positives to some extent) die by apoptosis (negative selection). Some, however, escape death and become Treg (sometimes designated c Treg, "c" for central) and are released to the periphery.

Another mechanism of T-cell negative selection occurs in the periphery (peripheral tolerance). This involves elimination of potentially self-reactive T cells that, for one reason or another, have escaped deletion in the thymus. Those cells circulate in the periphery and, upon encountering an APC offering the cognate peptide, interact but receive low co-stimulation from the APC (e.g., via B7 molecules). Lacking sufficient stimulation, they die of apoptosis.

Peripheral tolerance can be induced by parenteral administration of antigens under conditions that are not conducive to immune responses: for example, by solutions of proteins (lacking particulate matter) given without adjuvants. High doses and repeated injections are usually required. Attempts to induce peripheral tolerance to particulate antigens seldom succeed. Once established, peripheral tolerance to a given test antigen does not extend to the GALT.

Recall that feeding protein antigens or intragastric deposition leads to OT. A relatively short time (24 h or less) is required for the establishment of OT, and once established the tolerant state extends to the periphery. The same antigen, even when given orally together with the adjuvant, cholera toxin subunit B (CT-B), will not break the tolerant state.

Quantities of soluble protein in the milligram range will induce OT when given alone intragastrically. When given together with the adjuvant CT-B to untreated animals, vigorous immune responses to the antigen ensue. If the antigen is covalently linked to CT-B, OT can be induced with doses of antigen in the microgram range.[63] Giving antigen either way, separate or coupled to CD-B, leads to the same result; Treg appear in concert with establishment of tolerance. OT is effected by way of induced Treg that produce immunomodulatory cytokines: for example, Tr1 cells that secrete IL-10[64,65] and Th3 cells that secrete TGF-β.[66] The regulatory cells that have been most widely studied are those that express CD25. Treg that are CD25 + CD4+ may produce either IL-10 or TGF-β or both. However, CD25 is an unstable marker.[67] Another molecule, Foxp3, has been shown to be associated reliably with CD25+ CD4+ Treg.[68] Foxp3 was discovered as a result of a mutation in the *scurfin* gene, the murine ortholog of Foxp3, that results in a lethal autoimmune disorder in mice owing to severe depletion of CD25+ CD4+ Treg.[69–71]

CD25− CD4+ cells do not express Foxp3 and are not immunosuppressive. There is now abundant evidence that exposure to TGF-β, either in vitro [68,72] or in vivo [64,72,73] can induce naïve, CD25− CD4+ cells to convert to CD25+ CD4+ Treg. Moreover, mutant mice lacking a functional *tgfb1* gene develop lethal disease characterized by massive T-cell proliferation, extensive immunopathology, and activation of both Th1 and Th2 cells.[73] Transfer into those mice of Foxp3+ Treg inhibited differentiation of Th1 cells but promoted emergence of Th17 cells.[73] The latter are CD4+ (possibly CD8+)[74] cells that secrete IL-17, IL-6, and TNF-α. They are considered to be intimately involved in the onset of autoimmune disorders such as rheumatoid arthritis and multiple sclerosis.[75] Thus, TGF-β promotes development of Treg; but TGF-β along with IL-6 facilitates appearance of Th 17 cells.[75]

It is worthwhile to attempt a synthesis of the recent findings and to produce a sketch of the mechanism of Treg suppression of mucosal and peripheral immunity. When antigen is given orally, that which survives and reaches the jejunum and ileum may, in small amounts, traverse the epithelial barrier by transport into M cells and/or capture by DC extensions into the lumen. When antigen is given as an attachment to CT-B, the immunogenic potency of that which traverses the epithelium is enhanced, leading the tolerant state. The oral administration of whole cholera toxin will disrupt even the durable tolerant state.[65] It seems an oversight that so little attention has been given to the mechanism of CT-B adjuvanticity. What it might do vis-à-vis the intestinal epithelium could involve TGF-β. All three isoforms of TGF-β (1, 2, 3) are coexpressed in the epithelium of the mouse small intestine and colon.[76]

Antigen that traverses the follicle-associated epithelium (FAE) is picked up by the immature DC that reside in the SED (CD11b+ CD8α−) and express CCR6. Those Cd11b+ DC that express CCR6 are attracted to the SED by the CCL20, which is expressed by cells of the FAE.[77] Several substances including bacterial flagellin are able to induce CCL20 expression by the FAE. As the DC mature, they express CCR7 and migrate to the IFR. From there they migrate into the MLN via afferent lymph. What occurs within the MLN can be inferred from the results of studies in vitro, using epithelial cell monolayers, and in vivo, by use of TCR transgenic T cells. The interactions between entering DC, which now are mature APC, and naïve T cells within the interfollicular regions of the MLN generate CD25 + CD4+ Treg. TGF-β promotes the activation of the transcription factor Foxp3. The CD25+ CD4+ Treg suppress the functions of other T cells both by cell–cell contact and by secreting additional TGF-β and IL-10. Naïve CD4+ and CD8+ T cells are rendered anergic; they are unable to respond to cognate antigen or to stimulation via CD3. Upon optimum stimulation and costimulation, they neither proliferate nor secrete cytokines.

Exactly how the induction of OT in the GALT renders inactive the responses of peripheral tissues, spleen, and lymph nodes remains unresolved. Possibly, Treg and DC from the MLN infiltrate peripheral lymphoid tissues and exert their tolerizing influence. However, there are compelling findings that suggest that antigen is distributed from the LP not only to PP and MLN but to peripheral locales as well.[54,78] For example, after oral antigen, TCR transgenic T cells are found to be activated and proliferating concurrently in the MLN and spleen. Once tolerized, however, the transgenic T cells are unable to respond to antigen, or provide help to cognate B cells.

The description of the induction of tolerance provided in the preceding paragraphs pertains to rodents. Tolerance induced in humans and probably other mammals differs somewhat in that immunosuppressive Treg display CD25 and CD4, and also MHC class II molecules.[79] Thus, Treg in humans can be identified as CD25+ CD4+ DR+ and are also typified by expression of Foxp3. T cells of mice lack Class II molecules because they cannot transcribe CIITA which is necessary for Class II expression.[80]

Mechanisms of Innate Intestinal Immunity

A few years ago, writing a section on innate intestinal immunity would have been a short and simple task. It would have been impossible to draft even a few sentences concerned with aging of innate intestinal immunity. As will become evident, there is now considerable information about innate elements of gut immunity. However, there remains a dearth of insight regarding the effects of aging on those innate elements.

Toll-Like Receptors

One of the major recent advances in knowledge concerning innate immunity in general, not only that of the intestine, is the discovery and analysis of the Toll-like receptors (TLRs).[81,82] The TLRs are present on MP and DC consonant with their key role in the recognition of bacterial and viral pathogens. TLRs are present also on intestinal epithelial cells, both M cells and enterocytes, where they recognize

Table 9.2 Well-known Toll-like receptors and their ligands

TLR number (s)	Ligands	Human, mouse, or both
2/1	Bacterial lipoproteins	Both
2/6	Bacterial lipoproteins	Both
	Lipoteichoic acid	
	Yeast cell wall mannans	
2	GPI anchors	Both
	Bacterial porins	
3	ds RNA	Both
4	LPS, HSPs,	Both
	Some viral proteins	
5	Bacterial flagellin	Both
7	ss RNA (viral)	Both
8	ss RNA (viral)	Both
9	CpG containing DNA	Both

commensal organisms.[83–85] There are 13 known TLRs, each of them broadly specific for compound molecules present at the surface of viruses, bacteria, fungi, and parasites. A listing of TLRs and their ligands (if known) is provided in Table 9.2. Inspection of the list of ligands indicates that the TLRs recognize components of microorganisms rather than precise moieties. For that reason, the TLRs are called "pattern recognition receptors" (PRR) and collectively their ligands are termed "pathogen-associated molecular patterns" (PAMP).

There are excellent examples of the consequences of engagement of different TLRs on DC or MP. For example, association of bacterial lipoproteins with TLR-1 and TLR-2 (heterodimers) on myeloid DC triggers release of IL-10 but little IL-12. Immature CD4+ T cells are directed along the Th2 or Treg pathways. Conversely, occupancy of DC TLR-4 by bacterial lipopolysaccharide (LPS) or heat shock proteins (HSP 60/70) evinces secretion of IL-12p70 and IFN-α. Immature CD4+ T cells then mature along the Th1 pathway. Stimulation of DC or MP through TLR-4 offers a good example of the consequences of being dependent on the types of auxiliary (adaptor) proteins that associate with the TLR–ligand complex. If the signaling involves the adaptor MyD88, the DC or MP generates proinflammatory cytokines IL-12, IL-6, and TNF. The result includes attraction of microbicidal cells (neutrophils and others) to the location of the offensive pathogen. On the other hand, signal transmission via adaptor TRIF results in output of type 1 interferons, an antiviral response.

While the majority of TLRs appear to be expressed on the surface of DC or MP, at least two, TLR-7 and TLR-9, are located internally. The ligand for TLR-7 is a single-stranded RNA that is rich in G and U nucleotides often found in viruses. TLR-9 interacts best with CpG-rich DNA, also frequently found in viruses. The two types of receptors are located within intracellular endosomal vesicles. In that location, they have ready access to viral nucleic acids because many viruses enter host cells by way of endosomes.

The TLRs are considered to be phylogenetically ancient. TLR-7 and TLR-9 exemplify the conservation of receptors that are of great utility and their appropriation by modern mammals. They also reveal what a fine line separates protective innate immunity from destructive autoimmunity. Mammalian DNA and RNA can engage TLR-9 and TLR-7, respectively; however, they do so with much less avidity than the viral nucleic acids. Mammalian DNA, unlike prokaryotic DNA, contains CpG that are largely methylated. Similarly, many of the G/U nucleotides in eukaryotic RNA are methylated. Those molecular differences and other findings of a genetic nature[86] largely explain why autoimmune disorders such as lupus erythematosus are relatively rare. But the potential exists and could be manifested via the TLRs.

As noted, TLRs are present on cells of the intestinal epithelium.[83–85] TLR-2 is expressed by cells both in the FAE and the villus epithelium (VE). The introduction of ligands (e.g., peptidoglycan) into the intestinal lumen was seen to cause the rearrangement of TLR-2 on cells of the FAE but not the VE.[85] The M cells of the FAE were enhanced in their ability to transport indicator microparticles. Of particular interest was the movement of subepithelial DC into the FAE in response to TLR-2 activation. Similar events occurred in response to luminal LPS, suggesting TLR-4 stimulation.[85]

A detailed study of TLR-4 in intestinal epithelium revealed that PAF-R and $\alpha_5\beta_1$ integrin, in addition to TLR-4, are present on M cells.[87] TLR-4 is present on M cells in apical location but not on VE cells. PAF-R is equally distributed on M cells and VE cells. Both M and VE cells were capable of Gram-negative bacteria uptake but only M cells were capable of translocating bacteria. An important role of M cell-associated $\alpha_5\beta_1$ integrin in the translocation of bacteria was demonstrated. Recent evidence that TLR-4 present on enterocytes promotes binding and internalization of LPS[83,87] kindled interest in a study of enterocyte internalization and translocation of Gram-negative bacteria.[88] It was concluded that the translocation of bacteria involved a process of phagocytosis that did not include typical membrane ruffling and macropinocytosis. However, the types of cells that engaged in the postulated "novel" process of phagocytosis were not precisely identified; they may have been M cells or DC or MP.

Although TLR-2, TLR-4, TLR-5, and TLR-9 have been reported to be present in intestinal epithelium, attention has been given to TLR-4, as it, in particular, appears to play a significant role in experimental colitis.[89] A study performed in TLR-4 knockout mice (TLR-4−/−) revealed a severe deficiency in mobilization of inflammatory cells (MP, neutrophils) and in the release of chemokines. Live bacteria could be cultured from mesenteric lymph nodes. The onset of colitis was quicker and more severe than in control (TLR-4+/+) mice. Similar results obtained in MyD88−/− mice indicated that the signal from TLR-4 was transduced via the MyD88 pathway leading to elaboration of proinflammatory cytokines such as TNF and IL-1.

In addition to TLR-7 and TLR-9, there are other intracellular bacterial detectors of which the nucleotide oligomerization domain (NOD) family proteins are well known. There are three prominent members of the NOD family: NOD1, NOD2, and cryopyrin. All three recognize components of bacterial peptidoglycans. NOD1 is particularly suited for detecting components of Gram-negative bacteria, while

NOD2 and cryopyrin are sensitized by components of both Gram-positive and - negative bacteria (especially those that include muramyl dipeptide). Signaling initiated by occupancy of any of the three results in production of inflammatory cytokines. The cellular distribution of NOD1 is broad and includes intestinal epithelial cells. NOD2 is more restricted to MP, DC, and PC located in the intestinal crypts, where it is involved in activating production of α-defensins.

Microbicidal Peptides and Proteins

Some persons have considered the huge population of commensal organisms in the gut to be equivalent to a host organ. In some respects, that seems a reasonable idea. The problem with the idea is that the commensal population is pathogenic. The state of mutualism is one in which each partner derives benefit from the existence of the other; nevertheless, it is a state of armed truce. Early in the course of coevolution, each partner selected "weapons" with which to resist the aggressive tactics of the other. In the case of vertebrate hosts, it appears that the weapons selected were microbicidal peptides and a variety of proteins.

There is a large array of microbicidal peptides that exist in the vertebrate intestinal epithelium and in cells of myeloid origin.[90–92] The antimicrobial peptides disrupt the membranes of bacteria and fungi but ignore the membranes of self. The molecular basis of that discrimination is uncertain but probably centers around the existence of cholesterol in mammalian but not bacterial membranes.[93] Also, bacterial membranes are more highly negatively charged and may attract positively charged molecules of the antimicrobial peptides.

It is convenient to arrange the microbicidal peptides in three categories: α-defensins, β-defensins, and cathelicidins. Members of both categories of defensins are 29–35 amino acids in length and are folded in accord with three disulfide bonds into a three-stranded β-sheet structure. The cathelicidins are of similar length but differ in the manner of their folding.

It should be noted that the defensins are widely distributed among vertebrates. There appears to be a wider variety of the β- than of the α-defensins. There are differences between human and mouse defensins. The six α-defensins of the mouse are all generated by PC located near the bottoms of intestinal crypts. For that reason, the mouse α-defensins have been termed "*cryptdins*" (crypt defensins). In contrast, only two of the six human α-defensins are produced by intestinal crypts (HD-5 and HD-6). The other four (HD-1 through HD-4) are located in MP and neutrophils, especially the latter.

Human and mouse β-defensins are expressed in a variety of tissues including epithelial surfaces of the intestine, lung, trachea, and esophagus. In some sites they appear to be expressed constitutively but are inducible at other sites.[92] In the intestinal epithelium, at least some of the β-defensins are inducible by infection or by exposure to cytokines such as IL-1, IL-6, and TNF.

Defensins and corticostatins are closely related. Indeed, certain defensins may act as corticostatins. The latter antagonize the actions of ACTH. Both, defensins and corticostatins, are concentrated in leukocyte granules. In systems for studying the antagonism of ACTH, corticostatin activity is evident at concentrations in the micromolar range, whereas antibacterial activity is displayed in the millimolar range. For that reason, it has been speculated that the primary biological action of defensins could be endocrinological. However, defensins are quite abundant in neutrophils, accounting for some 5% of the neutrophil protein, which seems to confirm that they were selected for defense.

Several studies have demonstrated that certain defensins may serve as chemoattractants for DC, monocytes, or even T cells. For example, human β-defensins 1 and 2 attract immature DC and T cells that display CCR6.[94] The cathelicidin, LL-37, is chemotactic for human neutrophils, monocytes, and T cells.[95]

The elaboration of chemoattractant defensins or cathelicidins, whether by PC or myeloid cells, is considered to be an important phenomenon for controlling commensal bacteria. Moreover, the full potential of that mechanism is evident when the epithelial barrier is violated and the entrance of the commensals leads to IBD. In addition to the direct and indirect attacks of the defensins and cathelicidins on commensal organisms, yet another mechanism has emerged to control the pathological potential of these organisms. Neutrophils, in particular, respond to chemotactic peptides released by bacteria. Those peptides are small, only a few amino acids in length, and have formylated amino termini (e.g., formyl-Met-Leu-Phe) reflecting the use of N-formyl methionine by bacteria to initiate protein synthesis. When an inflammatory condition begins to develop, epithelial cells (especially in the colon and distal ileum) express a special apical receptor, hPepT1, for formylated peptides.[96,97] Entrance of those peptides into the epithelial cells triggers the release of cytokines and chemoattractants. The peptides themselves may be released into the LP at the basolateral face of the epithelial cells and by passage between the cells when the inflammation disrupts the tight junctions. The attraction exerted by the peptides may be so strong that the neutrophils follow the gradient of increasing peptide concentration right into the intestinal lumen.

To conclude this section on innate immune receptors, the C-type lectins should be mentioned. Reg 111γ is an example that is well suited for obstructing the transepithelial incursion of commensal microorganisms.[98] It is directly bactericidal toward Gram-positive organisms and reacts with peptidoglycan. Because it lacks a domain for interacting with components of the complement system, Reg 111γ of mouse and its human counterpart, HIP/PAP, are considered to be ancient, primitive forms of C-type lectins. Reg 111γ is located in the secretory granules of PC. Upon stimulation by luminal bacteria, the granules are secreted at the apical face of PC. The distribution of Reg 111γ along the intestine of the mouse is consonant with the distribution of crypts, viz., more frequent in the distal ileum following the numerical increase of intestinal microorganisms. Reg 111γ has a role in protecting the gut from invasion by commensals as suggested by (a) the substantial rise in concentration during weaning (postnatal days[17–22]) in conventional but not germ-free mice and (b) the marked increase in amount when the intestinal flora from conventional mice were introduced into germ-free recipients.

Crypts and Stem Cells

There are more than one million crypts in the small intestine of the mouse. They are located primarily in the ileum, the frequency increasing toward the junction with the colon. Normally there are few if any in the colon. There are approximately 250–300 cells per crypt.[99,100] About half of those cells are in the rapid cell cycle. Each crypt produces about 300 new cells per day which migrate to the villus tip and are sloughed into the lumen.[100]

Located near the bottom of the crypt is a group of stem cells which may vary in number per crypt but is most often 4–6. The stem cells are responsible for generating four lineages of progeny: enterocytes, goblet cells, enteroendocrine cells, and Paneth cells. Cells of three lineages are constantly migrating out of the crypt and up the villus but Paneth cells remain in the crypt at a location near the bottom.

Crypt stem cells have not attracted the attention they deserve primarily because of their inaccessibility. However, methods are being developed that will allow them to be obtained in adequate numbers. One of the key questions about stem cells has concerned their accumulation of mutations. That question has been answered in the case of mitochondrial DNA (mt DNA) of crypt stem cells.[101–103]

mt DNA is a small, self-replicating molecule present in many copies in the individual mitochondrion. Thus, there are thousands of copies of mt DNA in a single cell. The mt DNA encodes 13 essential proteins of the respiratory chain, 2 ribosomal RNA (rRNA) genes, and 22 transfer RNA (tRNA) genes which are utilized for mt protein synthesis. All other proteins of mt are encoded by nuclear genes. Mutations that occur in mt DNA can appear in all copies in a cell (termed *homoplasmy*), or a mixture of wild-type and mutated copies may be present (*heteroplasmy*). It is estimated that about 80% of the copies must be mutant before the functions of a cell are affected – such as defective oxidative phosphorylation. That is a fascinating example of physiological redundancy, which suggests that only 20% of the potential is required to maintain a normal level of function.

The results of some ingenious experiments, in which the detection and frequencies of wild-type and mutant elements of the respiratory chain were assessed, were reported recently.[101,103] Three types of crypts could be detected: those in which the mt DNA was entirely wild type, others in which the mt DNA was entirely mutant, and still others in which both wild-type and mutant mt DNA were present. Analysis of that situation showed the homoplasmic crypts resulted from clonal expansion of single stem cells that possessed either wild-type or mutant mt DNA. Heteroplasmic crypts resulted from the clonal expansion of two stem cells, one having predominantly the wild type the other predominantly mutant mt DNA. Thus, those experiments have demonstrated that mutations in the mitochondrial genome can occur in normal stem cells, which subsequently give rise to progeny that occupy the entire crypt.

Several investigators have adduced evidence that crypts can multiply by fission.[100,103,104] When they do, it appears that the daughter crypts display progeny of the same stem cell clone that dominated in the progenitor. Moreover, crypts that display a homoplasmic mutant genotype undergo repeated fission to form homo-plasmic clusters and even larger assemblages termed *patches*. In this manner, stem cell mt DNA mutations can spread in the lower intestine.

A particularly interesting finding emerged from the studies on mutations in mt DNA. It was found that mutant crypts increase with increasing age. This agrees with the observed spread of mutations in the intestine by crypt fission and congregation. The rate of mutation that occurs in mt DNA of these crypt stem cells was estimated to be approximately 5×10^{-5} per genome per day, which far exceeds that of nuclear DNA. One likely explanation for that is the proximity of the mt DNA to the generators of free radicals in mitochondria. The relationship between free radicals, mitochondria, and aging is at the forefront of theories of aging.

Adaptive Intestinal Immunity

For several reasons, some of which remain unknown, the GALT produces only IgA. The unique character of the local DC and the particular combination of cytokines and retinoic acid are partly responsible but not entirely. There are two varieties of IgA that are to some extent restricted in distribution. Most IgA present at epithelial surfaces (intestine, respiratory tract, female reproductive tract, salivary glands) is largely polymeric (pIgA), composed of two or more (usually two) complete mono-mers. Nearly all IgA of the blood is monomeric (mIgA). That is the situation in humans and mice but may differ in other mammalian species. In the case of the intestine, IgA is exclusively pIgA, reflecting its synthesis and the manner in which it is transported into the lumen. Very little of pIgA reaches the blood circulation.

In the human there are two subclasses of IgA: IgA1 and IgA2. In the mouse there is only 1, in rabbits 13.[105] However, one subclass and one constant-α gene is the usual condition. Both IgA1 and IgA2 human subclasses form multimers, generally dimers, in which two monomers associate via their constant regions and are joined by a small molecule known as the *J chain*. The complete molecules of pIgA that are secreted into the lumen of the intestine comprise two subunits of mIgA plus J chain and part of the polymeric IgA receptor (pIgAR) called the secretory component (SC). The secreted complex is termed secretory IgA (sIgA).

Antimicrobial Actions of IgA

Intestinal IgA molecules are synthesized by plasma cells located beneath the intestinal epithelium in the LP. The molecules are secreted as dimers joined by the J chains. They diffuse through the basement "membrane" and bind to the polyimmunoglobulin receptors (pIgR) that are displayed on the basolateral aspects of enterocytes.[106] The pIgA–J–R complexes are internalized and transported by endosomes to the apical faces of the enterocytes. Endosomal–apical membrane fusion occurs, and the pIgA–J–R complexes are displayed on the apical face of the enterocyte but still anchored to the enterocyte membrane via the C-terminal domain of the R. Release from the enterocyte is achieved by proteolytic cleavage near the C terminus of the R. The short C terminus remains behind, while the rest of the R, now known as SC, enters the lumen. The pIgR is adapted to accept pIgA with attached J chain but binds mIgA weakly if at all. A molecule of the pIgR is utilized for each molecule of pIgA–J complex that is transported into the intestinal lumen.[107] Therefore, the availability and efficiency of transport of the pIgR can determine the rate and amount of pIgA that reaches the surface. The availability and transport efficiency of the pIgR are determined, in part, by TLR-3 and TLR-4 on the intestinal epithelial cells.[108] It has been shown that the surface expression of pIgR is substantially elevated in response to signals transduced by dsRNA-stimulated TLR-3 or LPS-stimulated TLR-4.[108] The response to TLR-4 signaling was much lower than to TLR-3 and led to the interpretation that TLR-4 signaling induced by commensal microbiota might well be a homeostatic device.

Secretory IgA is capable of a variety of functions, not only after release at the luminal surface but during intraepithelial transport as well. During transport, the two antigen-binding sites on each mIgA are accessible and, therefore, may interact with cognate moieties that are in the enterocytes, e.g., neutralization of virions located in the same endosome in which the sIgA molecules are being transported[109,110] or, perhaps, intersection of the path of sIgA transcytosis with a pathway of virion assembly. Recycling of sIgA is known in which the M cells transport molecules back into the LP,[111] primarily into the SED of PP, where they associate with DC as well as with CD4+ T cells and B cells.[112] The small amount that is transported across the M cells (relative to the large amount that is present in the lumen) and its association with DC and CD4+ cells in the PP have suggested that this is a mechanism of limited sampling of commensal microbes for the purpose of maintaining the homeostatic condition. The receptor located on the luminal face of the enterocytes has not been characterized; it is neither the conventional FcαI (CD89) nor the sIgR.[111]

The principal functions of sIgA are the destruction of pathogens and the control of enteric commensal organisms. IgA conducts its activities in a noninflammatory manner; if it did not, the gut would be in a perpetual life-threatening, inflamed condition. The sIgA achieves its antipathogen objectives in three ways: (a) by serving as an opsonin to promote the ingestion and intracellular destruction of pathogens by phagocytes; (b) by direct neutralization as in the case of viruses and toxins; and (c) by blocking the attachment to and colonization of mucosal surfaces. It should be added that commensal organisms aid in the latter activity by occupying ecologically favorable niches and blocking their accessibility to pathogens. By preventing colonization, the latter are unable to establish biofilms that could protect the microbes from immunological destruction.[113]

Phagocytic destruction of pathogens is promoted through Fcα receptors (FcαR) on macrophages and polymorphonuclear cells (PMNs), primarily neutrophils. The binding element on sIgA involves both Cα2 and Cα3 domains. The FcαR number and activity on neutrophils are markedly enhanced by prior stimulation of the cells with TNF-α, IL-8, or GM-CSF.

The attachment of microbial pathogens and, to some extent, of commensals as well, is prevented by interaction with sIgA molecules. Compared to other Igs, a prodigious amount of IgA is synthesized in the GALT (3–5 g of sIgA per day) and transported into the lumen. As will be discussed, two types of B lymphocytes are involved in the production of intestinal IgA. One type (B1) generates progeny that produce IgA antibody of low affinity and specificity and, owing to its polyspecificity, may be the type that coats the commensal microbial population. The results may be a stabilization of the natural microbiota. The other, B2 type of cell, is the more familiar type that gives rise to progeny that produce antibodies of high specificity and affinity. This antibody eliminates pathogens in the ways already discussed, often termed "*immune exclusion*".[114]

Unlike immune complexes formed with IgG or IgM, complexes that involve IgA do not activate the complement (C) system either via the conventional or alternative pathways.[115] There is evidence that IgA–antigen complexes may suppress complement activation by complexes of IgG or IgM with antigen; thus, it has been suggested[114] that activation of IgA responses at sites of IgG- or IgM-mediated inflammation could be a method of mitigating inflammation. In any event, sIgA responses to intestinal pathogens do not trigger inflammation. That, presumably, is a fortunate selective event in the coevolution of host and intestinal commensal microorganisms.

Intraepithelial Lymphocytes

There is a myriad of different types and stages of B and T cells within the GALT.[116–119] Sorting them out and deciding what role, if any, each type may play in intestinal immune responses is a work in progress. To make matters worse, the last few years have witnessed a bewildering disclosure of the variations of DC according to specificity, function, and maturity. Some, located in the GALT, appear to be unusual compared to those in peripheral lymphoid tissues. Here we will first consider those types of T cells for which there appears to be an established role in the immunophysiology of the GALT.

Unlike the condition in peripheral lymphoid tissues, in the intestine there is a high proportion of γδ T cells, especially among the IEL. In mice 20–80% the IEL are γδ T cells; the proportion varies with the strain. In humans, an average of 30% of the IEL are γδ T cells. In the LP, the frequency is much lower, some 1–5% are of the γδ variety. According to the limited usage of the V-region genes, the specificity repertoire of these cells is quite limited. Furthermore, the dominant V gene expression varies among different tissues. For example, Vγ5 is common among dendritic epidermal T cells, Vγ6 among cells of vaginal epithelium, and Vγ7 among IEL. What are the functions of the γδ T cells located in the IEL? Much of the information has come from studies of *Listeria monocytogenes* in Vγ1 knock-out mice (Vγ1−/−) and involve the spleen. The involvement of Vγ1δ T cells in splenic immunity was studied in the absence of such cells.[120,121] It was demonstrated that the Vγ1δ T cells play no part in the direct killing of the bacteria. However, two important functions were identified, one occurring early in the course of the infection and one near the end as the infection was cured. The early wave of γδ T cells that entered the spleens on day 2 of the infected mice were active in producing cytokines that promote immune response to the bacteria (IL-4, IL-5, IL-10, IFN-γ, TNF-α). The output of those cytokines increased over the next few days preceding elimination of the infection. Cure of *L. monocytogenes*, which is an intracellular pathogen, involves destruction of the bacteria by host cells, primarily MP and neutrophils. These cells are fully activated as the infection reaches a climax, and from about day 8 onward to day 14, when the infection is cured, a sizeable population of aggressive cells becomes established. At this stage, a second wave of γδ T cells migrates into the spleen and proceeds to attack and kill those hostile MP and PMN and concurrently secrete immunosuppressants, especially TGF-β. That is how the inflammatory reaction is brought under control.

The studies of the functions of γδ T cells in *L. monocytogenes* infection provide insight into the probable actions of γδ T cells in the IEL. It is likely that they minimize inflammation that accompanies local responses to pathogens, especially responses that involve inflammatory MP, DC, or PMNs. Recently, it has been demonstrated that the γδ T cells, but few αβ T cells, of the IEL recognize and respond to selected phospholipids presented by CD1 (+) APC.[122] Because both epithelial cells and DC display CD1 surface molecules, it seems likely that they may collaborate with the γδ T cells to control inflammatory reactions triggered by phagocytic cells responding to microbial components and other noxious substances in the gut.

Possibly related to the function of γδ T cells in damping inflammation are the findings that γδ T cells are required for the establishment of OT by feeding antigen.[62,123] Data obtained from those studies led to postulate that enterocytes (which are known to display MHC class I and class II molecules) might present immunogenic peptides to neighboring γδ T cells. The latter, in response, might secrete cytokines that activate suppressor T cells (Tregs).[62]

The majority of T lymphocytes in the IEL express the CD8 α chain. Of those only some 20% express CD8 β chain. Both TCR αβ and TCR γδ cells can express CD8 αα, whereas CD8 αβ is found only in the TCRαβ cells. There is compelling evidence that T cells that display the CD8 αα homodimer are generated outside the thymus.[124] The progenitors are located in the numerous, small patches of cells (cryptopatches) distributed along the LP. Whether or not the progenitors are descendants of earlier cells that originated in the thymus has not been decided.

The local interactions in the epithelium between the CD8 αα (+) IEL and the epithelial cells (EC) have important consequences. As noted, EC display TLRs, and commensal microorganisms (as well as pathogens) produce agonists that can trigger signaling within the EC. Transduction of the signal along the MyD88 pathway results in release of IL-15. Only a few types of cells, including mono-cytes/macrophages and EC, can produce IL-15. The results of a recent, trenchant investigation revealed that the presence of IL-15 is essential for the maintenance of the CD8αα+ T cells, either TCRαβ (+) or TCRγδ (+).[125] An earlier study showed a similar requirement for IL-15 in the development of the IEL CD8αα subsets.[126] The authors of the recent report[125] concluded that the proper maintenance of the CD8 αα (+) IEL is required for intestinal epithelial homeostasis.

Nestled among the IEC are the T cells a high proportion of which are CD8 αα (+) and may have an extrathymic origin. These T cells include many that possess self-reactive TCR.[127,128] Moreover, those cells are not like thymus-derived T cells, most of which are naïve and in a resting state. Rather, they are considered to be in an activated state in that they do not require priming (i.e., exposure to the same antigen) prior to exercising their effector functions (e.g., killing target cells, secreting cytokines). They are, therefore, potentially dangerous, poised to kill epithelial cells and secrete inflammatory cytokines. Why, then, do they not do so? The answer seems to lie in the fact that the EC express a class I molecule called "thymus leukemia antigen" (TL), which is a ligand for CD8αα homodimer.[129] TL is found almost exclusively on EC of the small intestine. It binds to CD8αα receptor with high energy. The consequences of the interaction of TL on EC with CD8αα on the intraepithelial T cells (TCRαβ and TCRγδ) are (a) stimulation of cytokine release by the T cells (IL-2 and IFNγ) and (b) inhibition of the ability of the T cells to kill target cells and of their ability to proliferate. The stimulation of cytokine release was assessed only in the case of IL-2 and IFN-γ. Production of other cytokines was not evaluated but probably was enhanced, at least in the case of those that might favor continuous and rhythmic migration of enterocytes to the tips of the villi. The inhibition of CD8αα (+) proliferation and cytolytic ability clearly is designed to prevent excessive proliferation of IEL and killing of EC, both of which could destroy the epithelial barrier. Because none of the epithelial T cells is suited for interaction with APC and stimulation of B cells, the T cells that participate in IgA antibody production are located elsewhere, viz., in the LP, PP, and MLN.

Intestinal B Lymphocytes

Two types of B cells are known (B1 and B2) and both participate in generating intestinal IgA. However, it appears that cells of the B2 lineage, which originate in the bone marrow and require interaction with CD4+ T-helper cells, are active in IgA immunity against enteric pathogens. B1 cells are recruited primarily from the peritoneal cavity and produce IgA against enteric commensal organisms.[130]

The generation of anticommensal IgA is antigen driven,[130] i.e., the presence of microflora in the gut is required. The principal site where the encounter of micro-organism and B cell occurs is the MLN. Bacteria traverse the epithelium via M cells and are ingested by DC. They may survive for as long as 60 h in the DC, which is ample time for a productive encounter between DC and B1 cell. No live bacteria either free or in MP are found, either in PP or MLN.

IgA production initiated from B1 cells requires no T-cell help. Furthermore, mutant mice lacking organized follicular dendritic network or B-cell follicles develop near-normal numbers of B1-derived plasma cells to their microflora.

Experiments with mutant mice lacking PP and MLN revealed the need for lymphoid aggregates to serve as inductive sites, but further organization of follicles and GC where encounter with T cells might occur appears unnecessary.[130]

T-cell-dependent IgA antibody production occurs by IgA+ B cells that are derived from B220+ IgM precursors. Class switching (IgM to IgA by Ig-gene rearrangements) is thought to occur in the LP. Both naïve B cells, directly from bone marrow and not previously acquainted with the gut, and the so-called gut-primed B cells can migrate into the LP.[131] The former are attracted to the LP by a factor, NIK (NF-κB-inducing kinase), associated with stromal cells. These naïve B220+ IgM cells undergo class-switching and further differentiation to yield B220 (−) IgA (+) cells, possibly in the absence of organized follicles and GC. The second type of precursor, gut-primed, appears in the LP as a result of expressing the integrin $\alpha_4\beta_7$ (MadCAM), a homing molecule that was acquired upon previous exposure to the gut microenvironment. In either case, the B220 (−) IgA (+) cells upon activation and costimulation generate a population of IgA antibody-producing daughters.

We have seen that B1 cells drawn from the peritoneal cavity and B220 (+) cells that originated in bone marrow can generate IgA-producing progeny. In the case of B1 cells, no involvement of T cells is necessary. In the case of the B220 (+) IgM (+) precursors, one type migrates into the LP with the guidance of $\alpha_4\beta_7$ integrin, while the other is drawn through the actions of a stromal factor NIK. A recent, comprehensive study of gut-homing B cells seems to add another layer of complexity, while, at the same time, providing exciting new information.[118]

Isolated B cells from the spleens of mice were activated and incubated together with DC from PP. The B cells were induced to express gut-homing $\alpha_4\beta_7$ integrin molecules. The same thing occurred when the B cells were incubated with an appropriate amount of retinoic acid (RA) rather than the DC.[118] When tested in vivo, the RA-treated DC migrated to the small intestine. Further experiments with this system revealed that when activated B cells were cultured with PP-DC, they gave rise to progeny that secreted substantial amounts of IgA. That occurred in the absence of T cells. Addition of a combination of RA, IL-5, and IL-6 to cultures of activated B cells and PP–DC (or DC from other locations) resulted in a substantial elevation in the yield of IgA-producing cells. That effect was attributed to enhancement of B-cell class-switching rather than to expansion of already committed IgA-producing cells. None of the three substances added alone enhanced the formation of IgA-producing cells. Among DC from various tissues, only those from the GALT were capable of synthesizing RA.

It is clear that there exist B cells not derived from the conventional bone marrow source that require only contact with GALT-DC in order to give rise to IgA-producing daughters. RA is a major factor contributed by the DC but probably not the only one. No organized, lymphoid follicles or GC and no T cells are required for those B cells to generate IgA producing daughters.

The PP are populated largely with naïve IgM (dull)/IgD (bright) B2 cells. The nearby IFR contains both CD4+ and CD8+ T cells. DC transport antigen acquired from M cells from the SED to the IFR and thus all the components necessary for organization of GC would seem to be present. Class-switching and affinity maturation should ensue, leading to transport of dimeric IgA–J chain molecules through the enterocytes accompanied by the pIgR. However, a problem has appeared recently concerning the site where class-switching occurs.[132] Compelling evidence has been provided that excludes the LP, PP, and MLN as the sites of class-switching among B1 cells and doubt has been cast on the notion that B2 class-switching occurs at those sites. In the case of B1 cells, class-switching must occur outside of the GALT. Other investigators have raised doubt about IgM to IgA class-switching occurring in the LP.[133,134] Questions regarding class-switching are complex and the answers are tentative at present. In the case of B2 cells it may occur in the LP or, more likely, in the MLN. The presence of GALT–DC is required, and RA probably plays a key role. TGF-β derived from TLR-stimulated macrophages, or possibly enterocytes, is believed to stimulate class-switching (see later). However, in the case of B1 cells, class-switching occurs outside the intestine.

How significant is the contribution of IgA by B1-derived plasma cells? In the case of intact mice, the B1 contribution appears to be minor, perhaps 19–24% of the total in the gut.[135] It is possible that the contribution from B1 cells is conditioned by the quantity or quality (specificity, affinity) of the IgA produced by the existing population of B2 cells (see later).

Effects of Aging on the GALT

The five preceding sections present a selective survey of the structural and functional complexities of the GALT and related tissues. We trust that the preceding sections have revealed that the unique features of the GALT and its relationships to the central and systemic components of the immune system offer a "gold mine" of research opportunities for gerontologists and all others who have an interest in aging. From a different perspective, however, research concerned with aging of the GALT and the reasons for its existence, viz., to protect against the horde of potential pathogens that lie just one cell thickness away, might seem more of a "mine field." The complexities are bewildering, and choosing a site or system for productive investigation is more a matter of taste than rational decision. The following discussion is offered to aid in making the selection of research approaches somewhat more rational, simply as a result of organizing much of the information in a heuristic fashion.

Aging of the Intestinal Epithelium

Enterocytes

The enterocytes display both MHC class I and class II conventional molecules and several nonclassical MHCs as well (e.g., CD1, TL). They express several TLR: TLR-3 and TLR-4 in particular. They (i.e., the FAE) secrete chemokines CCL9 and

CCL20 and the key cytokine, IL-15. They secrete a neutrophil chemoattractant. They synthesize and express the pIgA R and transport pIgA into the gut lumen. They are intensely involved in maintaining a selectively penetrable barrier composed of tight junctions. In spite of – or perhaps because of – the extreme variety of functions, the enterocytes are a highly dynamic system, undergoing constant turnover. They arise from stem cells in the crypts, migrate up the villi, and after about 3–5 days are shed from the tips of the villi and succumb to apoptotic death (sometimes necrotic death). What do we know about the effects of senescence on the enterocytes? Very little. The rate of their migration from base to tip of the villi slows with age probably reflecting a reduced rate of generation from stem cells in the crypts.[136] They continue to present an effective barrier against the microbiota of the gut, although there is some evidence of "leakiness" of the epithelium among aging subjects.[137] This will be considered further in a discussion of "inflamma-ging" (below). The presence of pIgR on enterocytes appears to remain constant with age.[138,139] However, the amount of antigen-specific pIgA that is transported into the gut in response to specific intra-intestinal antigen challenge declines with age.[139]

Toll-Like Receptor

There appears to be a strong explanation for the age-associated decline in the amount of sIgA that appears in the gut; it centers on the effects of aging on the TLRs.[140–142] Each of the TLRs has been found to suffer the effects of senescence. A comprehensive study of macrophages (splenic and thioglycolate-elicited) of young and aged mice revealed that the surface expression of seven TLRs was substantially less in aged mice. Furthermore, stimulation of the macrophages with cognate ligands resulted in substantially lower secretion of IL-6 and TNF-α by macrophages from aged animals.[140] A study of the PBMC isolated from the blood of two groups of humans, aged 21–30 years or over 65 years, produced similar results.[141] Stimulation of the cells via TLR-1/2 resulted in a highly significant, reduced output of TNF-α and IL-6 by cells from aged subjects. In contrast, stimulation of young and aged cells via other TLRs revealed only minor differences. In a study of a murine model of Alzheimer's disease it was found that the frequencies of TLR-1, TLR-2, TLR-4, TLR-5, and TLR-7 were greater in brain tissue of aged compared to young mice.[142] Of that group, TLR-7 could be associated with mononuclear phagocytes. By comparison, the amount of TLR-3, TLR-6, and TLR-8 were the same in the two age groups, while TLR-9 was less in aged than in young mice.

It has been demonstrated[143] by use of a cell line of IEC that stimulation of enterocytes via TLR-3 (with dsRNA) or TLR-4 (with LPS) results in upregulation of the pIgR. That effect was found to involve signaling through NF-κB and enhanced transcription of pIgR mRNA. If, as has been claimed,[139] the age-associated deficiency in sIgA production is a reflection of defective pIgR, then the age-associated change is likely to be in the expression of enterocytic TLR or the mechanism of signal transduction. Given the variation in results reported in the three cited works, it seems likely that the frequency and functions of the TLRs vary among different tissues, cell types, and local environments; so, it may not be safe to generalize an effect of senescence on the TLRs per se.

Intraepithelial Lymphocytes

As discussed previously, a major concentration of $\gamma\delta$ T cells is in the intestinal epithelium. Some 70–80% of IEL in the mouse are $\gamma\delta$ T cells and, of those, nearly all express the CD8$\alpha\alpha$ (α homodimer). Among the $\alpha\beta$ T cells, about half express the CD8$\alpha\alpha$ while the other half are CD8$\alpha\beta$. Data concerning possible changes in those proportions with age are lacking. There is compelling evidence that a significant proportion of the IEL originate extra-thymically[124,143–146]; still, the thymus is the ultimate source for at least some of the IEL.[143] The CD8$\alpha\alpha$ IEL can be separated into two groups: CD4+ CD8$\alpha\alpha$ and CD4− CD8$\alpha\alpha$+. Cells with the CD4− CD8$\alpha\alpha$+ phenotype migrate out of the thymus of neonatal mice younger than 2 weeks of age. After 2 weeks of age of the newborn, the thymus releases almost exclusively CD4+ CD8$\alpha\alpha$+ cells. It should be informative to determine the phenotype of the IEL in aged mice when the residual thymus exports few cells. It should be relatively easy to determine whether the stem cells in the cryptopatches continue to produce the CD8$\alpha\alpha$ [CD4 (+) or (−)] IEL and whether senescence has affected those stem cells either qualitatively or quantitatively.

It has been demonstrated more than once that T cells having self-reactive capability are present in the neonatal but not the adult thymus of the mouse.[128] Moreover, negative selection to eliminate autoreactive $\alpha\beta$ and $\gamma\delta$ T cells is markedly inoperative early in ontogeny. As a result, potentially self-reactive $\gamma\delta$T cells are able to escape selection and "find sanctuary"[128] in the IEL where they enjoy a supportive environment. Those T cells are "primed" as a result of having been exposed to self-antigen in the thymus prior to their escape. As we have seen (op. cit.), there exists a mechanism for preventing those hostile cells from reacting against self-antigens in the intestinal epithelium; viz., the interaction between thymus leukemis (TL) antigen elaborated by enterocytes and the cognate receptor CD8$\alpha\alpha$.[129] A question that needs to be answered is this: what is the life-span of the IEL $\gamma\delta$ T cells and $\alpha\beta$ T cells that display CD8$\alpha\alpha$ and what is the source of their replacements? Another question is: how durable is the TL-mediated inhibition of the self-reactive CD8$\alpha\alpha$ cells; does the potential reactivity against self gradually appear and allow the barrier to be breached resulting in subclinical inflammation in the aged subject?

A compelling but unsubstantiated argument can be formulated to the effect that aging results in significant changes in the $\gamma\delta$ T cells of the intestinal epithelium. First, there is the evidence that $\gamma\delta$ T cells in the GALT, possibly in the epithelium, are required for development and maintenance of OT.[62,147] But the establishment of OT is severely impaired in the case of old animals.[148–150] Second, as we have seen, the frequency of TLRs and their signaling efficiency are affected by aging. A major signaling pathway initiated by engagement of several of the TLRs proceeds via

MyD88, an adaptor protein involved in activation of transcription of cytokine genes. Third, an important cytokine in maintaining γδ T cells in the intestinal epithelium is IL-15, which is produced by enterocytes of the epithelium. In the absence of intact signaling via MyD88, IL-15 production is severely impaired and the numbers of CD8αα TCRαβ and CD8αα TCRγδ intestinal epithelial cells are substantially reduced.[151] It is, therefore, reasonable to suggest that there occur senescent changes of enterocytes that affect either the surface density of TLRs or the pathways by which TLR signals are transduced. The amount or quality of IL-15 produced by the enterocytes might suffer and that, in turn, might result in failure to sustain the CD8αα TCRαβ and TCRγδ lymphocytes.

Although the suggestion developed in the preceding paragraph could account for age-related loss of IEL and deterioration of the intestinal barrier, there is also the possibility of senescent changes in the CD8αα TCRγδ cells themselves. Thus, it must be asked: do not those cells turn over and need to be replaced? Does the interaction between CD8αα and TL on the enterocytes markedly prolong their residence in the epithelium? If regular replacement does occur, where do the replacements originate? In the cryptopatches? If so, is there an effect of aging on the generative competence of the cryptopatches? All of those questions need to be answered.

GALT B cells and GC

The B lymphocyte population has been subdivided into categories in several ways: (a) homing propensities, (b) origins and anatomical locations, (c) time of appearance in neonatal life, and (d) expression of surface membrane molecules. Two broad categories are recognized, viz., B1 and B2. The latter are the conventional B cells that originate in the bone marrow. The B1 cells[152,153] originate early in neonatal life and escape negative selection. The B1 cells are located primarily in the peritoneal and pleural cavities. There are a few B1 cells in the spleen but hardly any in lymph nodes and peripheral blood. The B1 set is further subdivided into B1a and B1b subsets primarily on the basis of high (B1a) or low (B1b) expression of surface CD5. The surface CD5 receptors are inhibitory; they restrain the response of B1 cells to the antigens by which they were selected in the first place. B1 cells are capable of responding to self-antigens without the assistance of T cells or DC. They receive stimulation through cognate B cell receptors (BCR). They do, however, require co-stimulation, either by cytokines (IL-5 in particular) or via the TLR-4 which they display. When properly stimulated, B1 cells (which characteristically produce antibodies of the IgM isotype) may undergo immunoglobulin gene rearrangements and switch to producing plasma cells that generate IgG or IgA isotypes.

The current view of the generation of IgA-producing plasma cells from B2 precursors holds that the likely site where this occurs is the MLN. Antigen from commensal organisms is transported by special DC into the MLN. Those DC can harbor antigen (even live bacteria) for several hours because, unlike the local macrophages which are quite hostile, the DC are inefficient at destroying ingested material. Within the MLN it is envisioned that processed antigen is provided to conventional cognate T cells, which in turn provide help to B cells that have been activated via antigen bound to their receptors (BCR). Those interactions are presumed to occur in GC where class-switching from IgM to IgA, proliferation, and selection of stable plasma cells that produce antibodies of high affinity occur.

The preceding is a description of what may seem to be a tidy, well-understood component of the GALT immune response to intestinal microorganisms. It is not. There are numerous aspects of the preceding description that are not well documented and are controversial. We will discuss three in relation to the possible effects of senescence on the process of IgA antibody production, viz., (a) the participation of B1 and B2 cells in secretory antibody formation, (b) the mechanisms of IgA class-switching, and (c) intrinsic defects within the B subsets attributable to senescence.

We begin with a rather imprecise question: do B cells age? That is the way the question was phrased not so long ago. About a decade ago, it could be asserted[154] that aging is accompanied by a changing specificity repertoire and a broadening recognition of self-components. That seemed to occur in concert with a gradual shift in the set of B1 and B2 toward a prepondance of the former. Furthermore, there appeared to be a well-documented change – both qualitative and quantitative – in the formation of GC in response to antigenic challenge in aged subjects.[155] That GC deficiency was reflected by a decline in the efficiency of antibody class-switching and in the affinity of synthesized antibody. Those and a few other age-associated alterations were attributed in part to certain easily discerned modifications in T cells and in the bone marrow environment. The recent elucidation of the B-cell receptor (BCR), intracellular signal transduction, co-stimulation and the mechanisms of class-switching, and specificity repertoire selection have brought changes in the approaches to understanding B cell senescence.

The effects of aging on GALT immunity have barely been explored. Yet, the information that is required – some of it at least – seems rather obvious. First of all, there are questions about the homing of the B cells to the LP. The relevant homing receptors are $\alpha_4\beta_7$ integrin and the CCR9 chemokine receptor. Imprinting of those receptors is a consequence of exposure to RA provided by the specialized DC. Are all types of B cells equally imprinted or only a portion? Are both B1 and B2 imprinted by RA? And, in particular, is there a change with age in the type(s), numbers, and efficiency of imprinting of the B cells that can be enticed to home to the LP?

Second, information is needed about the formation of GC in the PP and the MLN of aged subjects. It is not clear that GC formation is impaired in the PP of aged subjects. Furthermore, as we have seen, the notion that GC formation is required or accompanies IgA class switching has been questioned.[132]

In addition to RA, at least two other substances have been implicated in IgA class switching; viz., TGF-β[156,157] and the cytokine, APRIL.[158] The effect of TGF-β occurs directly on B cells that are costimulated with LPS. The stimulation is more pronounced in the case of B1 than B2 cells.[159] Switching to isotypes other than IgA does not occur. As noted, TGF-β is present in the LP and probably in the intestinal epithelium as well. The recent finding that IL-15, which is a product of enterocytes, inhibits TGF-β-mediated signaling[160] offers a possible counteraction that can regulate TGF-β stimulation of B cell switching to the IgA isotype.

APRIL is a member of the TNF family that, like BAFF, acts on B cells, especially marginal-zone and follicular B2 cells. It particularly aids in marginal-zone responses to particulate antigens such as bacteria. It has now been found that intestinal epithelial cells release APRIL upon being stimulated through their TLRs. APRIL, then, promotes class-switching among the LP B cells.

Intriguing observations related to IgA isotype switching came from a study of B cells in GC of aged mice.[161] The numbers and phenotypes of activated B cells in PP GC of young and aged mice did not differ significantly. Of particular interest was the finding that the expected higher frequency of somatic mutations in the V-region genes of aged mice occurred with disproportionate frequency in the IgM isotype. An earlier report[162] revealed that serum immunoglobulins produced in response to "environmental antigens" (such as microorganisms) displayed a striking increase in somatic mutations correlated with aging. The frequency of mutations was substantially higher in the IgG compared to the IgM isotype. It should be fascinating to examine the somatic mutations in polymeric secreted IgA and compare with serum IgA. Moreover, comparing the mutations in sIgA generated by cells derived from B1 and B2 precursors could be quite informative given the evidence that the former experience class-switching outside the GALT and independent of GC.

A third major topic awaiting thorough study concerns the effects that age-modified TLRs may exert on B cells. We have discussed the influence of aging on TLRs and noted that the effect appears to vary with the tissue location. There are several different TLRs on enterocytes. In addition, both B cells (B1 and B2) and GALT DC express TLRs; signaling initiated by the TLRs can affect the functions of those cells. For example, B1 cells remain in the pleural and peritoneal cavities as long as they are not actively stimulated. They remain attached to the membranous linings of those cavities through the combined effects of integrins, ($\alpha_M\beta_2$ in particular) and CXCR5, the receptor for chemokine CXCL13. The introduction of LPS into those cavities results in a dramatic downregulation of the integrins and CXCR5[163] on B1 cells. As a consequence, the B1 cells are untethered and are free to migrate into other locations including the LP. That effect is caused by LPS stimulation via TLR-4.[163]

TLR-4 play an important role in the class-switch recombination that occurs in B cells leading to IgA production.[164] As noted, TGFβ1 stimulation of B cells triggers switching to IgA production.[118,165,166] Concurrent stimulation by LPS enhances the effect of TGF-β1. The effect of LPS is manifested in two ways[164]: (a) by stimulating the transcription of the key enzyme, activation-induced cytidine deaminase (AID) preceding the process of gene rearrangement and (b) by elevating the secretion of IgA after gene recombination. Experiments that produced these results were performed with splenic B cells. Presumably, the same results would be obtained with peritoneal B1 cells. However, the effect of LPS on class-switching in B1 cells should be examined because there is evidence[167] that LPS signaling may not be the same in B1 and B2 cells.

It is worth inquiring at what stage in the life history of B cells class-switch recombination occurs. Ingenious studies[168] have provided a clear answer. V (D) J recombinase is active in the common lymphoid progenitor (CLP) cells, i.e., in progenitors that retain, but typically never express, the potential to give rise to myeloid descendants.[168] The differentiative potentiality of CLP includes B, T, DC, and NK cells and it has been assumed that recombination events occur only in B- and T-lineage cells. The recent study[168] has demonstrated that recombination events occur in the CLP; moreover, early expression of *Erag*, an enhancer element that controls *rag* expression in B progenitors, appears to be a precocious indication that subsequent differentiation will follow the B-cell path.

The B2 population has received considerable attention vis-à-vis the effects of senescence. A recent study[169] has demonstrated that the effects of aging are apparent in all of the early stages of B2 cell development. Both B-lineage-committed pro-B cells and their immediate pluripotential progenitors were decreased in aged animals. All subsets of cells were defective in responsiveness to IL-7. The loss of responsiveness to IL-7 is important because all stages in B-cell development up to the antigen-responsive, immature B cell are stimulated to proliferate in response to IL-7. Defective display of IL-7R, or of IL-7R signaling, probably accounts for the age-associated deficiency of B2 cells, at least in the mouse. A second cytokine may be involved in human B2 cell development.

In addition to the differences between B1 and B2 cells described above, there are others that are being elucidated. For example, the frequency of receptors (CXCR5) is substantially higher on B1 than on B2 cells. As noted above, CXCR5 is the receptor for a chemokine known as B-lymphocyte chemokine (BLC; CXCL13), which is a chemoattractant for B cells.[170] The presence of CXCL13 in the peritoneal cavity is essential for the homing of B1 cells and expression of immunity in the cavity. CXCL13 is produced especially by myeloid DC [CD11b (+) CD11c (+)]. Those DC have been found to produce substantial amounts of CXCL13 at sites of autoimmune pathogenesis. In developing murine lupus nephritis, for example, concentrations of CXCL13-producing DC were found in kidney and thymus of mice of an autoimmune strain, and there was an accompanying accumulation of B1 cells.[171] Similarly, in a murine model of systemic lupus erythematosus, the distribution of B1 cells was influenced by the presence or absence of CXCL13-producing macrophages.[172] To our knowledge, the uncertainty concerning the production of CXCL13 by cells (DC or MP) in the LP has not been resolved.

Reports from different laboratories vary with regard to the numbers of B1 cells and their IgA-producing derivatives that are present in the LP. One of the most comprehensive reports[173] indicated that about half of the IgA-producing plasma cells were derived from self-replenishing B1 precursors of the peritoneal cavity. More recent reports generally concur[174] and, in addition, have stressed the key role of IL-5 in stimulating sIgA production by those cells. Considered from the perspective of aging, these and related reports suggest that fruitful lines of investigation could be (a) effects of senescence on the numbers, mobility, and phenotypic characteristics of peritoneal B1 cells and (b) availability of IL-5 in the peritoneal space and in GALT.

Homing of Cells to GALT and Associated Lymphoid Tissue

Both B and T cells are conveyed to the GALT and MLN by lymph and blood. They are extracted from the blood by the actions of homing receptors and chemokines. T cells in the blood which display $\alpha_4\beta_7$ integrin and L-selectin molecules are deterred by the presence of the mucosal addressin MadCAM-1 in the high endothelial venules of mucosal tissue. They then enter the lamina propria by diapedesis and adhere to the basolateral faces of the intestinal epithelial cells. Adherence in the small intestine is achieved by interactions of $\alpha_E\beta_7$ and CCR9 on the T cells with, respectively, E-cadherin and CCL25 on the epithelial cells. In the large intestine, adherence involves CCR10 on the T cells and CCL28 on epithelial cells.

The attraction of B lymphocytes, both B1 and B2, to the LP and MLN is a subject in need of investigation. Three molecules appear to be involved: $\alpha_4\beta_7$ integrin, L-selectin, and LFA-1 on B cells which react with their counterparts MadCAM-1 and ICAM-1 on high endothelial venules. It has been reported that in the LP, MadCAM-1 does not display saccharide moieties that are recognized by L-selectin. That and the low level of $\alpha_4\beta_7$ on naïve lymphocytes suggest that the naïve B cells may not readily migrate into the intestinal mucosa.[175] Chemokines that might be involved have not been clearly established. In a review article[176] it was stated: "Identifying the physiologic factors responsible for activating firm adhesion and arrest in lymphocyte homing to mucosal lymphoid organs, determining whether such activation is required for lymphocyte recruitment via lamina propria venules, and analysis of the extent to which this activation step contributes to the selectivity of mucosal lymphocyte trafficking are important areas for future investigation." Future investigation is needed, particularly in the case of B1 cells. The effects of aging on lymphocyte homing to the LP and MLN have not been studied. Some important changes are likely to be found.

Knowledge concerning the homing of immunoblast cells to the lamina propria is more advanced than in the case of early B cells. Three recent publications are in agreement that the chemokines, CCL25 (TECK), and CCL28 (MEC) are instrumental in the sequestration of IgA(+) plasmablasts by the LP.[177–179] CCL25 is produced by epithelial cells and readily attracts IgA(+) cells that express CCR9 in the PP and MLN. When those IgA(+) cells migrate to the LP, they display much less CCR9 and remain in the LP.[177] It was noted[178] that CCL25 is present in significantly higher levels in epithelial cells at mucosal sites than at other locations in the "common mucosal immune system" (mammary gland, salivary gland, colon, lung, trachea). It was postulated and demonstrated that a second chemokine, CCL28 (MEC), was involved in the efficient attraction of immunoblasts to the other sites. It was clear that CCR9 and CCR10 are responsible for the settling of IgA(+) plasmablasts in the small intestine. However, the homing of IgA(+) plasmablasts to the colon was more efficiently achieved by CCL28 and CXCL12.[179] The epithelial cells of the colon were found to express CCL28 and CXCL12, and the IgA(+) blasts in the colon displayed CCR10 and CXCR4.

The results presented in those publications reveal that the cells prepared for IgA production in the MLN, and perhaps in less-organized locations in the LP, will return to subepithelial locations in the small and large intestine. From the perspective of aging, three key questions come to mind. First, the chemokines are secreted largely by epithelial cells; because there are effects of senescence on the epithelial cells (e.g., changes in TLRs), there may be quantitative and qualitative changes in the chemokines they secrete. Second, there may be differences between IgA(+) plasmablasts that arise from B1 compared to conventional B2 precursors: recall that the proportion of B1 precursors increases with advancing age. It is reasonable to question whether or not the chemokine receptors or the adhesion molecules on the IgA(+) blasts are affected by aging. Third, there are unconfirmed reports that lymphocyte homing is disturbed in aged animals as a result of changes in the expression and distribution of homing receptors.

Finally, we consider the type of cell that is perhaps most in need of attention vis-à-vis immunosenescence, viz., the DC. In recent years, information concerning the variety of DC and their functions has blurred the traditional distinction between lymphoid and myeloid DC. In the GALT there are two prominent types of DC as noted previously; viz., CD11b (hi) CD11c (hi) CD8α (−), and CD11b (lo) CD11c (hi) CD8α (+). One, or perhaps both, of them has the unique ability to ingest debris from dying epithelial cells and transport it to the MLN where it is presented to T cells. The latter are induced to secrete IL-4 and IL-10: in short, to promote a noninflammatory type of immune response.[180] It is reasoned that the debris includes antigenic materials as from luminal microorganisms.

The migration of the DC from LP to MLN involves the chemokines CCL21 and/or CCL19 and the CCR7 on the surface of the DC.[180] Additional insight concerning the migration of DC from LP to MLN has been gained by experiments that utilized DC collected from thoracic duct of rats that, first, had the MLN removed surgically (MLN lymphadenectomy).[181] Those DC had not experienced any tissue microenvironment after leaving the LP. They were found to express ICAM-1, CD11c, CD11b, CD80, CD86, and MHC class II molecules. Their immaturity when freshly isolated was indicated by their phagocytic ability. Both immature and mature preparations of DC were provided to recipient rats by injection into the subserosa of the small intestine, and the accumulation of the DC in the MLN was monitored. In that manner, it was demonstrated that accumulation of mature DC was dependent on attraction of CCR7 surface molecules to chemokine CCL21. Accumulation of immature DC, on the other hand, depended on the attraction between surface molecules of CCR6 and chemokine CCL20.

The distribution of TLRs on DC varies among the various subsets/populations of DC. The CD11b(+) CD11c (+) DC of the LP express TLR-7 and, therefore, are responsive to the synthetic agonist, R-848. The effects of stimulating the DC via TLR-7 on their migration to MLN have been examined. The factors involved in the accumulation of DC in the MLN[182] have been identified. Rodents were subjected to mesenteric lymphadenectomy, and then stimulated orally with R848. Cells were collected from the thoracic duct and analyzed. In both experiments, intact animals were given R-848, and MLN and other tissues examined histologically. Treatment with R-848 essentially depleted the LP of DC. Many of those cells were accumulated in the MLN. Furthermore, feeding R-848 stimulated a marked output of IL-6, IL-12p 70, TNF-α and IFN-α. A substantial portion of those cytokines was produced in the MLN by plasmacytoid DC, not by CD11b(+) or CD11b(−) DC. The plasmacytoid DC (pDC) were the exclusive source of IFN-α following TLR-7/8 stimulation. Experiments to determine what factors were responsible for MLN accumulation of the R-848-mobilized DC revealed that TNF-α was primarily responsible for accumulation of the DC and that IFN-α induced activation of the accumulated DC. Both of those cytokines were produced by pDC located in the MLN.

The so-called "steady-state" intestinal DC (those not strongly stimulated) are immature in certain respects. They display substantial levels of MHC class II and CCR7. Their migration to the MLN is dependent on cytokines CCL20 and CCL19, as we have seen,[180,181] which are likely produced by local DC. In contrast, strong stimulation of the DC (LP and others) via TLRs may trigger an emergency response that involves the pDC. It should be noted that the latter are unique among DC in that they circulate in the blood, are not phagocytic, and respond vigorously to viruses by secreting type 1 IFNs. They express high levels of TLR-7 and TLR-9, which makes them well suited for responding to viral nucleic acids.

We have provided some details of the studies on migration of DC from LP to MLN[181,182] because (a) this is a system that appears to be susceptible to the effects of aging and (b) the experimental procedure involving mesenteric lymphadenectomy is well suited for application to aged animals. The effects of aging on TLRs that appear to be so common may be strongly manifested on the TLRs of the enterocytes, the CD11b (hi) CD8α(−) and CD11b (lo) CD8α (+) DC, and especially the plasmacytoid DC of the MLN.

Exploring Examples of GALT Aging

Evidence that intestinal immune competence declines with age is impressive but not overwhelming. No single cause is evident – nor is it to be expected. Rather, the effects of aging will be found in a number of systems, processes, and events that comprise intestinal mucosal immunity. We have attempted to focus attention on some of the major elements that are likely to be altered by senescence but, for the most part, have not been adequately studied. Included are elements of both innate and adaptive immune operations. As a final brief summary of our efforts to identify fruitful lines of investigation of the effects of senescence, we suggest the following two schemes.

Manning the Barrier: Aging and the Intestinal Epithelium

Enterocytes perform a large number of functions that possibly are susceptible to senescence. They include pIgA transcytosis, maintenance of tight junctions, selective permeability to prospective antigens, production of chemokines and cytokines, and responsiveness to various signals such as those from the TLRs. They produce IL-15 and display TL for controlling CD8αα+ T cells. Perhaps the most important gap in available information is the lack of information concerning the precise effects and consequences of aging of the epithelial cell TLRs. Another critical gap is the dearth of information about the status of the epithelial barrier. Does the integrity of the barrier remain intact with advancing age? Or does it become more fragile as a result of changes in the rate or mechanisms of epithelial cell turnover and replacement? Or of poor maintenance of tight junctions? The elderly experience normal (occasionally abnormal) decline in hydrochloric acid production and more alkaline conditions in the proximal small intestine. Changes in bacterial number and species often result. Both in the ileum and colon there may be changes in the microflora as a consequence of aberrant nutrition, which is fairly common in the elderly. Such changes in the enteric microbial population may upset homeostasis in various locations and result in spots of inflammation. It is frequently stated that a substantial proportion of elderly humans suffer from chronic, subclinical intestinal inflammation, which has led to the expression "inflammaging." That condition is likely to reflect disruption of the barrier at vulnerable "spots" or loci rather than along an extensive segment of the intestine. What might create those loci of inflammation? Possibly local concentrations (colonies) of certain bacteria that secrete enzymes capable of attacking tight junctions, or perhaps groups of activated cells that secrete high levels of IFN-γ with or without TNF-α, resulting in disruption of tight junctions.

An intriguing prospect is that the intestinal epithelium of the elderly might differ from that of the young adult as a consequence of a reduced rate of enterocyte turnover. The rate of ascent of the villi by maturing enterocytes is reduced in the elderly and the rate of apoptotic cell death is lower. Thus, the transit time of enterocyte from crypt to villus tip is longer and those cells live longer. Whether or not that change could affect the durability of the barrier is uncertain, but it is an issue worthy of investigation.

Peering into the Crypt: An Aging Effect in Want of an Explanation

The effect is as follows: (a) with advancing age there is an increasing rate of mutation in mtDNA in the stem cells; (b) there is a propensity for formation of homoplasmic crypts – either all mutant mtDNA or wild-type mtDNA; (c) at least 80% of the mtDNA in a cell must be mutated before there is any effect on the function of the cell (a remarkable example of "physiological redundancy"); (d) in parallel with the increased rate of mutation of mtDNA with age there is an increase in the tendency of crypts to aggregate and to form patches of crypts (Fig. 9.3). This phenomenon requires investigation from the perspective of acquiring new information such as the following: (a) Is the high rate of mutation due to the proximity of

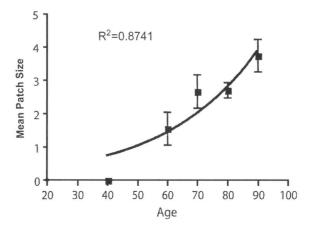

Fig. 9.3 The increasing size of colonic crypt patches associated with aging, reflecting aggregation of defective crypts with age (from Ref. 103 with permission)

the DNA to the source of free radicals (the electron transport cascade)? (b) Does the high rate occur only in the stem cells of the crypt and, if so, why? (c) Is the excessively high rate of mutation in stem cells of crypts of elderly subjects reflected in highly mutated enterocyte progeny and are the functions of the latter affected by their load of mutations? (d) Are the stem cells in the crypts of aged subjects killed as a result of accumulated mutations and are aggregates and patches of crypts composed of "dead crypts?" Those are only a few questions pertaining to the fascinating crypts and the effects of senescence on them.

Finally, it should be stressed that the effects of senescence on intestinal mucosal immunity will not be easy to identify and study by experimental approaches that involve simply comparing a system or process in intact young and aged subjects. That is because subjects of the two ages are likely to possess physiological (immunological) potential far in excess of that required for an acute response or action. Virtually every organ or system bears excess potential: liver, kidney, central nervous, muscle. Remove, say, half of the potential, and there is little noticeable effect – except in case of trauma when the excess may be needed. To illustrate the point in the case of the systemic immune system, it was only with the introduction of the adoptive transfer method that the effects of aging on the immune system could clearly be detected and quantified. Thus, in order to generate a given level of immune response in irradiated recipient animals, 5–10 times more cells from aged than from young donors had to be transferred. Merely assessing the response to equal doses of antigen generated in intact young and aged animals showed that there was no difference; in other words, it appeared that aging was without effect on the immune system. Irradiated recipient animals were employed in the early days of adoptive transfer experiments. Today, nude and SCID as well as other mutant strains of animals (mice) are likely to be used.

To complete the preceding line of thought, we recommend experiments to test whether or not B1 and B2 cells from young and aged differ; in other words, has senescence affected the cells from aged mice? The experimental design might be to compare both types of B cells (B1 and B2) from donors of different age (young adult, old) with respect to their ability to settle in the PP of immunodeficient recipients (SCID, SCID-Rag−/−) and to produce sIgA. Previous studies in which the homing of B1 and B2 were compared gave inconsistent results. Direct transfer experiments into SCID or irradiated recipients of peritoneal B1 and bone marrow B2 cells indicated that a considerable proportion of the total sIgA was derived from B1 precursors.[183] In contrast, experiments performed with intact mice in which sIgA derived from B1 or B2 precursors could be tracked by Ig allotype markers showed that very little sIgA was derived from B1 precursors.[184] It was argued that the latter design of the experiment provided more physiologically realistic conditions and an optimum chance for both types of B cells to "compete" for occupancy of the PP. The term "compete" is the critical word. It may be necessary for the B2 cells to differentiate in the marrow before they are free to migrate to the PP, whereas B1 cells require no further maturation. Therefore, B2 cells might be at a selective disadvantage in the SCID recipient's environment. It can be argued that the B1 cells are also hampered by the fact that they may become "tethered" in the peritoneal cavity by the action of B-lymphocyte chemokine (BLC/CXCL13).[185]

In any event, the approach illustrated by the two methods outlined in the preceding paragraph offers an excellent opportunity to study the effects of aging on B1 and B2 cells: both qualitative and quantitative. It should be fascinating to determine whether or not there is a finite volume available for B-cell-derived plasmablasts in the PP and LP. If the space is filled with B2 and their progeny, B1 cells might be unable to settle there and vice versa. Is there a different volume available to B cells (either B1 or B2) in the PP and LP of the aged animal compared to the young adult?

New questions to be answered and new territory to be explored in the province of aging and mucosal immunity have no limit. We have asked our share of questions. Perhaps they will energize others to explore the territory in the quest for answers.

References

1. Saltzman JR, Russell TM. The aging gut: nutritional issues. Gastroenterol Clin North Am 1998;27:309–324.
2. Wolf JL, Rubin DH, Finberg R, Kauffman RS, Sharpe AH, Trier JS, Fields BN. Intestinal M cells: a pathway for entry of reovirus into the host. Science 1981;212:471–472.
3. Kraehenbuhl J-P, Neutra MR. Epithelial M cells: differentiation and function. Annu Rev Cell Dev Biol 2000;16:301–332.
4. Shreedhar VK, Kelsall BL, Neutra MR. Cholera toxin induces migration of dendritic cells from the subepithelial dome region to T- and B-cell areas of Peyer's patches. Infect Immun 2003;71:504–509.
5. Kelsall BL, Strober W. Distinct populations of dendritic cells are present in the subepithelial dome and T cell regions of the murine Peyer's patch. J Exp Med 1996;183:237–247.

6. Iwasaki A, Kelsall BL. Localization of distinct Peyer's patch dendritic cell subsets and their recruitment by chemokines macrophage inflammatory protein MIP-3α, MIP-3β, and secondary lymphoid organ chemokine. J Exp Med 2000;191:1381–1393.
7. Zhao X, Sato A, Dela Cruz CS, Lineham M, Luegering A, Kucharzik T, Shirakawa A-K, Marquez G, Farber JM, Williams I, Iwasaki A. CCL9 is secreted by the follicle-associated epithelium and recruits dome region Peyer's patch CD11b+ dendritic cells. J Immunol 2003;171:2797–2803.
8. Alberts B, Bray D, Hopkin K, Johnson A, Lewis J, Raff M, Roberts K, Walter P. Essential Cell Biology, 2nd ed. London: Garland Science, 2004;711:722.
9. Macpherson AJ, Smith K. Mesenteric lymph nodes at the center of immune anatomy. J Exp Med 2006;203:497–500.
10. Ley RE, Peterson DA, Gordon JI. Ecological and evolutionaary forces shaping microbial diversity in the human intestine. Cell 2006;124:837–848.
11. Simon GL, Gorbach SL. Intestinal flora in health and disease. Gastroenterology 1984;86:174–193.
12. Sterzl J, Silverstein AM. Developmental aspects of immunity. Adv Immunol 1967;6:337–459.
13. Cebra JJ, Jiang H-Q, Sterzl J, Tlaskalova-Hogenova H. The role of mucosal microbiota in the development and maintenance of the mucosal immune system. In: Ogra PL, Mestecky J, Lamm ME, Strober W, Bienenstock J, McGhee J, eds. Mucosal Immunology, 2nd ed. New York: Academic Press, 1999, pp. 267–280.
14. Moreau M, Ducluzeau R, Guy-Grand D, Muller MA. Increase in the population of duodenal immunoglobulin A plasmocytes in axenic mice associated with different living or dead bacterial strains of intestinal origin. Infect Immun 1978;21:532–539.
15. Leidy J. On the existence of entophyta in healthy animals as a natural condition. Proc Acad Natl Sci Phila 1849;4:225–233.
16. Klaasen HLBM, Van den Heijden PJ, Stock W, Poelma FGJ, Koopman JP, Van den Brink ME, Bakker MH, Eling WMC, Beynen AC. Apathogenic, intestinal, segmented, filamentous bacteria stimulate the mucosal immune system of mice. Infect Immun 1993;61:303–306.
17. Tyrer P, Foxwell AR, Cripps AW, Apicella MA, Kyd JM. Microbial pattern recognition receptors mediate M-cell uptake of a Gram-negative bacterium. Infect Immun 2006;74:625–631.
18. Yamanaka T, Straumfors A, Morton HC, Fausa O, Brandtzaeg P, Farstad IN. M cell pockets of human Peyer's patches are specialized extensions of germinal centers. Eur J Immunol 2001;31:107–116.
19. Yamanaka T, Helgeland L, Farstad IN, Fukushima H, Midtvedt T, Brandtzaeg P. Microbial colonization drives lymphocyte accumulation and differentiation in the follicle-associated epithelium of Peyer's patches. J Immunol 2003;170:816–822.
20. Borghesi C, Bertelli E, Regoli M, Nicoletti C. Modifications of the FAE by short term exposure to a non-intestinal bacterium. J Pathol 1996;180:326–332.
21. Man AL, Prieto-Garcia ME, Nicoletti C. Improving M cell mediated transport across mucosal barriers: do certain bacteria hold the keys? Immunology 2004;113:15–22.
22. Neutra MR, Phillips TL, Mayer EL, Fishkind DJ. Transport of membrane-bound macromolecules by M cells in the FAE of rabbit Peyer's patches. Cell Tissue Res 1987;247:536–546.
23. Meng G, Wei X, Wu X, Sellers MT, Decker JM, Moldoveanu Z, Orenstein JM, Graham MF, Kappes JC, Mestecky J, Shaw GM, Smith PD. Primary intestinal epithelial cells selectively transfer R5 HIV-1 to CCR5+ cells. Nat Med 2002;8:150–156.
24. Gebert A. The role of M cells in the protection of mucosal membrane. Histochem Cell Biol 1997;108:455–470.
25. Finzi G, Cornaggia M, Capella C, Fiocca R, Bosi F, Solcia E, Samloff IM. Cathepsin E in follicle-associated epithelium of intestine and tonsils: localization to M cells and possible role in antigen processing. Histochemistry 1993;99:201–211.
26. Jones BD, Ghori N, Falkow S. *Salmonella typhimurium* initiates murine infection by penetrating and destroying the specialized epithelial M cells of the Peyer's patches. J Exp Med 1994;180:15–23.

27. Perdomo JL, Cavaillon JM, Huerre M, Ohayon H, Gounon P, Sansonetti PJ. Acute inflammation causes epithelial invasion and mucosal destruction in experimental shigellosis. J Exp Med 1994;180:1307–1319.
28. Grutzkau A, Hanski C, Hahn H, Riecken EO. Invasion of Peyer's patch: a common mechanism shared by *Yersinia enterocolitica* and other entero-invasive bacteria. Gut 1990;3: 1011–1015.
29. Meynell HM, Thomas NW, James PS, Holland J, Taussig MJ, Nicolletti C. Up-regulation of microsphere transport across the follicle-associated epithelium of Peyer's patch by exposure to *S. pneumoniae* R36a. FASEB J 1999;13:611–619.
30. Borghesi C, Taussig MJ, Nicoletti C. Rapid appearance of M cells after microbial challenge is restricted at the periphery of the follicle-associated epithelium of Peyer's patch. Lab Invest 1999;79:1391–1410.
31. Gebert A, Steinmetz I, Fassbender S, Wendlandt KH. Antigen transport in Peyer's patches: increased uptake by constant numbers of M cells. Am J Pathol 2004;64:65–72.
32. Neutra MR, Pringault E, Kraehenbuhl JP. Antigen sampling across epithelial barriers and induction of mucosal immune responses. Annu Rev Immunol 1996;14:275–300.
33. Chieppa M, Rescigno M, Huang AY, Germain RN. Dynamic imaging of dendritic cell extension into the small bowel lumen in response to epithelial cell TLR engagement. J Exp Med 2006;203:2841–2852.
34. Evans EA, Calderwood DA. Forces and bond dynamics in cell adhesion. Science 2007;316:1148–1153.
35. Mitic LL, Van Itallie CM, Anderson JM. Molecular physiology and pathophysiology of tight junctions I. Tight junction structure and function: lessons from mutant animals and proteins. Am J Physiol Gastrointest Liver Physiol 2000;279:G250–G254.
36. Schneeberger EE, Lynch RD. The tight junction: a multifunctional complex. Am J Physiol Cell Physiol 2004;286:C1213–C1228.
37. Connolly JL, Rodgers SE, Clarke P, Ballard DW, Kerr LD, Tyler KL, Dermody TS. Reovirus-induced apoptosis requires activation of transcription factor NFκB. J Virol 2000;74: 2981–2989.
38. Sonoda N, Furuse M, Sasaki H, Yonemura S, Katahira J, Horiguchi Y, Tsukita S. *Clostridium perfringens* enterotoxin fragment removes specific claudins from tight junction strands: evidence for direct involvement of claudins in tight junction barrier. J Cell Biol 1999;147:195–204.
39. Wang F, Graham WV, Wang Y, Witkowski ED, Schwarz BT, Turner JR. Interferon-γ and tumor necrosis factor-α synergize to induce intestinal epithelial barrier dysfunction by up-regulating myosin light chain kinase expression. Am J Pathol 2005;166:409–419.
40. Utech M, Ivanov AI, Samarin SN, Bruewer M, Turner JR, Mrsny RJ, Parkos CA, Nusrat A. Mechanism of IFN-β-induced endocytosis of tight junction proteins: myosin II-dependent vacuolarization of the apical plasma membrane. Mol Biol Cell 2005;16:5040–5050.
41. Clark E, Hoare C, Tanianis-Hughes J, Carlson GL, Warhurst G. Interferon gamma induces translocation of commensal *Escherichia coli* across gut epithelial cells via a lipid raft-mediated process. Gastroenterology 2005;128:1258–1267.
42. Moriez R, Salvador-Cartier C, Theodoru V, Fioramonti J, Eutamene H, Bueno L. Myosin light chain kinase is involved in lipopolysaccharide-induced disruption of colonic epithelial barrier and bacterial translocation in rats. Am J Pathol 2005;167:1071–1079.
43. Cunliffe RN, Mahida YR. Expression and regulation of antimicrobial peptides in the gastrointestinal tract. J Leukoc Biol 2004;75:49–58.
44. Mowat A McI. The role of antigen recognition and suppressor cells in mice with oral tolerance to ovalbumin. Immunology 1985;56:253–260.
45. Mowat AM. Dendritic cells and immune responses to orally administered antigens. Vaccine 2005;23:1797–1799.
46. Husby S, Mestecky J, Moldoveanu Z, Holland S, Elson CO. Oral tolerance in humans. T cell but not B cell tolerance after antigen feeding. J Immunol 1994;152:4663–4670.

47. Macpherson AJ, Smith K. Mesenteric lymph nodes at the center of immune anatomy. J Exp Med 2006;203:497–500.
48. Mowat AM, Weiner HL. Oral tolerance: physiological basis and clinical applications. In: Ogra PL, Mestecky J, Lamm ME, Strober W, Bienestock J, McGhee JR, eds. Mucosal Immunology, 2nd ed. New York: Academic Press, 1999, pp. 587–618.
49. Kato H, Fujihashi K, Kato R, Yuki Y, McGhee JR. Oral tolerance revisited: prior oral tolerization abrogates cholera toxin-induced mucosal IgA responses. J Immunol 2001;166:3114–3121.
50. Strobel S, Ferguson A. Persistence of oral tolerance in mice fed ovalbumin is different for humoral and cell-mediated immune responses. Immunology 1987;60:317–318.
51. Ke Y, Kapp JA. Oral antigen inhibits priming of CD8+ CTL, CD4+ T cells and antibody responses while activating CD8+ suppressor T cells. J Immunol 1996;156:916–921.
52. Friedman A, Weiner HL. Induction of anergy or active suppression following oral tolerance is determined by antigen dosage. Proc Natl Acad Sci USA 1994;91:6688–6694.
53. Chen Y, Inobe J, Marks R, Gonnella P, Kuchroo VK, Weiner HL. Peripheral deletion of antigen-reactive T cells in oral tolerance. Nature 1995;376:177–180.
54. Worbs T, Bode U, Yan S, Hoffmann MW, Hintzen G, Bernhardt G, Forster R, Pabst O. Oral tolerance originates in the intestinal immune system and relies on antigen carriage by dendritic cells. J Exp Med 2006;203:519–527.
55. Brinkmann V, Cyster JG, Hla T. FTY720: sphingosine 1-phosphate receptor-1 in the control of lymphocyte egress and endothelial barrier function. Am J Transplant 2004;4:1019–1025.
56. Spahn TW, Fontana A, Faria AM, Slavin AJ, Eugster HP, Zhang X, Koni PA, Ruddle NH, Flavell RA, Rennert PD, Weiner HL. Induction of oral tolerance to cellular immune responses in the absence of Peyer's patches. Eur J Immunol 2001;31:1278–1287.
57. Spahn TW, Weiner HL, Rennert PD, Lugering N, Fontana A, Domschke W, Kucharzik T. Eur J Immunol 2002;32:1109–1113.
58. Kraus TA, Brimnes J, Muong C, Liu J-H, Moran TM, Tappenden KA, Boros P, Mayer L. Induction of mucosal tolerance in Peyer's patch-deficient, ligated small bowel loops. J Clin Invest 2005;115:2234–2243.
59. Shreedhar VK, Kelsall BL, Neutra MR. Cholera toxin induces migration of dendritic cells from the subepithelial dome region to T- and B-cell area of Peyer's patches. Infect Immun 2003;71:504–509.
60. Milling SW, Yrlid U, Jenkins C, Richards CM, Williams NA, Mac Pherson G, Regulation of intestinal immunity: effects of the oral adjuvant *Escherichia coli* heat-labile enterotoxin on migrating dendritic cells. Eur J Immunol 2007;37:87–99.
61. Jang MH, Sougawa N, Tonaka T, Hirata T, Hiroi T, Tohya K, Guo Z, Umemoto E, Ebisuno Y, Yang BG, Seoh JY, Lipp M, Kiyono H, Miyasaka M. CCR7 is critically important for migration of dendritic cells in intestinal lamina propria to mesenteric lymph nodes. J Immunol 2006;176:803–810.
62. Ke Y, Pearce K, Lake JP, Ziegler HK, Kapp JA. γδ lymphocytes regulate the induction of oral tolerance. J Immunol 1997;158:3610–3618.
63. Sun J-B, Holmgren J, Czerkinsky C. Cholera toxin B subunit: an efficient transmucosal carrier-delivery system for induction of peripheral immunological tolerance. Proc Natl Acad Sci USA 1994;91:10795–10799.
64. Groux H, O'Garra A, Bigler M, Rouleau M, Antonenko S, de Vries JE, Roncarolo MG. A CD4+ T cell subset inhibits antigen-specific T cell responses and prevents colitis. Nature 1997; 389:737–742.
65. Kamanaka M, Kim ST, Wan YY, Sutterwala FS, Lara-Tejero M, Galan JE, Harhaj E, Flavell RA. Expression of interleukin-10 intestinal lymphocytes detected by an interleukin-10 receptor knockin tiger mouse. Immunity 2006;25:941–952.
66. Belkaid Y, Rouse BT. Natural regulatory T cells in infectious disease. Nat Immunol 2005;6:353–360.

67. Wan YY, Flavell RA. Identifying Foxp3-expressing suppressor T cells with a bicistronic reporter. Proc Natl Acad Sci USA 2005;102:5126–5131.
68. Khattri R, Cox T, Yasayko SA, Ramsdell F. An essential role for Scurfin in CD4(+) CD25(+) T regulatory cells. Nat Immunol 2003;4:337–342.
69. Hori S, Nomura T, Sakaguchi S. Control of regulatory T cell development by the transcription factor Foxp3. Science 2003;299:1057–1061.
70. Fontenot JD, Gavin MA, Rudensky AY. Foxp3 programs the development and function of CD4(+) CD25(+) regulatory T cells. Nat Immunol 2003;4:330–336.
71. Chen WJ, Jin W, Hardegen N, Lei K, Li L, Marinos N, McGrady G, Wahl SM. Conversion of peripheral CD4+ CD25− naïve T cells to CD4+ CD25+ regulatory T cells by TGF-β induction of transcription factor Foxp3. J Exp Med 2003;198:1875–1886.
72. Huber S, Schramm C, Lehr HA, Mann A, Schmitt S, Becker C, Protschka M, Galle PR, Neurath MF, Blessing M. Cutting edge: TGF-β signaling is required for the in vivo expansion and immunosuppressive capacity of regulatory CD4+ CD25+ T cells. J Immunol 2004; 173:6526–6531.
73. Li MO, wan YY, Flavell RA. T cell-produced transforming growth factor-beta 1 controls T cell tolerance and regulates T1- and Th 17-cell differentiation. Immunity 2007;26(5):579–591.
74. Liu S-J, Tsai J-P, Shen C-R, Sher Y-P, Hsieh C-L, Yeh Y-C, Chou A-H, Chang S-R, Hsiao K-N, Yu F-W, Chen H-W. Induction of a distinct CD8 Tnc 17 subset by transforming growth factor-β and interleukin-6. J Leukoc Biol 2007;82(2):354–360.
75. Gutcher I, Becher B. APC-derived cytokines and T cell polarization in autoimmune inflammation. J Clin Invest 2007;117:1119–1127.
76. Barnard JA, Warwick GJ, Gold LI. Localization of transforming growth factor beta isoforms in the normal murine small intestine and colon. Gastroenterology 1993;105:67–73.
77. Rumbo M, Anderle P, Didierlaurent A, Sierro F, Debard N, Sirard J-C, Finike D, Kraehenbuhl J-P. How the gut links innate and adaptive immunity. Ann NY Acad Sci 2004;1029:16–21.
78. Garside P, Millington O, Smith KM. The anatomy of mucosal immune responses. Ann NY Acad Sci 2004;1029:9–15.
79. Baecher-Allan C, Wolf E, Hafler DA. MHC Class II expression identifies functionally distinct human regulatory T cells. J Immunol 2006;176:4622–4631.
80. Chang CH, Hong SC, Hughes CC, Janeway CA Jr, Flavell RA. CIITA activates the expression of MHC class II genes in mouse T cells. Int Immunol 1995;7:1515–1518.
81. Janeway CA Jr, Medzhitov R. Innate immune recognition. Annu Rev Immunol 2002;20: 197–216.
82. Germain RN. An innately interesting decade of research in immunology. Nat Med 2004; 10:1307–1320.
83. Cario E, Brown D, Mckee M, Lynch-Devaney K, Gerken G, Podolsky DK. Commensal-associated molecular patterns induce selective Toll-like receptor trafficking from apical membrane to cytoplasmic compartments in polarized intestinal epithelium. Am J Pathol 2002;160:165–173.
84. Bambou JC, Giraud A, Menard S, Begue B, Rakotobe S, Heyman M, Taddei F, Cerf-Bensussan N, Gaboriau-Routhiau V. In vitro and ex vivo activation of the TLR5 signaling pathway in intestinal epithelial cells by a commensal Escherichia coli strain. J Biol Chem 2004;279:42984–42992.
85. Chabot S, Wagner JS, Farrant S, Neutra MR. TLRs regulate the gatekeeping functions of the intestinal follicle-associated epithelium. J Immunol 2006;176:4275–4283.
86. Goodnow CC. Discriminating microbe from self suffers a double toll. Science 2006; 312:1606–1608.
87. Otte J-M, Cario E, Podolsky D. Mechanisms of cross hyporesponsiveness to Toll-like receptor bacterial ligands in intestinal epithelial cells. Gastroenterology 2004;126:1054–1070.
88. Neal MD, Leaphart C, Levy R, Prince J, Billiar TR, Watkins S, Li J, Cetin S, Ford H, Schreiber A, Hackam D. Enterocyte TLR4 mediates phagocytosis and translocation of bacteria across the intestinal barrier. J Immunol 2006;176:3070–3079.

89. Fukata M, Michelsen KS, Eri R, Thomas LS, Hu B, Lukasek K, Nast CC, Lechago J, Xu R, Naiki Y, Soliman A, Arditi M, Abreu MT. Toll-like receptor-4 is required for intestinal response to epithelial injury and limiting bacterial translocation in a murine model of acute colitis. Am J Physiol Gastrointest Liver Physiol 2005;288:G1055-G1065.

90. Cunliffe RN, Mahida YR. Expression and regulation of antimicrobial peptides in the gastrointestinal tract. J Leukoc Biol 2004;75:49–58.

91. Sansonetti PJ. War and peace at mucosal surfaces. Nat Rev Immunol 2004;4:953–964.

92. Mahida YR, Cunliffe RN. Defensins and mucosal protection. Novartis Found Symp 2004;263:71–77.

93. Mani R, Cady SD, Tang M, Waring AJ, Lehrer RI, Hong M. Membrane-dependent oligomeric structure and pore formation of a β-hairpin antimicrobial peptide in lipid bilayers from solid-state NMR. Proc Natl Acad Sci USA 2006;103:16242–16247.

94. Yang D, Chertov O, Bykovskaia SN, Chen Q, Buffo MJ, Shogan J, Anderson M, Schroder JM, Wang JM, Howard OM, Oppenheim JJ. Beta-defensins: linking innate and adaptive immunity through dendritic and T cell CCR6. Science 1999;286:525–528.

95. De Y, Chen Q, Schmidt AP, Anderson GM, Wang JM, Wooters J, Oppenheim JJ, Chertov O. LL-37, the neutrophil granule-and epithelial cell-derived cathelicidin, utilizes formyl peptide receptor to chemoattract human peripheral blood neutrophils, monocytes, and T cells. J Exp Med 2000;192:1069–1074.

96. Steel A, Nussberger S, Romero MF, Boron WF, Boyd CA, Hediger MA. Stoichiometry and pH dependence of rabbit proton-dependent oligopeptide transporter PepT1. J Physiol 1997;498:563–569.

97. Charrier L, Merlin D. The oligopeptide transporter hPepT1: gateway to the innate immune response. Lab Invest 2006;86:538–546.

98. Cash HL, Whitham CV, Behrendt CL, Hooper LV. Symbiotic bacteria direct expression of an intestinal bactericidal lectin. Science 2006;313:1126–1130.

99. Hagemann RF, Sigdestad CP, Lesher S. A quantitative description of the intestinal epithelium of the mouse. Am J Anat 1970;129:41–52.

100. Li YQ, Roberts SA, Paulus U, Loeffler M, Potten CS. The crypt cycle in mouse small intestinal epithelium. J Cell Sci 1994;107:3271–3279.

101. Taylor RW, Barron MJ, Borthwick GM, Gospel A, Chinnery PF, Samuels DC, Talor GA, Plusa SM, Needham S, Greaves LC, Kirkwood TBL, Turnbull DM. Mitochondrial DNA mutations in human colonic crypt stem cells. J Clin Invest 2003;112:1351–1360.

102. Schon EA. Tales from the crypt. J Clin Invest 2003;112:1312–1316.

103. Greaves LC, Preston SL, Tadrous PJ, Talor RW, Barron MJ, Oukrif D, Leedham SJ, Deheragoda M, Sasieni P, Novelli MR, Jankowski JAZ, Turnbull DM, Wright NA, McDonald SAC. Mitochondrial DNA mutations are established in human colonic stem cells, and mutated clones expand by crypt fission. Proc Natl Acad Sci USA 2006;103:714–719.

104. Park HS, Goodlad RA, Wright NA. Crypt fission in the small intestine and colon: a mechanism for the emergence of G6PD locus-mutated crypts after treatment with mutagens. Am J Pathol 1995;147:1416–1427.

105. Knight KL, Winstead CR. Organization and expression of genes encoding IgA heavy chain, polymeric immunoglobulin, and J chain. In: Ogra PL, Mestecky J, Lamm ME, Strober W, Bienenstock J, McGhee JR, eds. Mucosal Immunology, 2nd ed. New York: Academic Press, 1999, pp. 153–162.

106. Mostov K, Kaetzel CS. Immunoglobulin transport and the polymeric immunoglobulin receptor. In: Ogra PL, Mestecky J, Lamm ME, Strober W, Bienenstock J, McGhee JR, eds. Mucosal Immunology, 2nd ed. New York: Academic Press, 1999, pp. 181–211.

107. Hempen PM, Phillips KM, Conway PS, Sandoval KH, Schneeman TA, Wu H-J, Kaetzel CS. Transcriptional regulation of the human polymeric Ig receptor gene: analysis of basal promoter elements. J Immunol 2002;169:1912–1921.

108. Scheeman TA, Bruno MEC, Schjerven H, Johansen F-E, Chady L, Kaetzel CS. Regulation of the polymeric Ig receptor by signaling through TLRs 3 and 4: linking innate and adaptive immune responses. J Immunol 2005;175:376–384.

109. Mazanec MB, Kaetzel CS, Lamm ME, Fletcher D, Nedrud JG. Intracellular neutralization of virus by immunoglobulin A antibodies. Proc Natl Acad Sci USA 1992;89:6901–6905.

110. Mazanec MB, Coudret CL, Fleetcher DR. Intracellular neutralization of influenza virus by immunoglobulin A anti-hemaglultinin monoclonal antibodies. J Virol 1995;69:1339–1343.

111. Mantis NJ, Cheung MC, Chintalacharuvu KR, Rey J, Corthesy B, Neutra MR. Selective adherence of IgA to murine Peyer's patch M cells: evidence for a novel IgA receptor. J Immunol 2002;169:1844–1851.

112. Rey J, Garin N, Speertini F, Corthesy B. Targeting of secretory IgA to Peyer's patch dendritic and T cells after transport by intestinal M cells. J Immunol 2004;172:3026–3033.

113. Costerton JW, Stewart PS, Greenberg EP. Bacterial biofilms: a common cause of persistent infections. Science 1999;284:1318–1322.

114. Mestecky J, Russell MW, Elson CO. Intestinal IgA: novel views on its function in the defence of the largest mucosal surface. Gut 1999;44:2–5.

115. Russell MW, Mansa B. Complement-fixing properties of human IgA antibodies: alternative pathway complement activation by plastic-bound, but not by specific antigen-bound IgA. Scand J Immunol 1989;30:175–183.

116. Lefrancois L, Puddington L. Basic aspects of intraepithelial lymphocyte immunobiology. In: Ogra PL, Mestecky J, Lamm ME, Strober W, Bienenstock J, McGhee JR, eds. Mucosal Immunology, 2nd ed. New York: Academic Press, 1999, pp. 413–428.

117. Lambolez F, Kronenberg M, Cheroutre H. Thymic differentiation of TCR alpha beta (+) CD8 alpha alpha (+) IELs. Immunol Rev 2007;215:178–188.

118. Mora JR, Iwata M, Eksteen B, Song S-Y, Junt T, Senman B, Otipoby KL, Yokota A, Takeuchi H, Ricciardi-Castagnoli P, Rajewsky K, Adams DA, von Andrian UH. Generation of gut-homing IgA-secreting B cells by intestinal dendritic cells. Science 2006;314:1157–1160.

119. Pulendran B, Palucka K, Banchereau J. Sensing pathogens and tuning immune responses. Science 2001;293:253–256.

120. Andrew EM, Newton DJ, Dalton JE, Egan CE, Goodwin SJ, Tramonti D, Scott P, Carding SR. Delineation of the function of a major $\gamma\delta$ T cell subset during infection. J Immunol 2005;175:1741–1750.

121. Newton DJ, Andrew EM, Dalton JE, Mears R, Carding SR. Identification of novel $\gamma\delta$ T-cell subsets following bacterial infection in the absence of V γ 1+ T cells: homeostatic control of $\gamma\delta$ T-cell responses to pathogen infection by V γ 1+ T cells. Infect Immun 2006;74:1097–1105.

122. Russano AM, Bassotti G, Agea E, Bistoni O, Mazzochi A, Morelli A, Porcelli SA, Spinozzi F. CD1-restricted recognition of exogenous and self-lipid antigens by duodenal $\gamma\delta$ + T lymphocytes. J Immunol 2007;178:3620–3626.

123. Mengel J, Cardillo F, Aroeira LS, Williams O, Vaz NM. Anti-$\gamma\delta$ T cell antibody blocks the induction and maintenance of oral tolerance to ovalbumin in mice. Immunol Lett 1995;48:97–102.

124. Saito H, Kanamori Y, Takemori T, Nariuchi H, Kubota E, Takahashi-Iwanaga H, Iwanaga T, Ishikawa H. Generation of intestinal T cells from progenitors residing in gut cryptopaatches. Science 1998;280:275–278.

125. Yu Q, Tang C, Xun S, Yajima T, Takeda K, Yoshikai Y. MyD88-dependent signaling for IL-15 production plays an important role in maintenance of CD8$\alpha\alpha$ TCR$\alpha\beta$ and TCR$\gamma\delta$ intestinal intraepithelial lymphocytes. J Immunol 2006;176:6180–6185.

126. Schluns KS, Nowak EC, Cabrera-Hernandez A, Puddington L, Lefrancois L, Aguida HL. Distinct cell types control lymphoid subset development by means of IL-15 and IL-15 receptor α expression. Proc Natl Acad Sci USA 2004;101:5616–5621.

127. Rocha B, von Boehmer H, Guy-Grand D. Selection of intraepithelial lymphocytes with CD8α/α co-receptors by self-antigen in the murine gut. Proc Natl Acad Sci USA 1992;89:5336–5340.

128. Lin T, Yoshida H, Matsuzaki G, Guehler SR, Nomoto K, Barrett TA, Green DR. Auto-specific γδ thymocytes that escape negative selection find sanctuary in the intestine. J Clin Invest 1999;104:1297–1305.

129. Leishman AJ, Naidenko OV, Attinger A, Konig F, Lena CJ, Xiong Y, Chang H-C, Reinherz E, Kronenberg M, Cheroutre H. T cell responses modulated through interaction between CD8 and the nonclassical MHC Class I molecule, TL. Science 2001;294:1936–1939.

130. Macpherson AJ, Gatto D, Sainsbury E, Harriman GR, Hengartner H, Zinkernagel RM. A primitive T cell-independent mechanism of intestinal mucosal IgA responses to commensal bacteria. Science 2000;288:2222–2226.

131. Suzuki K, Meek B, Doi Y, Honjo T, Fagarasan S. Two distinctive pathways for recruitment of naive and primed IgM+ B cells to the gut lamina propria. Proc Natl Acad Sci USA 2005;102:2482–2486.

132. Bergqvist P, Gardby E, Stennson A, Bemark M, Lycke NY. Gut IgA class switch recombination in the absence of CD40 does not occur in lamina propria and is independent of germinal centers. J Immunol 2006;177:7772–7783.

133. Shikina T, Hiroi T, Iwatanik K, Jang MH, Fukuyama S, Tamura M, Kubo T, Ishikawa H, Kiyono H. IgA class switch occurs in the organized nasopharynx – and gut – associated lymphoid tissue, but not in the diffuse lamina propria of airways and gut. J Immunol 204;172:6259–6264.

134. Macpherson AJ, Uhr T. Induction of protective IgA by intestinal dendritic cells carrying commensal bacteria. Science 2004;303:1662–1665.

135. Thurnheer MC, Zuercher AW, Cebra JJ, Bos NA. B1 cells contribute to serum IgM, but not to intestinal IgA, production in gnotobiotic Ig allotype chimeric mice. J Immunol 2003;170:4564–4571.

136. Li YQ, Roberts SA, Paulus U, Locffler M, Potten CS. The crypt cycle in mouse small intestinal epithelium. J Cell Sci 1994;107:33271–3279.

137. Berg RD, Bacterial translocation from the gastrointestinal tract. In: Paul PS, Francis DH, eds. Mechanisms in the Pathogenesis of Enteric Diseases 2. New York: Plenum Press, 1999, pp. 11–30.

138. Daniels CK, Schmucker DL, Bazin H, Jones AL. Immunoglobulin A receptor of rat small intestinal enterocytes is unaffected by aging. Gastroenterology 1988;94:1432–1439.

139. Taylor LD, Daniels CK, Schmucker DL. Aging compromises gastrointestinal mucosal immune response in the rhesus monkey. Immunology 1992;75:614–618.

140. Renshaw M, Rockwell J, Engleman C, Gewirtz A, Katz J, Sambhara S. Cutting edge: impaired Toll-like receptor expression and function in aging. J Immunol 2002;169:4697–4701.

141. van Duin D, Mohanaty S, Thomas V, Ginter S, Montgomery RR, Fikrig E, Allore HG, Medzhitov R, Shaw AC. Age-associated defect in human TLR-function. J Immunol 2007;178:970–975.

142. Letiembre M, Hao W, Liu Y, Walter S, Mihaljevic I, Rivest S, Hartmann T, Fassbeender K. Innate immune receptor expression in normal brain aging. Neuroscience 2007;146:248–254.

143. Lin T, Matsuzaki G, Kenai H, Nomoto K. Extrathymic and thymic origin of IEL: are most IEL in euthymic mice derived from the thymus? Immunol Cell Biol 1995;73:469–473.

144. Lefrancois L, Le Corre R, Mayo J, Bluestone JA, Goodman T. Extrathymic selection of TCR gamma delta + T cells by class II major histocompatibilitty complex molecules. Cell 1990;63:333–340.

145. Bandeira A, Itohara S, Bonneville M, Burlen-Defranoux O, Mota-Santos T, Coutinho A, Tonegawa S. Extrathymic origin of intestinal intraepithelial lymphocytes bearing T-cell antigen receptor gamma delta. Proc Natl Acad Sci USA 1991;88:43–47.

146. Kanameri T, Ishimaru K, Nanno M, Maki K, Ikuta K, Nariuchi H, Ishikawa H. Identification of novel lymphoid tissues in murine intestinal mucosa where clusters of c-kit+ IL-7R+ Thy1 + lympho-hemopoietic progenitors develop. J Exp Med 1996;184:1449–1459.

147. Locke NR, Stankovic S, Funda DP, Harrison LC. TCR γδ intraepithelial lymphocytes are required for self-tolerance. J Immunol 2006;176:6553–6559.

148. Kato H, Fujihashi K, Kato R, Dohi T, Fujihashi K, Hagiwara Y, Kataoka K, Kobayashi R, McGhee JR. Lack of oral tolerance in aging is due to sequential loss of Peyer's patch cell interactions. Int Immunol 2003;15:145–158.

149. Fujihashi K, McGhee JR. Mucosal immunity and tolerance in the elderly. Mech Ageing Dev 2004;125:889–898.

150. Wakabayashi A, Utsuuyama M, Hosodda T, Sato K, Takahashi H, Hirokawa K. Induction of immunological tolerance by oral, but not intravenous and intraportal, administration of ovalbumin and the difference between young and old mice. J Nutr Health Aging 2006;10:183–191.

151. Yu Q, Tang C, Xun S, Yajima T, Takeda K, Yoshikai Y. MyD88-dependenet signaling for IL-15 production plays an important role in maintenance of CD8αα TCRαβ and TCRγδ intestinal intraepithelial lymphocytes. J Immunol 2006;176:6180–6185.

152. Martin F, Kearney JF. B1 cells: similarities and differences with other B cell subsets. Curr Opin Immunol 2001;13:195–201.

153. Berland R, Wortis HH. Origins and functions of B1 cells with notes on the role of CD5. Annu Rev Immunol 22002;20:253–300.

154. Weksler ME. Changes in the B-cell repertoire with age. Vaccine 2000;18:1624–1628.

155. Zheng B, Han S, Takahashi Y, Kelsoe G. Immunosenescence and germinal center reaction. Immunol Rev 1997;160:63–77.

156. Lebman DA, Lee FD, Coffman RL. Mechanism for transforming growth factor beta and IL-2 enhancement of IgA expression in lipopolysaccharide-stimulated B cell cultures. J Immunol 1990;144:952–959.

157. Kim PH, Kagnoff MF. Transforming growth factor β 1 increases IgA isotype switching at the clonal level. J Immunol 1990;145:3773–3778.

158. He B, Xu W, Santini PA, Polydorides AD, Chir A, Estrella J, Shan M, Chadburn A, Villanacci V, Plebani A, Knowles DM, Rescigno M, Cerrutti A. Intestinal bacteria trigger T cell-independent immunoglobulin A(2) class switching by inducing epithelial-cell secretion of the cytokine APRIL. Immunity 2007;26:812–826.

159. Kaminski DA, Stavnezer J. Enhanced IgA class switching in marginal zone and B1 B cells relative to follicular/B2 cells. J Immunol 2006;177:6025–6029.

160. Benahmed M, Meresse B, Arnulf B, Barbe U, Mention JJ, Verkarre V, Allez M, Cellier C, Hermine O, Cerf-Bensussan N. Inhibition of TGF-beta signaling by IL-15: a new role for IL-15 in the loss of immune homeostasis in celiac disease. Gastroenterology 2007;132: 994–1008.

161. Rogerson BJ, Harris DP, Swain SL, Burgess DO. Germinal center B cells in Peyer's patches of aged mice exhibit a normal activation phenotype and highly mutated IgM genes. Mech Ageing Dev 2003;124:155–165.

162. Williams GT, Jolly CJ, Kohler J, Neuberger MS. The contribution of somatic hypermutation to the diversity of serum immunoglobulin: dramatic increase with age, Immunity 2000;13:409–417.

163. Ha S, Tsuji M, Suzuki K, Meek B, Yasuda N, Kaisho T, Fagarasan S. Regulation of B1 cell migration by signals through Toll-like receptors. J Exp Med 2006;203:2541–2550.

164. Park S-R, Kim H-A, Chun S-K, Park J-B, Kim P-H. Mechanisms underlying the effects of LPS and activation-induced cytidine deaminase on IgA isotype expression. Mol Cells 2005;19:445–451.

165. Shockett P, Stavnezer J. Effect of cytokines on switching to IgA and alpha germline transcripts in the B lymphoma 1.29mu. Transforming growth factor-beta activates transcription of the unrearranged C alpha gene. J Immunol 1991;147:4374–4383.

166. van Vlasselaer P, Punnonen J, deVries JE. Transforming growth factor-beta directs IgA switching in human B cells. J Immunol 1992;148:2062–2067.

167. Koide N, Morikawa A, Ito H, Sugiyama T, Hassan F, Islam S, Tumurkhuu G, Mori I, Yoshida T, Yokochi T. Defective responsiveness of CD5+ B1 cells to lipopolysaccharide in cytokine production. J Endotoxin Res 2006;12:346–351.

168. Borghesi L, Hsu L-Y, Miller JP, Anderson M, Herzenberg L, Herzenberg L, Schlissel MS, Allman D, Gerstein RM. B lineage-specific regulation of V (D) J recombinase activity is established in common lymphoid progenitors. J Exp Med 2004;199:491–502.

169. Miller JP, Allman D. The decline in B lymphopoiesis in aged mice reflects loss of very early B-lineage precursors. J Immunol 2003;171:2326–2330.

170. Ansel KM, Harris RBS, Cyster JG. CXCL13 is required for B1 cell homing, natural antibody production, and body cavity immunity. Immunity 2002;16:67–76.

171. Ishikawa S, Sato T, Abe M, Nagai S, Onai N, Yoneyama H, Zhang Y, Suzuki T, Hashimoto S, Shirai T, Lipp M, Matsushima K. Aberrant high expression of B lymphocyte chemokine (BLC/CXCL13) by CD11b+ CD11c+ dendritic cells in murine lupus and preferential chemotaxis of B1 cells toward BLC. J Exp Med 2001;193:1393–1402.

172. Ito T, Ishikawa S, Sato T, Akadegawa K, Yurino H, Kitabatake M, Hontsu S, Ezaki T, Kimura H, Maatsushima K. Defective B1 cell homing to the peritoneal cavity and preferential recruitment of B1 cells in the target organs in a murine model for systemic lupus erythematosus. J Immunol 2004;172:3628–3634.

173. Kroese FG, Butcher EC, Stall AM, Lalor PA, Adams S, Herzenberg LA. Many of the IgA producing plasma cells in murine gut are derived from self-replenishing precursors in the peritoneal cavity. Int Immunol 1989;1:75–86.

174. Moon B, Takaki S, Miyake K, Takatsu K. The role of IL-5 for mature B-1 cells in homeostatic proliferation, cell survival, and Ig production. J Immunol 2004;172:6020–6029.

175. Poupon V, Cerf-Bensussan N. Adhesion molecules on mucosal lymphocytes. In: Ogra PL, Mestecky J, Lamm ME, Strober W, Bienenstock J, McGhee JR, eds. Mucosal Immunology, 2nd ed. New York: Academic Press, 1999, pp. 523–540.

176. Butcher EC. Lymphocyte homing and intestinal immunity. In: Ogra PL, Mestecky J, Lamm ME, Strober W, Bienenstock J, McGhee JR, eds. Mucosal Immunology, 2nd ed. New York: Academic Press, 1999, pp. 507–522.

177. Pabst O, Ohl L, Wendland M, Wurbel M-A, Kremmer E, Malissen B, Foster R. Chemokine receptor CCR9 contributes to the localization of plasma cells to the small intestine. J Exp Med 2004;199:411–416.

178. Lazarus NH, Kunkel EJ, Johnston B, Wilson E, Youngman KR, Butcher EC. A common mucosal chemokine (mucosae-associated epithelial chemokine/CCL28) selectively attracts IgA plasmablasts. J Immunol 2003;170:3799–3805.

179. Hieshima K, Kawasaki Y, Hanamoto H, Nakayama T, Nagakubo D, Kanamaru A, Hoshie O. CC chemokine ligands 25 and 28 play essential roles in intestinal extravasation of IgA antibody-secreting cells. J Immunol 2004;173:3668–3675.

180. Jang MH, Sougawa N, Tanaka T, Hirata T, Hiroi T, Tohya K, Guo Z, Umemoto E, Ebisuno Y, Yang B-G, Seoh J-Y, Lipp M, Kiyono H, Miyasaka M. CCR7 is critically important for migration of dendritic cells in intestinal lamina propria to mesenteric lymph nodes. J Immunol 2006;176:803–810.

181. Kobayashi H, Miura S, Nagata H, Tsuzuki Y, Hokari R, Ogino T, Watanabe C, Azuma T, Ishii H. In situ demonstration of dendritic cell migration from rat intestine to mesenteric lymph nodes: relationships to maturation and role of chemokines. J Leukoc Biol 2004;75:434–442.

182. Yrlid U, Milling SWF, Miller JL, Cartland S, Jenkins CD, MacPherson GG. Regulation of intestinal dendritic cell migration and activation by plasmacytoid dendritic cells, TNFα and type 1 IFNs after feeding a TLR7/8 ligand. J Immunol 2006;176:5205–5212.

183. Kroese FGM, Ammerlaan WAM, Kantor AB. Evidence that intestinal IgA plasma cells in μ, κ transgenic mice are derived from B-1 (Ly – 1B) cells. Int Immunol 1993;5:1317–1325.

184. Thurnheer MC, Zuercher AW, Cebra JJ, Bos NA. B1 cells contribute to serum IgM, but not to intestinal IgA, production in gnotobiotic Ig allotype chimeric mice. J Immunol 2003;170:4564–4571.

185. Ishikawa S, Sato T, Abe M, Nagai S, Onai N, Yoneyama H, Zhang Y, Suzuki T, Hashimoto S, Shirai T, Lipp M, Matsushima K. Aberrant high expression of B lymphocyte chemokine (BLC/CXCL13) by CD11b+ CD11c+ dendritic cells in murine lupus and preferential chemotaxis of B1 cells towards BLC. J Exp Med 2001;193:1393–1402.

Chapter 10
Clostridium and The Ageing Gut

Sarah Connor and Steven L. Percival

Introduction

As mentioned in previous chapters, humans live in close association with vast numbers of organisms that are present on the skin, in the mouth, and in the gastrointestinal (GI) tract. Following birth there is a progressive formation of a complex intestinal microflora, which develops into a host–bacterial mutualism in the human intestine. This development is significant to the host initiating its own immune system. Also, initial colonizing intestinal microflora is considered to have a significant effect on the health and well-being of the individual with advancing age.

The greatest concentration of indigenous organisms is found within the GI tract, with a community in excess of 500 species of bacteria, fungi, and occasional protozoa. If the conditions in the microbial habitat remain constant, the composition of the intestinal flora remains relatively stable throughout life. The ecosystem responsible for this composition depends on numerous factors including local immune mechanisms, interactions between different microbial species, substrates supplied by the mucosa and by the diet, gut transit times, pH, and local supply of oxygen.

A stable intestinal flora and immune system act as a barrier against colonization of potentially pathogenic microorganisms and against overgrowth of already present opportunistic organisms (colonization resistance). Indigenous bacteria may influence local expression of cytokines and therefore have a significant influence on functional parameters such as immunoglobulin (Ig) E levels, macrophage activation, and antibody production (IgA).

Intestinal Flora and Disease

Several factors decrease resistance to disease and predispose the intestine to infectious inflammatory, degenerative, and neoplastic conditions in both infants

S. Connor and S.L. Percival
Department of Microbiology, Leeds General Infirmary, Leeds, UK

S.L. Percival (ed.), *Microbiology and Aging.*
DOI: 10.1007/978-1-59745-327-1_10, © Springer Science + Business Media, LLC 2009

and adults.[1] Diarrhoea, the passage of frequent or abnormally formed faeces, remains one of the most frequently presented symptoms of disease in all age groups with attack rates estimated at 2–12 episodes per person annually worldwide.[2]

In a normal situation, the gut will always exert a low-level immune response to invading microorganisms in combination with normal uptake of nutrients.[3] When the immune responses in the gut are no longer controlled, clinical gastrointestinal problems ranging from food allergies and irritable bowel syndrome (IBS) to inflammatory bowel disease (IBD) may occur.[4] However, the most common cause of gastroenteritis in the community is due to infection by foodborne enteric pathogens such as *Campylobacter* spp., *Salmonella* spp., *Shigella* spp., *E. coli* O157, and Rotavirus.[3,2] Nearly all hospitalized patients, generally those of advanced age, infected with such enteric pathogens will therefore have been admitted with diarrhoea. Nosocomial diarrhoea (ND – the onset of two or more loose or watery stools per day for more than 2 days at least 72 h after hospital admission) is therefore less likely to be caused by such organisms as above.[5] In contrast with community-acquired diarrhoea (CSD), non-infectious causes are most common.[6] Multiple non-infectious aetiologies are linked to ND, including medication intolerance or abuse medical procedures, hyperalimentation, and diarrhoea associated with other medical conditions (diabetic neuropathy, ureamia, etc.).[5]

Most significantly, the use of antibiotics, immunosuppressive therapy, and irradiation, among other forms of treatment, has been shown to cause significant alteration in the composition and effect of the gut flora leading to diarrhoea.[1,7] Their effects may be independent of antimicrobial activity – erythromycin acts as a motion receptor antagonist and accelerates the rate of gastric emptying.[8]

However, the disturbance in normal gut ecology and subsequent change in the balance of gut organisms may also dysregulate normal homeostatic immune responses or provide an ideal ecological niche for microbes with pathogenic potential.[3,8,9]

Outbreaks of infectious intestinal disease (IID) in hospitals have a considerable impact on public health with an average of over 100 outbreaks, affecting in excess of 3,000 patients and staff each year.[10] Mortality in these vulnerable populations is avoidable, yet the rates remain higher than for outbreaks in any other setting. In the United Kingdom, deaths due to nosocomial infections have been estimated to be more frequent than mortality due to road traffic accidents.

Noscomial diarrhoea is therefore a substantial burden on the health service both in terms of direct costs, longer hospital stay, and possible ward closure.[11] Consequently, it should be important to document both the incidence and the impact of hospital-acquired infection in an attempt to encourage the release of resources.[12] However, the absence of standardized protocols for the conduct of the laboratory investigation of nosocomial diarrhoea militates against understanding the true burden of disease. A survey by Meakins et al. found that in almost a quarter of infectious outbreaks, aetiology was not confirmed by laboratory investigation.[10]

Antibiotic-Associated Diarrhoea, Differential Diagnosis, and Spectrum of Disease

Antibiotic-associated diarrhoea (AAD) may be defined as an otherwise unexplained diarrhoea that occurs in association with the administration of antibiotics.[8]

While symptoms may develop from anything between a few hours to up to 2 months after antibiotic intake, the spectrum of clinical manifestations observed in cases of AAD differ greatly.[13] Symptoms may range from nuisance diarrhoea, defined as frequent loose and watery stools with no other complications, to Pseudomembranous enterocolitis (PMEC) characterized by the presence of pseudomembranes on the intestinal mucosa on endoscopic examination.[14] In these cases, lesions may be located either on the small bowel (Pseudomembranous enteritis (PME)), the colon (Pseudomembranous colitis (PMC)), or both (PME and PMC). In addition, PMC and PME have similar characteristics of clinical presentation with watery diarrhoea, fever, and leucocytosis occurring in 80% of patients.[8,15] Severe, potentially fatal complications of PMEC include toxic megacolon perforation and shock.[16]

The mechanisms by which antibiotics lead to AAD include disturbances of the composition and function of the normal intestinal flora overgrowth by pathogenic microorganisms and allergic and toxic effects of antibiotics on intestinal mucosa or pharmacological effects on motility.[13] As previously discussed, symptoms are induced either by the effects of the antibiotic itself or another non-antibiotic treatment in approximately 70–80% of cases.

However, particular signs and symptoms have been demonstrated to have a strong association with AAD of an infectious cause. For example, studies have demonstrated that the presence of faecal leucocytes is strongly indicative of AAD with an infectious origin and that the majority of colonoscopically proven PMC cases are caused by *C. difficile*[6,8,14,15] (see Table 10.1).

Since the link between antibiotic-associated colitis and *Clostridium* spp. was firmly established in the late 1970s, both interest and incidence of *C. difficile*-associated diarrhoea has greatly increased.[17] However, while *Clostridium difficile* is the most commonly identified pathogen in hospital-acquired infective diarrhoea, it only accounts for approximately 20% of cases. Therefore, for most cases (up to 80%) the organism responsible remains undiagnosed.[18] While is has been suggested that AAD is clinically significant only when there are three or more mushy or watery stools per day, current control strategies for infective AAD depend on early identification through appropriate specimen collection and laboratory investigation.[19]

The challenge for physicians should therefore be to assess the clinical features of the AAD with host-related risk factors and alert both clinicians and the laboratory to potentially infectious and therefore potentially transmissible preventable cases.[13]

Aetiology of Infectious AAD

The extent to which antimicrobial agents will disturb the ecological balance between host and microorganisms depends on age, the spectrum of the agent, the dose, the route of administration, pharmokinetic and pharmacodynamic properties, and in vivo inactivation of the agent.[20]

Table 10.1 A comparison of some common characteristics from antibiotic-associated diarrhoea due to infectious and non-infectious aetiologies

Characteristic	AAD with infectious aetiology	AAD from other causes
Most commonly implicated antibiotics	Clindamycin, cephalosporins, penicillins	Clindamycin, cephalosporins, amoxicillin-clavulanate, erythromycin, neomycin
History	No relevant history of antibiotic intolerance	History of diarrhoea with antibiotic therapy common
Diarrhoea	May be florrid; evidence of colitis with cramps, fever, and faecal leucocytes common	Usually moderate in severity (i.e. "nuisance diarrhoea")
CT[a] or endoscopy	Evidence of colitis (not enteritis) common; pseudomembranous lesions	Usually normal
Complications	Hypoalbuminaemia, anasarca, toxic megacolon fulminant colitis	Usually none except dehydration
Epidemiological pattern	May be epidemic or endemic in hospital ward or long-term-care facility	Sporadic
Withdrawal of implicated antibiotic	May resolve but often persists or progresses	Usually resolves
Antiperistaltic agents	Contraindicated	Often useful
Oral metronidazole or vancomycin	Prompt response although relapses with treatment with metronidazole or vancomycin common with *C. difficile*	Not indicated

Adapted from Ref. 8
[a]*CT* denotes computed tomotography

Nearly all antibiotics have been implicated in the suppression of some component of the microflora, leading therefore to an altered susceptibility to infection.[21] Antibiotics may then select the overgrowth or colonization of an organism with either intrinsic resistance or one that has acquired resistance via plasmid-mediated transfer in vivo.

In recent years, discussions of infectious AAD have centred on *C. difficile*-associated diarrhoea (CDAD).[13] However, in 1984 Borriello and colleagues demonstrated that some *C. difficile*-negative cases of AAD were accounted to enterotoxigenic strains of *C. perfringens* type A.[16,22] However, given antimicrobial pressure, any organism with the opportunity and potential may multiply liberating toxins and other pathogenic factors causing the symptoms associated with AAD. Various organisms have thus been reported to be associated with disease, although their exact role in the pathogenesis of diarrhoea is still debated because most of them are considered to be usual indigenous bacteria of the gut flora.[16]

Staphylococcus aureus

Although it is occasionally a normal inhabitant of the GI tract, *S. aureus* is rarely considered a cause of gastoenteritis.[23] However, in pre-antibiotic days this organism was implicated as the chief cause of pseudomembranous enterocolitis. During this time, terms such as pseudomembranous colitis, postoperative enterocolitis, antibiotic-associated colitis, and staphylococcal enterocolitis were used interchangeably.[14]

The change in opinion came in 1953 when an editorial in the *New England Journal of Medicine* discussed the relationship between staphylococcus enteritis and pseudomembranous enterocolitis and postulated that these may be separate entities. Over the ensuing decades, little attention was paid to the organism's role in AAD, with many authors concluding that any previous associations were confused with unrecognized pseudomembranous enterocolitis due to *C. difficile*.[23]

In 1982, a study at The Royal Melbourne Hospital Australia reported ten cases of AAD observed over a 12-month period thought to be caused by methicillin-resistant *S. aureus* (MRSA).[24] Each patient had severe underlying disease and had been treated with broad-spectrum antibiotics. Diagnosis was made on distinctive Gram-stain appearance of faecal smears along with a heavy growth of methicillin-resistant *S. aureus* from stool culture in the absence of other bowel pathogens (including *C. difficile*). In-patients whose condition responded to vancomycin, or bacitracin stools were clear of Staphylococci post treatment. Many more cases of MRSA enterocolitis after post-surgical antibiotic therapy have appeared in Japanese literature, although in one such report 23 out of 55 cases were also positive for concurrent *C. difficile* infection.[25,26] In an American review, Schiller et al. reported a case of MRSA enterocolitis as a nosocomial infection in a patient with a prior hemigastrostomy who had been receiving broad-spectrum antibiotics.[23] In this case, no other gastrointestinal aetiology was identified, and the patient responded promptly to vancomycin after 3 days of treatment. The authors in this study postulated that it is the use of broad-spectrum antibiotics following gastrostomy that selects the colonization and subsequent overgrowth of MRSA that may produce toxins causing enterocolitis.

Salmonella spp

Although well known as a common cause of food poisoning in the United States, *Salmonella* spp. constitutes the second most common aetiological agent of infectious ND.[5] Although this data does not compare with that reported in the UK, *Salmonella* spp. has been reported as causing enteritis after antibiotic therapy, occasionally presenting as pseudomembranous colitis.[27]

In a recent review, Levy suggested that the instigating factor associated with reports of systemic salmonellosis in chronic Salmonella carriers was loss of gastrointestinal barrier function following antimicrobial treatment.[21] From patients with acute Salmonella infection, previous antimicrobial therapy was observed to have prolonged the duration of the carrier state.

Antibiotics have also been demonstrated to facilitate the selection of resistant mutants and in vivo acquisition of resistance plasmids by Salmonella.[21] Multi-drug-resistant *Salmonella newport* from contaminated beef was implicated in an nosocomial outbreak of diarrhoea among patients who had taken ampicillin, while fluoroquinolone-resistant enteric disease caused by Salmonella has been reported in patients previously treated with fluroquinolones.[28,29]

Candida spp

While a selection of studies suggest *Candida* spp. may cause AAD, many authorities question the validity of reports in view of conflicting evidence.[8,30]

In a recent polish study, Rokosz and co-workers cultured massive fungal growths from 50 out of 100 faecal samples from hospitalized patients with AAD.[30] Although *C. difficile* toxins were also detected in 38 of the samples, the authors concluded that in some cases fungal strains are responsible for the symptoms of AAD and that patients should be concurrently treated with antifungal agents.

In 2002, Krause and colleagues reported results of a Scandinavian study to assess the role of Candida-secreted phospholipase in AAD.[31] Forty-three Candida isolates obtained from faecal samples of patients with AAD, and controls, were tested on egg yolk agar for the production of phospholipase. Phospholipase zones did not differ between the isolates from patients with AAD and the controls, indicating that this fungal virulence factor is not responsible for AAD in adults.

In a later study, Krause and his team reported that significantly higher *Candida albicans* counts were found in stool fluids from AAD patients than from healthy subjects.[32] The author suggested that this increase may have been due to reduced soluble Candida inhibitors and increased availability of growth factors and nutrients.

Other Organisms

Acute segmental haemorrhagic colitis is a rare complication characterized by an acute haemorrhagic diarrhoea and abdominal cramps starting approximately 4 days post treatment with oral penicillin or penicillin derivatives.[13] While pseudomembranes are not found with this condition, colonoscopy findings include submucosal haemorrhage, diffuse mucosal oedema, and in some cases erosions or ulcerations in the colon. Although previously attributed to penicillin hypersensitivity, studies revealed high levels of cytotoxin-producing *Klebsiella oxytoca* in the gut during the acute phase of the disease, suggesting overgrowth during therapy.[33] Minami et al. found that these ampicillin-resistant organisms induced fluid accumulation in the colon and bloody fluid in the rabbit intestinal-loop model.[34] While the toxin alone induced the same effects, non-toxin-producing strains of *K. oxytoca* did not.

Kim and colleagues reported seven cases of nosocomial diarrhoea presumably caused by *Pseudomonas aeruginosa*, which was the predominant organism isolated from stool cultures.[35] All patients had underlying diseases and had been receiving antibiotics for which the Pseudomonas isolates were resistant before diarrhoea onset. Diarrhoea stopped 3 days after withdrawal of the offending antibiotics in two patients, while the remaining five patients were successfully treated with antipseudomonal agents.

Although rarely considered as an enteric pathogen, enterotoxic *B. fragilis* was isolated from 4 out of 30 faecal samples taken from polish children with AAD.[36] While toxigenic *C. difficile* was also isolated from three of the samples, enterotoxinogenic *B. fragilis* was the only organism cultured in one AAD case and the authors suggested its role in the pathogenesis of the disease.

Although the organisms mentioned above are not routinely screened for and considered, when investigating the aetiology of AAD, given the evidence provided it would be prudent that for patients with severe diarrhoea and underlying disease but with negative *C. difficile* and *C. perfringens* toxin tests, examination for other possible causative agents should be undertaken.

Clostridium Difficile

Microbiological History

Clostridium difficile, a spore-forming Gram-positive anaerobic bacillus, was first isolated in 1935 by Hall and O'Toole following isolation from the meconium, and stools of infants.[37,38] Today over 100 different strains of *C. difficile* exist. Initially, Hall and O'Toole termed *C. difficile*, *Bacillus difficilis*, so named because it was difficult to isolate.[39] Together with Snyder, they successfully demonstrated the "toxic effect" of the organism when injected into laboratory animals and postulated that *B. difficilis* toxins liberated in the infant gut could play a role in diarrhoea.[40,41]

In 1974, Tedesco and colleagues reported an association between pseudomembranous colitis and patients receiving clindamycin.[42] In an independent study, Green described a cytotoxin present in the stools of guinea pigs treated with penicillin.[43] The organism shown to produce this cytotoxin was later confirmed as *C. difficile*.[40]

C. difficile is now recognized as a cause of a wide spectrum of enteric diseases ranging from mild episodes of diarrhoea to extreme explosive diarrhoea.[39] It is the ability of *C. difficile* to inhabit the bowel of a small percentage of asymptomatic patients while disseminating to cause serious illness in others that has allowed it to remain the most common cause of nosocomial AAD in the developed world.

Natural History

C. difficile, either as vegetative organisms or as spores, can be readily isolated from many environmental samples such as soil, water, raw vegetables, farm/pet animal faeces, and in addition general surfaces in homes and veterinary clinics.[39,40] Environmental contamination is especially common in hospitals and facilities that provide long-term care.[14] In 2001, Verity and colleagues reported that, over a 4-week period, approximately one quarter of all environmental sites in a large hospitals side rooms were contaminated with C. difficile.[44]

While vegetative forms of C. difficile are easily killed by exposure to air, the spores are resistant to most commonly used disinfectants.[39] For example, Wilcox and colleagues reported widespread environmental contamination of C. difficile in medical wards for the elderly. Levels of spores increased when detergent-based cleaners were used.[45] Contaminations in some environmental sites were significantly more persistent, with commodes, toilet floors, and bed frames found to be C. difficile positive on more than 50% of occasions.

As C. difficile can survive on fomites and other surfaces for months, it can be easily transmitted via colonized patients or healthcare personnel when they make contact with other patients.[14,45] Hospitalized patients therefore often acquire C. difficile as a nosocomial infection, which originate from another patient's stool.[14] Today the most toxigenic strain of C. difficile in the UK is strain 027.

Asymtomatic Human Carriage

Asymptomatic carriage of C. difficile, as demonstrated in the preliminary studies of Hall and O'Toole, has been the subject of many studies.[37,40] Carriage appears to be influenced by a number of factors including age, exposure to antibiotics, and the environment to which the subject is exposed. As a consequence, reports of prevalence rates vary considerably.[40]

Infants

In 1984 Bolton et al. cultured the faeces from 66 babies born in a single maternity unit in the first week of life and found C. difficile present in 47%.[46] In 1982, Larson et al. demonstrated that the acquisition of the organism in neonates was not uniform even within the same institution and found patient carriage rates between wards varying from 2 to 52%.[47] Further studies have demonstrated that in many asymptomatic neonates these C. difficile isolates are toxigenic strains and produce detectable toxins associated with disease. This was confirmed in a study by Wongwanish and coworkers who found that of 235 asymptomatic infant outpatients 21.1% carried *C. difficile* two of which were toxigenic strains.[48]

Acquisition of *C. difficile* by neonates is believed to be from the hospital environment itself, with many workers isolating *C. difficile* from inanimate objects on neonatal wards.[46,47,49] However, some studies have suggested maternal transmission via vaginal delivery and breast feeding to be associated with infants acquiring cytotoxin-positive stools.[40,50,51]

The resistance to disease exhibited by neonates and infants, even with high levels of toxins A and B detected in the gut, remains unexplained. Hypotheses proposed include the possibly that there are few or no receptors in the newborn gut for the toxins. In addition, the development of normal gut flora is considered to have a role to play, which is important for colonization resistance.[52]

Adults

Various studies have detected *C. difficile* in the guts of healthy adults suggesting a subclinical carrier state.[53,54] In the community, asymptomatic carriage of *C. difficile* has been reported between 0 and 5%.[55,56] In patients exposed to antibiotics, carriage, in the absence of diarrhoea, rises to approximately 10–25%, although rates of up to 65% have been reported in some hospitals and nursing homes.[13,14]

While *C. difficile* spores may persist in the adult GI tract for many years, their presence is often transient and there is still debate as to whether *C. difficile* permanently colonizes the healthy adult gut.[53] Various in vitro experiments have confirmed that an abnormal gastrointestinal flora is required before *C. difficile* can flourish, and the organism is therefore never considered part of the 'normal' microbiota.[14]

Pathogenicity

C. difficile is ingested from the environment via the faecal-oral route. The heat- and acid-resistant spores survive the acidic environment of the stomach and are later converted to vegetative forms in the colon.[14,53] When it is present in the colon, the organism is suppressed by other components of the intestinal indigenous microbiota and produces no clinical symptoms.[57] However, agents that produce alterations in the intestinal flora and amino acid content will make the bowel more susceptible to infection. In addition, reduced colonic ion secretion and depressed motor function of the mucosa are also implicated to encourage the overgrowth of AAD-inducing microorganisms.

C. difficile colitis is primarily a toxin-mediated disease without evidence of microbial invasion of the colonic lumen or its epithelium.[14] However, a number of virulence factors contribute to the pathology associated with infection either directly, or simply enable *C. difficile* to colonize the human intestinal tissue.

Adherence

There have been many attempts to identify the significant adhesins of *C. difficile*.[58] Two independent adhesion studies using human gut cells identified a heat-stimulated protein or heat-shock protein (Hsp) that appeared to be involved in adhesion.[59,60] Waligora et al. reported that this was likely to be GroEL, a member of the Hsp60 family of chaperons.[61] The groESL operon of *C. difficile* contains groES and groEL, the latter encoding a 58-kDa surface-exposed adhesin mediating adherence to cultured cells. In the same laboratory, Henequin et al. later analysed expression of groEL of *C. difficile* in response to stress following heat, acid, or osmotic shock; iron deprivation; or presence of a subinhibitory concentration of ampicillin.[62] All these stresses increased transcription of groEL and production of groEL to various degrees, and the authors postulated that after destroying the barrier flora antibiotics have secondary effects of favouring *C. difficile* attachment to cells by increasing transcription of groEL or other adhesins.

Early studies also implicated a role for toxin A itself, showing that on human biopsy material co-administration of toxin-A, with a non-pathogenic strain, raised adhesion by the latter compared to that seen for the highly virulent strain.[63]

More recently, studies undertaken at the Imperial College of Science, London, UK, have investigated tissue-binding of *C. difficile* surface layer proteins (SLPs), which are the predominant outer surface components.[64] Previous work had shown these to consist mainly of two components – a high molecular weight subunit and a low molecular weight subunit, both resulting from the cleavage of a precursor encoded by the *slp*A gene.[64] On immunohistochemical analysis, Calabi and his team revealed strong binding of *C. difficile* to lumen surface epithelium lining the digestive cavities and to subjacent lamina propria.[65] Fluorescence-activated cell sorter analysis and enzyme-linked immunoabsorbent assay studies have shown that antibodies to the high molecular weight SLP inhibited this adherence.

The ability of *C. difficile* to adhere to gut receptors is also enhanced by the presence of flagella, which enable the bacteria to move from the lumen to the chemo attractant gut mucus.[66] However, whether or not the flagella or pili of *C. difficile* directly function as adhesins remains to be determined.[52]

Capsules

As with all pathogens, not all strains of *C. difficile* are equally virulent. A study in 1990 correlated the detection of a polysaccharide capsule with increased virulence and toxicity in *C. difficile*-associated PMC.[67] The authors concluded that as opsonization of capsulated *C. difficile* would be necessary for significant phagocytosis to occur, the accumulation of polymorphonuclear cells in the gut tissue in PMC may contribute to the tissue damage seen in these more severe cases. However, conflicting evidence regarding the significance of capsulated strains has led to the suggestion that there may be a difference in the production of extracellular material in vivo and in vitro.[68] The conditions required for its production are as yet unknown.

Enzymes

C. difficile has been shown to produce various tissue-degradative enzymes.[69] Steffen and Hentges demonstrated enzymes such as collagenases, heparinidase, and hyaluronidase to be more active in highly virulent strains than less virulent strains.[70] Although such hydrolytic enzymes are thought to be produced for the nutritional advantage of the organism, it has been postulated that they probably contribute to the observed pathology by further compromising gut integrity and fluid accumulation.[69]

Toxins

C. difficile produces two types of toxins, enterotoxin (A) and cytotoxin (B). Both these toxins are responsible for colitis. Since early studies first established the toxigenic nature of *C. difficile*, it has been generally accepted that although putative virulence factors play an important role in energy production and survival, it is toxins rather than the organism that leads to CDAD.[71] While several toxins have been reported in association with *C. difficile*, their existence is often random and strain specific, and their action and importance in relation to AAD remains unknown.[72] Molecular and genetic characterization of pathogenic strains shows that *C. difficile* contains the majority of the genetic material responsible for causing disease within a 19.6-kb region termed the *toxigenic element* or *toxicon*.[73] This element contains the genes for two very large clostridial cytotoxins (LCTs), known as *toxin A* (TcdA) and *toxin B* (TcdB) along with three other smaller genes.[74] The two major proteins, which were originally designated toxins A and B because of their elution profile on anion exchange resins, are considered to be the major virulence determinants of the organism.[75] One of the smaller genes, termed *txeR*, expresses a protein that co-ordinately turns on high-level production of the toxins. The function of the other two genes is as yet unknown.

Controversy remains regarding physical and biological properties of the LCTs and the individual contribution to the disease state.[72] Early molecular studies found that TcdA and TcdB demonstrated no sequence similarity to any other characterized bacterial toxin gene. However, they do show homology to each other, and it is generally assumed that when produced together they act synergistically.[76]

Toxin A (MW 308 kDa) is a large, tissue-damaging enterotoxin (with some cytotoxic activity), which in rabbit ilieal loop tests produces a haemorrhagic and viscous fluid unlike that seen in any other bacterial toxins.[77,78] Cloning and sequencing of toxin A cDNA predicts a single peptide (in contrast to other enterotoxins) with a 38 repeating peptide sequence at the carboxy terminal representing the binding portion of this toxin.[77] Lyerly et al. purified a recominant peptide consisting of 33 of the 38 repeating units and found the peptide readily agglutinates rabbit erythrocytes, confirming a functional role in the binding of toxin A to its receptor.[79] Southern blot analysis with a toxin A probe also suggested that although toxigenic strains of *C. difficile* may vary in the amount of toxin A produced, there is no difference in the gene copy number – all strains possess a single gene.[75] Enterotoxin A is thought to bind to the human colonic brush-border via a glycoprotein receptor, which leads to internalization of toxin into the cell by endocytosis.[77]

Toxin B cDNA also predicts a single peptide but with a molecular weight of 270 kDa and containing a 24 repeat-unit binding portion.[80] Toxin B is an extremely potent cytotoxin causing damage to cells in culture in amounts of less than 1 pg. Although inactive when administered orally, toxin B becomes lethal after surgical manipulation of the intestine or in combination with sub-lethal doses of toxin A.[78] This observation led the authors to suggest that in vivo loss of mucosal integrity may be necessary to facilitate the action of toxin B alone, whereas together both toxins act on the intestine synergistically (toxin A primarily binds and initializes tissue damage, which provides toxin B with access to sensitive tissues).[75,78]

However, in 1988 in vitro studies demonstrated that both toxins A and B individually abolished the paracellular permeability or transepithelial resistance (TER) across cultured monolayers of epithelial T84 cells within 6–8 h.[81] The authors suggested that the effect of the toxins on epithelial barrier function resulted from redistribution of filamentous actin (F-actin) that indirectly altered tight junctions leading to visible cell rounding and loss of barrier function. The mechanism of actin disaggregation involves monoglycosylation of the Rho family of signalling proteins (RhoA Rac and Cdc 42) that control stress fibre development and stabilization.[82,83] Both toxins A and B have been reported to act as cation-dependent UDP glucose hydrolases exerting cellular toxicity through their ability to monoglycosylate. The glycosylation of Rho proteins leads to their inactivation and subsequent collapse of the actin cytoskeleton.[82]

Both LCTs of C. difficile have also been shown to promote cellular injury through pathways independent of their effect on actin rearrangement.[82] Chen et al. demonstrated that toxin A activates membrane and cysolic protein kinases (PKC), which decrease transepithelial electrical resistance and provide additional paracellular permeability changes distinct from dephosphorylation and cell rounding.[84] Many workers have also suggested that the release of neuropeptides and other cytokines from epithelium monocytes macrophages and neuroimmune cells of the lamina propria contribute significantly to the toxin-mediated inflammation and damage of the colonic mucosa.[83] Both toxins are capable of producing neutrophil chemotaxis and chemokinases and stimulating the production of inflammatory mediators in vitro.[77] Supporting evidence suggests that interleukin-1 (IL-1) plays an important role in mediating the outcome of C. difficile-associated AAD. In 1997 Steiner et al. demonstrated that stool samples from patients who had developed C. difficile colitis contained high concentrations of IL-1β.[85] The mediator presumably released from intestinal inflammatory cells appeared to correlate with clinical severity of disease. While toxin B did not stimulate IL-1β, both toxins induced the genesis of the oedemic TNF-α from the cells.[86]

The close proximity of the toxin genes may provide an explanation for the co-production of the toxins observed among the majority of toxigenic C. difficile strains. Sequence analysis of the toxin genes and flanking DNA demonstrated that the 3'-end of the toxin B gene is located 1,350 bp upstream from the toxin A translation site, providing physical evidence that the toxins are co-regulated.[75] Early DNA-probe and PCR studies have also demonstrated that most non-toxigenic strains appeared to lack both toxin genes A and B, suggesting a large chromosomal deletion.[87] More recently, strains of *C. difficile* that have defective deletions in the TcdA gene alone have been described. Rupnik et al. reported that strains that have deletions in the toxin A gene of greater than 800 bp have no detectable toxin A.[88] However, Von Eichel-Steiber et al. reported that some strains produce a truncated form of toxin A product that is non-functional because of lack of the binding region and so undetectable in tight-junction assays.[89] While toxin B was demonstrated to produce dose-dependent morphological changes in human colonic mucosa in vitro, for many years these toxin A negative isolates were not believed to be associated with clinically significant nosocomial disease.[90]

However, toxin A−/B+ isolates are recurrently associated with human disease across Euope, Asia, and America, including two nosocomial outbreaks (first in a Canadian tertiary hospital and more recently in the Netherlands).[90,91] Characterization of 48 strains from distinct geographical sites revealed that while all isolates lacked a functional toxin A gene product, the toxin B contained sequence variations downstream of the active site resulting in an extended glycosylation spectrum to R-Ras. In vivo studies showed that in addition to typical cell rounding and detachment, this variant toxin B resulted in an atypical cytopathic effect with the production of filopodia-like structures mediated by a transient activation of RhoA.[92] However, the similarity of the CPE produced by such strains and *C. sordelli* raises questions as to whether the toxin B in these strains is actually a hybrid between TcdB and the *C. sordelli* lethal toxin.[91]

The increasing number of accounts of strains lacking detectable toxin A and yet producing the full spectrum of clinical manifestations associated with CDAD suggests these variant strains are more common instigators of AAD than previously supposed.[90,93]

Clinical Aspects of *C. difficile* Infection

C. difficile-associated disease (CDAD) specifically refers to patients with symptomatic illness caused by *C. difficile*, and for the majority of patients diarrhoea is the most prominent symptom.[14] It is predominantly the most common cause of acute-care-hospital-acquired diarrhoea. In fact it has been estimated that over 300,000 cases of diarrhoea in the acute setting has been due to *C. difficile*. CDAD is associated with 15–25% of antibiotic diarrhoea, 50–75% of antibiotic-associated colitis, and 90–100% of cases of PMC.[94] PMC may be accompanied by toxic megacolon electrolyte imbalance and occasionally bowel perforation leading to death.[58] Hospitals around Europe and North America have outbreaks due to *C. difficile* as high as 39.9 cases per 1,000 admissions to hospital. The most prevalent strains have been identified as the epidemic strains, BI, the North American PGFE type 1 (NAPI), and strain 027. The NAP1 strain has been shown to be highly resistant to fluoroquinolone.

Antibiotic-Associated Diarrhoea

In most cases, AAD caused by *C. difficile* is watery, often containing mucus and rarely associated with blood.[77] Sigmoidoscopic examination in most patients reveals normal colonic mucosa, but in some mild oedema or hyperaemia of the rectum may be present. Systemic symptoms are usually absent and in the majority of patients, and diarrhoea stops when antibiotics are discontinued.

Antibiotic-Associated *C. difficile* Colitis

C. difficile may also cause a non-specific colitis characterised by watery diarrhoea up to 10–20 times a day and lower abdominal cramps. High fever, abdominal tenderness and leukocytosis may occur. Hypalbuminemia, electrolyte imbalance and dehydration may also be present in protracted cases. Sigmoidoscopic examination reveals a non-specific diffuse or patchy colitis without pseudomembranes frequently involving the proximal colon.[77]

Antibiotic-Associated *C. difficile* Pseudomembranous Colitis

Whilst the clinical features of PMC resemble those seen in *C. difficile* colitis the classic pathological feature of PMC is the presence of yellow or white plaque like pseudomembranes interspersed between normal mucosa observed on sigmoidoscopy.[14,7] Plaques are generally 2–4 mm in diameter and are composed of layers of mucus, dead mucosa, fibrinous exudates and leukocytes.[14] In severe cases pseudomembranes may become confluent giving the appearance of a shaggy membrane overlying the inflamed epithelium.[77] Histological examination reveals a typical summit lesion an outpouring of inflammatory exudates from the ulcerated epithelium that resembles a volcanic eruption. Although lesions affect the rectum in 77% of cases Tedesco et al. reported that rectal sparing is not uncommon with *C. difficile* colitis, and disease process can be confined to the right colon.[95]

Fulminant Colitis

Fulminant *C. difficile* colitis occurs mostly in elderly patients with underlying disease and may masquerade as post-operative fever or sepsis.[77] The patient appears toxic and may show signs of hypovolemic shock sepsis and paralytic ileus. Fever, tachycardia, localized tenderness, decreased bowel signs, and signs of toxaemia are present. Paralytic ileus may appear to improve diarrhoea without any corresponding improvement in the patient's condition. Without prompt treatment perforation, peritonitis, septicaemia, and renal failure may ensue.

Other CDAD Associations

Whilst GI disease therefore remains the main focus of *C. difficile* infection, the organism has also been demonstrated in clinical material other than faeces. Reports of *C. difficile* in the urogenital tract and in abdominal wounds are of doubtful clinical significance, as the organism is usually found at these sites as part of the polymicrobial flora.[96] In a recent report, Gravisse et al. reported a case of brain empyema that occurred after the recurrent intestinal carriage of both toxigenic and non-toxigenic strains of *C. difficile*.[97] In addition, cases of patients with recurrent severe sepsis and bacteremia due to *C. difficile* infection with no other identifiable aetiology have been documented.[15,98] Toxin B has also been demonstrated in the blood and ascites of children who developed fatal cases of PMC with underlying disease.[99] Such reports highlight the consequences of the increased intestinal permeability induced by *C. difficile* toxins and hence the potential of both organism and toxin to translocate the intestinal barrier and cause serious systemic toxicity and disease.

Clinical History and Risk Factors

A study comparing symptomatic *C. difficile*-infected patients with *C. difficile* carriers demonstrated that patients who have more than three underlying diseases or at least 20 days of antibiotic treatment have a higher risk of developing symptomatic *C. difficile* infection.[100] Although several classes of antibiotics have been implicated in the acquisition of *C. difficile*, the factors responsible for the rise in incidence have not been reliably identified.[101] The frequency of carriage of epidemic strains of *C. difficle*, particularly the NAP1 strains, is presently unknown. However, about two-thirds of patients that are colonized with *C. difficile* do become asymptomatic faecal carriers, and a number of studies have shown that asymptomatic carriers play a minor role in the transmission of the disease. A prospective study of patients has also shown that *C. difficile* frequently contaminates multiple skin sites, including groin, chest, abdomen, forearms, and hands, and was easily acquired on investigators' hands. Skin contamination often persisted on patients' chest and abdomen after resolution of diarrhoea.

Age-Related Susceptibility

Although the incidence of asymtomatic *C. difficile* carriage is highest in neonates, the incidence of CDAD increases with age.[102] Over a 3.5-year period in a paediatric hospital in Pennsylvania, USA, Spivack et al. reported a total of 22 *C.*

difficile-positive patients but no reported cases of CDAD.[103] As previously discussed, controversy exists about the pathogenicity of this organism in the infant population due to their high colonization rate.[104] However, in children greater than 2 years of age the epidemiology is similar to that seen in adults.[47,105]

Nash et al. reported that 62% of symptomatic patients were aged 60 years and over, thus supporting the earlier observations of Anand et al. who found in a 2-year study that the majority of patients with CDAD were over 65 years old and had underlying medical problems.[106,107] Neither group found any connection between age and mortality, although in a recent review Andrews et al. found that 75% of patients with severe CDAD were over 70 years old and had more co-morbid diseases.[108] Anand et al. also suggested that any perceived increase in mortality was associated with co-morbidity.[107] In a further retrospective study performed over 2 years, others have reported a rise in incidence of CDAD. However, this was despite a reduction in the number of elderly patients admitted into hospital, and the authors therefore concluded that while *C. difficile* predominantly affects the elderly, other factors appear to have contributed to the observed rise in incidence.

The rates of carriage of *C. difficile* in neonates, both in Europe and the US, range from 13 to 70%, with longer stays in hospitals increasing this colonization rate. A recent study has shown that carriage rates of *C. difficile* in infants under 2 years was 84.4%, with children 2 years of age and over with a carriage rate of 30.3%. The reasons for carriage rate in older infants are to date unclear, but it is probable that the microbes that form part of the indigenous microbiota of the developed intestine inhibit colonization of *C. difficile*. In fact, a number of workers have found that high densities of enterococci in the gut are related to colonization with *C. difficile*. The acquisition in neonates is considered to occur mainly in the hospital environment, although a number of studies have suggested maternal transmission as a route. One study has suggested that neonates that are born to mothers carrying *C. difficile* in the rectum or vagina also carried *C. difficile*.

Antibiotic-Associated Usage

It has been clearly demonstrated that nearly all elderly patients with CDAD have been treated with antibiotics in the preceding 3 months and most within 14 days to 4 weeks.[109] As previously discussed, exposure to antibiotics, particularly those adversely affecting gut flora, appear to create a niche which is exploited by *C. difficile*. An interesting observation was reported by McGowan and Kader in 1999,[104] who noted that because they continually receive antibiotics and are frequently hospitalized, children with cystic fibrosis (CF) would appear to be prime candidates for *C. difficile*-associated diarrhoea. Yet, despite the risk factors, prospective studies have shown that disease with *C. difficile* is unusual in children with CF. However, as many as 22% of children with CF are unsymptomatically colonized with strains of *C. difficile*, producing detectable toxin. While the reason for this is as yet unknown, the authors observed that normal stool samples from children with CF are much more likely to include organisms that are known to have inhibitory effects of *C. difficile* such as pseudomonas, staphylococcus, lactobacillus, and enterococcus.

Although there is much reporting of the propensity of various antibiotics, antibiotic classes, or components of their administration to induce CDAD, many such studies are based on retrospective studies.[110] The only prospective, comparative study of antibiotics found a significantly higher risk of CDAD after empirical treatment with ceotaxime compared with pipercillin-tazobactam.[111] In a recent systemic review, studies that investigated the association of antibiotics with hospital-acquired *C. difficile*-associated diarrhoea were analysed to summarize the strength of the evidence for this relationship.[112] Although the majority of studies found an association with various antibiotics, antibiotic classes, or components of administration, Thomas and Riley[112] found that most were limited in their ability to establish a causal relationship by the use of incorrect control groups, the presence of bias, and inadequate control of confounding and small sample sizes. While these limitations therefore prevented the authors pooling results for a meta-analysis, they concluded that two studies were found to provide reliable estimates of the strength of association.

In the first, McFarland et al. found an increased risk for CDAD after cephlosporin exposure for up to 1 week and penicillin exposure for between 1 and 2 weeks, adjusted for age and severity of disease using the Horn's index.[113] Several retrospective and intervention studies have indicated that third-generation cephalosporins have a high propensity to induce CDAD, claims supported by the reduced incidence of CDAD when antibiotic prescribing policies restrict their use.[114] A second moderately large cross-sectional study by Chang and Nelson provided precise estimates of effects for clindamycin and increased numbers of antibiotics.[115] There was also evidence of a dose effect relating to antibiotic duration and the use of multiple antibiotics in relation to *C. difficile*-associated disease.

Therefore, broad-specrum (particularly anti-anaerobic) agents should be those most associated with CDAD.[110] However, antimicrobial therapy itself can be largely affected by factors such as drug penetration into the gut lumen, specific and non-specific antibody binding, and gut and pH redox potential.

Chemotherapy and Neoplastic Agents

In his 2002 review, Dr John Bartlett noted that on occasion cases of *C. difficile* follow treatment with methotrexate or paclitaxel given for cancer chemotherapy.[8,116] Dr Perimen, a medical oncologist from the Harrington cancer centre, USA, replied to Bartlett in a letter to the *New England Journal of Medicine*.[117] He stated that while he had encountered many cases of diarrhoea associated with *C. difficile* infection in patients who had received broad-spectrum antibiotics because of neutropenic fever, he had yet to document a case after chemotherapy in the absence of antibiotic chemotherapy. However, some cases of *C. difficile* AAD due to cancer chemotherapy without a history of antibiotic treatment have been reported.[118,119] In a recent outbreak of *C. difficile*-related diarrhoea in an adult oncology unit in France, Blot et al. reported that chemotherapy but not antibiotics was found to be a risk factor for developing toxigenic *C. difficile*-related diarrhoea.[118] Odds ratios confirmed that chemotherapy was a risk factor for toxigenic *C. difficile* infection and antibiotic consumption significantly increased the risk for toxigenic *C. difficile*-related diarrhoea. While Hussain et al. had previously reported that higher doses of paclitaxel were more frequently associated with this complication than lower doses, Blot and his team found no statistical link between particular chemotherapy agents or regimes and risk of infection.[118,119]

While studies have therefore shown that adults receiving chemotherapy for cancer are at increased risk of acquiring *C. difficile*-associated diarrhoea, this does not appear to be true in paediatric oncology patients.[104] The reasons for this difference in susceptibility by age are not yet understood.

Immunosupression and Other Causes

Host factors are increasingly recognized as critical determinants of CDAD expression. However, the evidence for CDAD risk factors other than antibiotics is less clear, with certain factors often giving discrepant results between different studies.[120] For example, a retrospective Italian study of CDAD in AIDS patients cited a number of reports indicating that infection with HIV was not in itself an intrinsic risk factor for *C. difficile*.[121] However, patients with HIV appeared to be at an increased risk because of other predisposing factors such as antibiotic usage. The findings led the authors to conclude that CDAD was a major problem in AIDS patients and was associated with high morbidity. In contrast, a french study to determine the prevalence of *C. difficile* found that the carriage was low and did not differ from non-HIV infected patients regardless of treatment with multiple antibiotic regimes.[122]

The gut barrier can be adversely affected under a number of pathological conditions including burn trauma, haemorrhagic shock, and surgical stress.[123] In paediatric patients, most cases of enterocolitis associated with Hirschrung's disease are caused by *C. difficile*.[104] It has also been well known since the early 1980s that patients with idiopathic IBD or Crohn's disease are more prone to colonization with *C. difficile* than the general population.[124] However, the latter is most probably provoked by antibiotics that are used frequently in these populations of patients.[124] Freiler et al. also raised the issue of whether *C. difficile* colitis can occur in the residual segments after either a partial or total colectomy.[125] Kyne et al. performed a retrospective cohort study of 252 adult patients admitted to the hospital and receiving antibiotics.[126] At the time of hospital admission, disease was rated by clinicians as mild, moderate, severe, or extremely severe using a modified Horn's index. Clinical risk factors in addition to antibiotic therapy were assessed in a primary cohort and included GI or genital tract surgery, mechanical bowel preparation, naso-gastric tubing, anti-ulcer medication, and neonatal necrotising enterocolitis. In conclusion, the authors found that patients with severe to extremely severe disease at the time of admission may benefit from careful monitoring of antibiotic prescribing and early attention to infection control issues.

The Frequency of C. difficile-*Associated Diarrhoea*

Community

A British study investigated the frequency and aetiology of intestinal disease in patients in the community and attending their general practitioners. It found *C. difficile* to be responsible for 21 adult of cases who presented to general practitioners with diarrhoea associated with prior use of antibiotics.[127,128] The role of *C. difficile* diarrhoeal disease in general practice is poorly documented yet should not be underestimated.[129] Andrews et al. reviewed cases of CDAD presenting to the emergency department of St. Paul's Hospital, Vancouver, Canada.[108] The objective of the study was to determine predictors of severity in patients presenting from the community. From 153 patients, 44% had community-acquired CDAD and the remainder had hospital-acquired disease.

A prospective study of CDAD in Sweden found that 28% of all cases were community acquired as defined by their criteria of onset of symptoms outside the hospital without hospitalization within the preceding 4 weeks.[130] The investigators found that the annual incidence of community-acquired CDAD ranged from 5 to 47 per 100,000 inhabitants with a median of 20 per 100,000. The authors reported a sixfold increase in the use of cephalosporins since 1980 in Sweden, and suggested that minimizing antibiotic use in general would be one factor in the control of CDAD. This finding was also reflected when a reported rise in CDAD infection followed the introduction of British guidelines suggesting amoxicillin and clarithromycin therapy for the treatment of community-acquired pneumonia.[101] The authors suggested that antibiotic policies that promote the use of alternative drugs such as trimethoprim, aminoglycosides, and 4-quinolones appear the most likely to make an impact on the incidence of *C. difficile* infection.

Nosocomial

Over the last decade, hospitals in the UK have seen a marked increase in the incidence of *C. difficile* infection.[101] This is also reflected in Europe – in one Swedish hospital 62.5% of patients with AAD and 33.8% of asymptomatic patients were positive for *C. difficile* cytotoxin B.[131] In a recent study, hospitals in the UK were second only to residential homes as a setting for outbreaks of infectious intestinal disease.[10] The same report commissioned by the Public Health Laboratory Service (PHLS) Communicable Disease Surveillance Centre (CDSC) found that although the majority of cases were of viral aetiology, *C. difficile* was the second pathogen (12.6%) reported as the cause of nosocomial outbreaks.[10]

Reduced standards of hygiene, increasing numbers of elderly patients in hospital, greater use of cephalosporins, and increased stay have each been considered to be responsible. In a recent study, Khan and Cheesbrough found that while a policy of restricted prescribing reduced the incidence of CDAD within their hospital, it took 6 months to have a significant effect.[11] The authors postulated that this delay in the decline of CDAD after the virtual withdrawal of cephalosporins may be reflective of the high environmental reservoir of *C. difficile*. Hand hygiene still remains significant and as such an additional environmental reservoir of *Clostridium difficile*.[132] In a study addressing possible routes of infection, 49% of the rooms of patients with diarrhoea and 29% of the rooms of asymptomatic patients were confirmed to be contaminated with *C. difficile*.[133] *C. difficile* could be cultured from the hands of 20% of the hospital staff caring for these patients. In the same study, 21% of 399 hospitalized patients had acquired *C. difficile* during the hospital stay.

The risk of becoming colonized with the organism seems to increase progressively with the length of the hospital episode. One study showed that for patients hospitalized for 1–2 weeks the rate of colonization was 13%, rising to 50% for those hospitalized for >4 weeks. Other studies have found the colonization rate for adults, hospitalized for >1 week, to be >20%.[134,135]

As previously discussed, the majority of patients colonized with *C. difficile* will remain asymptomatic. It has been shown that these asymptomatic excretors are not at an increased risk of subsequent CDAD, and, indeed, it has been suggested that primary asymptomatic colonized patients may be at decreased risk of subsequent CDAD.[136] However, results of a number of studies indicate that although asymptomatic excretors are themselves not at any increased risk of CDAD, they are a significant reservoir for transmission of the organism to other patients.[133,134,137] The last 20 years has seen a higher level of use of high-risk antibiotics, an increase in asymptomatic carriage, and an increase in environmental contamination associated with the movement of patients within hospital units. The importance of such carriers discharged from acute-care hospitals to long-stay-care facilities introducing *C. difficile* into that population has been postulated.[138] This is supported by the results of Mcfarland et al., who found that 82% of such patients were still excreting *C. difficile* when they were discharged from hospital.[133]

Clostridium perfringens

Microbiological History

Clostridium perfringens (previously known as *C. welchii*) is a box-car-shaped, Gram-positive, aerotolerant, anaerobic bacillus that produces at least 15 different protein toxins.[139] Through the production of these toxins it causes many of the diseases that were among the first described during the modern era of clinical bacteriology.[140] Each individual *C. perfringens* isolate expresses only a defined subset of the toxin repertoire, allowing strains of to be subdivided into types A–E (see Table 10.2) depending on the combination of toxins generated.[141]

Table 10.2 Distribution of toxins among the different types of *Clostridium perfringens*

	Toxins produced				
Type	α	β	ε	τ	Enterotoxin
A	+	–	–	–	+
B	+	+	+	–	–
C	+	+	–	–	Rare
D	+	–	+	–	Rare
E	+	–	–	+	Rare

Table adapted from Ref. [140]

About 2–5% of all *C. perfringens* isolates, mostly belonging to type A, produce *C. perfringens* enterotoxin (CPEnt).[139] Traditionally, these bacteria are most recognized as the cause of *C. perfringens* Type A food poisoning, which although first documented in 1895 was not a confirmed aetiology until 1977.[139,141] This intestinal disorder caused by CPEnt is the result of the consumption of contaminated pre-cooked food that has been inadequately stored or reheated. During the First World War, the role of *C. perfringens* in the production of gas gangrene was also significant. However, in the early 1980s the first reports of CPEnt causing a spontaneous and antibiotic-associated diarrhoea unrelated to food poisoning began to appear.[140,141]

In 1984, Borriello et al. published a report in the *Lancet* from the CDC, Harrow, Middlesex, UK.[142] The study examined faecal specimens from patients with diarrhoea following antibiotic therapy. Specimens were screened by tissue culture assay for *C. perfringens* type A enterotoxin, and positive results were later confirmed using an in-house enzyme immunoabsorbant assay (ELISA). The study revealed high faecal counts of *C. perfringens* in all cases of patients with diarrhoea, and CPEnt was detected in 11 of the diarrhoeic stools. All positive samples cultured enterotoxic *C. perfringens* strains of a serotype not commonly associated with food poisoning. Blood was also noted to be present in the faeces of four of these patients, a symptom not typical of food poisoning associated with *C. perfringens*. From these findings the authors concluded that enterotoxigenic *C. perfringens* was a possible cause of AAD – observations later confirmed in another 39 patients when the study was continued.[13] Furthermore, Borriello et al. later described the successful treatment of such a CPEnt-positive AAD cases with metronidazole.[143]

Since this first report, evidence has mounted supporting the role of *C. perfringens* in the aetiology of AAD.[140] While *C. difficile* is therefore responsible for about 20% of antibiotic-associated diarrhoea in humans, about 5–10% are thought to be caused by CPEnt.[141]

Natural History

The natural habitat of *C. perfringens* is faeces, and its spores are ubiquitous in soil dust and air.[141] Type A is most often found in the lower gut of humans and other animals, making up 0.6% of the total human faecal flora, and is regularly present on humans skin especially in the region of the perineum buttocks and thighs.[140,144] It is the most common *Clostridium* species in the faeces of humans and pigs and has also been reported from dogs and reptiles.[141,145] In veterinary science workers often culture type A from samples of gangrenous animal muscle tissue, while gastric overgrowth in dogs and primates will inflate the stomachs of affected animals (hydrogen production) in a condition known as *acute gastric dilation*.[141]

Unlike *C. difficile*, *C. perfringens* does not sporulate readily and only does so under natural conditions: for example, in the bowel.[141] Its secondary habitats are usually those contaminated with faeces, e.g. sewage pasture, river and lake sedimentations, etc.[140,141] *C. perfringens* spores are able to resist the action of routinely used disinfectants, antiseptics, and wastewater treatment practices, and for that reason are often used as an indicator for faecal pollution of water.

Epidemiological data taken during a nosocomial outbreak of *C. perfringens* diarrhoea showed that infecting serotypes were present in the hospital environment (57% of areas sampled were positive), representing a high level recovery of spores. Infecting serotypes were also detected on the hands of infected patients, thus representing a potentially significant cross-infection problem.[18]

Asymptomatic Human Carriage

Unlike *C. difficile*, *C. perfringens* is regarded part of the normal flora of the many animals, although in virtually all instances only type A strains are found in healthy individuals regardless of age and circumstances.[141] In the human large intestine, *C. perfringens* ranges in incidence between 25 and 35%. The level of carriage, however, appears like *C. difficile* to be influenced by a number of factors including age, exposure to antibiotics, and the environment to which the subject is exposed. Early workers reported using a wide range of selective and differential techniques, and as a consequence reports of prevalence rates once again vary considerably.[141] In general, they found that while *C. perfringens* spores can be obtained in patients of all ages without symptoms, it is elderly, often institutionalized patients, that yield more spores than younger adults.[141] In neonates levels vary widely, and ill health may be more frequent in those carrying high numbers.[141]

In northern Mexico, studies have shown carriage of *C. perfringens* from a sub-population of healthy individuals using DNA probe analysis. *C. perfringens* was found in 200 faecal samples at an average of 7.4×10^3 spores per gram, with the elderly population showing the highest levels. Dot blot analysis using dig-labelled probes specific for the enterotoxin gene showed that 7% of the samples had isolates with toxigenic potential. Other workers have found that faecal counts of greater than 10^6 spores can be obtained in patients without symptoms, although diarrhoea has never been noted to occur in patients carrying less than 107.7/g of faeces.

Pathogenicity

While the natural habitat of *C. perfringens* is well known, there has been a continuation of the paucity of data relating to the pathogenesis of *C. perfringens* AAD. *C. perfringens* itself does not invade healthy cells but produces various toxins and enzymes that are responsible for the associated lesions and symptoms.[146] In cases of food poisoning, a single bolus of spores are ingested that germinate in the bowel, releasing CPEnt and leading to a transient self-limiting diarrhoea.[141] With AAD, it is thought that the bacterium replicates and sporulates in the gut (colonizes), leading to the extended presence of enterotoxin and prolongation of symptoms.[141] While the use of antibiotics in elderly or immunocompromised patients is considered the major risk factor for acquisition of this disease, it is not known whether antibiotic exposure primarily permits the proliferation of small numbers of resident *C. perfringens* or allows acquisition of ingested enterotoxogenic strains as a result of impaired colonization resistance. In studies with clostridal mobilisable transposons, Adams et al. found that elements containing antimicrobial resistance determinants such as chloramphenicol, erythromycin, and tetracycline resistance are capable of interspecies transfer, potentially an additional virulence factor in the antibiotic-treated gut.[147]

Adhesion

The determinants involved in *C. perfringens* colonization are unconfirmed.[146] In contrast to *C. difficile*, no specific adhesion factor has been discovered in *C. perfringens*. As various *C. perfringens* types have derived extrachromosomal elements from the type A pathovar, mobile elements may also share regulatory genes that assist rapid colonization in certain hosts.[146] It has been reported that in *C. perfringens* type C adheres to intestinal villi possibly by means of capsule polysaccharides.[148] Other suggestions for adherence determinants are surface loci containing the β-galactosidase proteins, already shown to be critical for *Bacteroides* sp. digestive tract colonization.[149]

Capsules

C. perfringens has been shown to have the ability to survive in amurine macrophage-like cell line J774–33 even under aerobic conditions.[150] The recent study investigated J774–33 cells in which *C. perfringens* can escape the phagosome and gain access to the cytoplasm. Since the receptor that is used for phagocytosis can determine the fate of an intracellular bacterium, the researchers used a variety of inhibitors of specific receptors to identify those used to phagocytose *C. perfringens*. It was found that the scavenger receptor and mannose receptor(s) were involved in this phagocytosis. In the presence of complement, the complement receptor was also involved in the binding. Carbohydrate analysis of *C. perfringens* type A strain 13 extracellular polysaccharide has confirmed the presence of mannose and negatively charged residues of glucuronic acid, which may provide the moieties that promote binding to the mannose and scavenger receptors, respectively.

Enzymes

C. perfringens secretes a wide range of hydrolytic enzymes that degrade extracellular substrates and components resulting from cell lysis.[146] Some of these factors are not truly toxic and have no known role in pathogenicity, although some are common to more than one group: neurotoxins lethal toxins lecithinases, haemolysins, ADP-ribosyltransferases.[151] Virulence factors such as haemolysin, collagenase/gelatinase, and a neuraminadase (encoded by pfoA, colA, and nan, respectively) are positively regulated by the same transcriptional regulation as α-toxin (VirR/VirS).[146] Such factors are well documented in gangrenous lesions by favouring the degradation of extracellular and lysed cell substrates and providing nutrients for growth.[152–154] However, the environmental signals triggering transcription is as yet unknown and their significance in the pathology of AAD has not been reported.

Toxins

As previously discussed, *C. perfringens* is characterized by its ability to produce numerous extracellular toxins including α-toxin, phospholipase C, [θ]-toxin or perfringolysin O, κ-toxin or collagenase, as well as the sporulation-associated enterotoxin.[155] The four major toxins are secreted into the medium during the exponential growth phase, and kill mice when the culture supernatant is injected peritoneally. Each type of toxin induces a specific syndrome.[146] *C. perfringens* type A causing gas gangrene in humans is a disease mediated primarily by α-toxin and secondarily by hydrolytic enzymes.[146] However, while it is only those producing a significant level of CPEnt that are associated with food poisoning and AAD, non-enterotoxogenic *C. perfringens* type A CPEnt negative strains have been isolated from animals with enterotoxaemia or enteritis.[151,156] While α-toxin had not previously been known to cause intestinal lesions in animals, the enteropathogenicity of these strains might result from high levels of α-toxin production from molecular variants that are more stable to protease digestion or are more active or from differing host sensitivity to α-toxin.[157,158] Historically, however, no difference in the production of α-toxin between type A strains isolated from clinical cases of gas gangrene and abdominal wounds and those isolated from faecal samples from healthy persons has been found. As previously discussed, the environmental signal triggering transcription of α-toxin via VirR/VirS is unknown, and as yet no association with the pathology of antibiotic associated diarrhoea has been documented.

The toxicosis associated with both food-borne illness and both sporadic and antibiotic-associated diarrhoea results from the production and gastrointestinal absorption of the protein enterotoxin discussed previously as CPEnt.[159] The CPE protein consists of a single 35-kDa polypeptide with a C-terminal receptor-binding region and an N-terminal toxicity domain. The regulation, expression, and mechanism of action of CPEnt have generated considerable interest, as the protein is unique with no significant homology to any other enterotoxin.[159,160]

Sarker et al. evaluated the importance of CPE in the pathogenesis of clostridial GI disease using allelic exchange to construct a CPE knock-out mutant of F4969 – a known CPE-positive type A strain.[161] When the virulence of a wild-type and mutant strains were compared in the rabbit ileal loop model, it was found that sporulating (but not vegetative) isolates of the wild-type strain induced significant ileal loop fluid accumulation and histopathological damage. However, neither the sporulating nor vegetative culture lysates of the CPE knock-out mutants induced these intestinal effects. The authors concluded that as CPE expression is necessary for CPE-positive *C. perfringens* type A human disease isolates to cause GI effects in the ileal loop model, this supports CPE as an important virulence factor in GI disease. This study also highlighted the observation that CPEnt is associated with sporulation of *C. perfringens* type A and not vegetative cells.

It is generally accepted that CPE expression is sporulation associated. While sporulation is hard to induce in vitro, spores readily form in the small bowel following ingestion and especially well in the antibiotically treated gut.[141] Although some enterotoxin is formed during exponential growth, the transcriptional factors activating the sporulation genes also upregulate the CPE gene. However, the environmental factor triggering sporulation is as yet unknown.

When the spores germinate, enterotoxin, formed under co-ordinate regulation with spores, is released. In 1991, Heredia et al. performed a study on the growth and sporulation of *C. perfringens* type A in the presence of human bile salts.[161] The researchers found that while human bile juice completely inhibited the growth of all the strains, a distinct stimulatory effect of the bile salts on sporulation was observed with a subsequent increase in enterotoxin concentration in cell extracts.

In food-borne illness, strains both the genes for spore formation and CPE are located on the bacterial chromosome.[159] However, non-food-borne human GI disease isolates carry the gene for CPEnt on a large plasmid. Sarker et al. found that isolates with chromosomal CPE have cells and spores possessing a higher degree of heat resistance than episomal CPE, which may explain their strong association with food poisoning isolates.[162]

The three promoter sites responsible for the sporulation-associated synthesis of CPEnt have been reported to be similar in consensus to the SigK and SigE sporulation promoters (known to be active in the mother cell compartment of sporulating cells of *Bacillus subtilis*). This is the same compartment in which enterotoxin is synthesized in *C. perfringens*. Although the genes encoding the α- and [θ]-toxin are located on the chromosome, the genes encoding many of the other extracellular toxins are also located on large plasmids.[155] Recently it has been suggested that because the VirR/VirS system has evolved to regulate both chromo- somal toxin gene and plasmid-encoded virulence factors, a similar global regulator may promote CPEnt production and sporulation.[163]

In a Norweigian study, Brynestad et al. used a strain of *C. perfringens* carrying the chloramphemicol-resistant mutant plasmid pMRS49969 to evaluate whether the CPE plasmid could conjugatively transfer to a CPE negative isolate.[164] The results demonstrated that the entire plasmid had been transferred to the recipient strain. The transfer required cell-to-cell contact and was DNAse resistant, indicating that transfer occurred by a conjugative mechanism.

In his recent studies, Miyamoto reported that the CPE plasmid of many type A isolates originated from the integration of a CPE-containing genetic element from the chromosomal locus.[165] The author also concluded that the observed similarity of the plasmid CPE locus is consistent with horizontal transfer of a common CPE plasmid among *C. perfringens* type A strains.

The clinical significance of both these studies is that if conjugative transfer of the CPE plasmid occurred in vivo, it would have the potential to convert CPE-negative *C. perfringens* strains in normal intestinal flora into strains capable of causing gastrointestinal disease.

Primarily, CPEnt exerts a cytotoxic effect through the formation of an approxi- mately 155-kDa CPE-containing complex corresponding to a pore.[166] This process is an innate property of CPEnt demonstrated by formation of pores in a synthetic phospholipid membrane in the absence of surface proteins.[160] The resulting cellular damage causes an increase in ionic permeability (excluding any paracellular per- meability), providing CPEnt access to intestinal epithelial cell tight junction (TJ) structural components including claudins and occludin. The specific binding of CPEnt to these structural proteins affects TJ structure and function thereby causing diarrhoea. The presence of these receptors has been reported to also be expressed at high levels in the lungs, liver, and kidneys, and at low levels in the heart and skeletal muscle.[167] While the authors expressed concern regarding further pathogenic potential of CPEnt, other researchers have turned attention to target the cytotoxicity of CPEnt as a potential new therapeutic for specific cancers.[168] However, a recent American study has demonstrated that death pathways activated in CaCo-2 cells by CPEnt suggest that both oncosis and apoptosis may also occur in the intestines during CPE-associated GI disease.[169]

C. Perfringens Enterotoxin-Associated Disease

As previously discussed, even in the absence of typical food poisoning, *C. perfrin- gens* enterotoxin can be produced in vivo resulting in diarrhoea. Just as the symptoms of food-borne botulism differ from those seen in infants with in vivo toxication, the clinical features of *C. perfringens* food poisoning and antibiotic- associated disease also differ.

Antibiotic-Associated CPEnt Diarrhoea

The clinical course of CPEnt AAD is different to that observed in food poisoning cases caused by the same toxin. The diarrhoea is more profuse (average 10 days although it can last for more than 2 weeks), and blood and mucous are frequently present. Abdominal pain also occurs more frequently. Histological examination of rectal mucosa reveals mild oedema, thereby implying that there may be more severe lesions in proximal regions of the gut that account for faecal blood.

Antibiotic-Associated CPEnt Colitis

To date, no reports of proven CPEnt AAD cases have documented evidence of colitis. However, while Borriello described an elderly patient with CPEnt AAD whose findings on sigmoidoscopy were normal, he concluded that as rectal sparing has been described in cases of PMC due to *C. difficile*, the excretion of blood and mucus in this patient may be indicative of more proximal colonic involement.[143] In Borriellos first study although three patients suffered bloody stools, the four patients who underwent colonoscopy showed no evidence of PMC.

Other CPEnt Associations

As with *C. difficile*, diarrhoea associated with *C. perfringens* can also occur spontaneously or in the absence of antibiotics.[141] This sporadic diarrhoea presents as with CPEnt AAD but without the antibiotic association. Although it is usually self-limiting, sufferers are likely to visit their GP because of its severity. *C. perfringens* type A has also been isolated from an abdominal abscess in a patient with AIDS. While it is not known whether this isolate was CPEnt positive, the predisposing factor of the infection was believed to be antibiotic therapy. The authors of this study also highlighted the relationship between clostridial infections and malignancies of the gastrointestinal tract (in particular Karposi's sarcoma) in patients with AIDS. CPEnt itself has been associated with sudden infant death syndrome (SIDS) because of its superantigenic nature.

Clinical History and Risk Factors

Reports of symptomatic CPEnt-positive, hospitalized patients appear to present a similar clinical background as for patients with *C. difficile* AAD.

Antibiotics

In most reports of *C. perfringens* enterotoxin-associated diarrhoea, the significance of antibiotic association is suggested. As with *C. difficile* diarrhoea, many drugs are thought to predispose patients to CPEnt AAD including those that are used to treat this diarrhoea and other infections with *C. perfringens*.[141] Implicated antibiotics have included penicillins, cephalosporins, augamentin, erythromycintrimethoprim, nitrofluorantoin, and cotrimoxazole.

Age-Related Susceptibility

While food poisoning from CPEnt occurs in all age groups, the majority of cases of infectious diarrhoea and AAD are in patients aged over 60 years. Many outbreaks and clusters of cases have been reported in geriatric wards and units where the early recognition of AAD in a highly vulnerable population is stressed. Reports to the public health laboratory between 1990 and 1996 concluded that the top three locations for outbreaks of infectious diarrhoea caused by *C. perfringnes* were homes for the elderly and geriatric and psychogeriatric hospitals.

Like *C. difficile*, the incidence of both asymptomatic carriage and of CPEnt AAD appears to increase with age. However, while this explains the higher incidence of sporadic, non-antibiotic cases in this age group, it does not explain the age distribution in antibiotic-associated ones.

Immunosupression

In his 1997 review, Carman also stated that the majority of patients with CPEnt antibiotic-associated diarrhoea are immunocompromised. Such patients include transplant recipients, burn victims, AIDS sufferers, and Hepatitis patients.[141]

Others

Although reports of the individual risk factors pre-empting CPEnt AAD are scarce, previous data suggests that any factors proven to predispose the patient to *C. difficile* AAD have the potential to play a significant role in the pathology of the *C. perfringens* gastroenteritis.

The Frequency of *C. Perfringens*-Associated Diarrhoea

While *C. difficile* is the most commonly identified pathogen in hospital-acquired infective diarrhoea, it only accounts for approximately 20% of cases. Therefore, for most cases (up to 80%) the organism responsible remains undiagnosed. The incidence of CPEnt AAD appears to vary between sites and may be higher during epidemics in hospitals and in institutions housing the elderly.[141]

Community

Previous studies that include cases of diarrhoea from the community, as well as hospital in-patients, have reported positive rates for CPEnt in faecal specimens ranging from 3.5 to 18.0%.

Nosocomial

In 1995, Allen et al. presented the findings of a large study to the Society of Anaerobic Microbiology, Cambridge.[170] The investigation spanned over a 30-month period investigating hospitalized cases of AAD. CPEnt-positive strains were cultured and serotyped. It was found that the causal serotypes were the most abundant in the environment while patients in that ward were having diarrhoea. The frequency of isolation dropped dramatically once treatment was begun. The data strongly suggested that CPEnt causes infectious nosocomial AAD. Samuel et al. studied the incidence of CPEnt AAD in the elderly and found a clear association of C. perfringnes diarrhoea in hospital in-patients most of who had received antibiotics before onset of symptoms.[171] More recent studies have investigated the prevalence of C. perfringnes AAD in contrast to that of C. difficile AAD. The incidence and significance of C. perfringnes, as an alternative to C. difficile and as a cause of AAD, has been investigated among groups of hospital in-patients.[172] The groups were defined according to the presence of diarrhoea and antibiotic usage. In a group of 94 patients with both diarrhoea and a past history of antibiotic therapy, 21 (22.3%) were C. difficile positive and 15 (15.9%) were CPEnt positive. While serotyping was not available, descriptive epidemiology was used to confirm cross-infection of CPEnt cases on the basis of geographical clustering. The author concluded, therefore, that in this study C. perfringens appeared to cause a similar incidence of AAD to C. diffiicle and had the potential to cause similar cross-infection problems. In a recent European study, Abraho et al. also reported a similar frequency of detection of CPEnt and C. difficile toxins in patients with AAD.[173] However, in September 2002 the results of a major UK trial were presented at the Edinburgh Hospital Infection Society meeting. The authors reflected the figures of Borriellos early studies, finding that from 200 in-patients with AAD, 8% were positive for CPEnt, 16% were positive for C. difficile cytoxins, and 2% gave positive results in both assays.[174] To contribute to the debate, Carney et al. published the results of a survey of the incidence of C. perfringens enterotoxin in a letter to the Journal of Clinical Pathology.[175] The researchers found that of 249 in patients with diarrhoea, 9.6% were positive for C. difficile cytoxins and only 1.6% were positive for CPEnt. The authors concluded that the low incidence of CPEnt suggests that screening for the toxin would not be justified. However, it is interesting to note that the seemingly low prevalence in this small study was in fact representative of in-patients with loose stools and mild symptoms, many of whom had no history of antibiotic usage.

Table 10.3 A table of evidence that suggests other pathogens as causing antibiotic-associated diarrhoea

Organism	Evidence	Reference
Salmonella spp.	Enteritis after antibiotic therapy; occasionally presenting as pseudomembranous colitis	5, 21, 27–29
	Outbreaks of multidrug resistance strains after penicillin therapy	
	Antibiotics enhance susceptibility of mice to *Salmonella* spp. by 1,000,000-fold	
Candida spp.	Massive fungal growths from 50/100 in-patients with AAD	30–32
	High Candida counts in stool fluids from patients with AAD – due to reduced soluble Candida inhibitors and increased availability of growth factors	
Klebsiella oxytoca	High levels of cytotoxin produced by ampicillin resistant *K. oxytoca* during acute phase of disease suggests overgrowth during therapy.	33,34
	Toxin producing *K. oxytoca* causes fluid accumulation in rabbit intestinal loop model – non-toxin-producing strains did not	
Pseudomonas spp.	*P. aeruginosa* – predominant organism isolated from seven patients stools, with nosocomial diarrhoea. Diarrhoea stopped in two patients after withdrawal of antibiotics to which pseudomonas were resistant; five patients responded to antipseudomonal therapy	35
Campylobacter sp.	*Campylobacter* involved in antibiotic associated diarrhoea	180
Staphylococcus aureus	Prevalence of enterotoxin producing *Staphylococcus aureus* in stools of patients with nosocomial diarrhoea	179

Conclusion

Colonizing intestinal microflora is considered to have a significant effect on the health and well-being of humans with advancing age.[176,177] This is particularly relevant when we consider the administration of antibiotics[178] and the development of AAD. AAD may be defined as an otherwise unexplained diarrhoea that occurs in association with the administration of antibiotics. AAD has been associated with a vast array of bacteria either by themselves or in synergy with other bacteria (see Table 10.3 [179,180]). But, to date, by far the most significant bacteria associated with AAD is Clostridium. Clostridia are important bacteria in the adult human gut and are considered to have a significant pathogenicity. Contrary to this, within neonates the effects of Clostridium are less apparent. *C. difficile* is recognized as the most significant human Clostridium species and a major cause of nosocomial infectious diarrhoea in the elderly population.[181–185] Current data from the Centres for Disease Control has confirmed that the incidence of *C. difficile* has doubled in recent years and accounts for over 3 million cases of diarrhoea and colitis annually. Older adults are at a higher risk for this infection particularly due to the changes in faecal flora and host immune response together with co-morbidities.

Asymptomatic carriers of epidemic and non-epidemic *C. difficile* strains contribute significantly to disease transmission in long-term-care facilities.[55] Neonates and infants, particularly in European countries and the US, have high frequencies of carriage of *C. difficile* and many neonates have been found to be infected with this organism after birth following short stays in the hospital. It seems plausible to accept, on the basis of the vast array of published material in this area, that as the gut ages, susceptibility to the effects of certain bacteria, e.g. *C. difficile*, becomes more significant, and it has been shown that antibiotic-induced diarrhoea occurs in up to 25% of patients that receive antibiotics and 15% of these are due to *C. difficile*.[186]

Hospitals around Europe and North America have outbreaks due to *C. difficile* with the species accounting for 39.9 cases per 1,000 admissions to hospital.[187,188] The most prevalent strains of *Clostridium difficile* include the epidemic strains, BI, the North American PGFE type 1 (NAPI), and strain 027.[189] The NAP1 strain has been shown to be highly resistant to fluoroquinolone.[190] Susceptibility to *C. difficile*, as well as other enteric bacteria, seems to increase with age.

References

1. Alvarez-Olmos MI, Oberhelman A. Probiotic agents and infectious diseases: a modern perspective on a traditional therapy. Clin Infect Dis 2001;32:1567–1576.
2. Rohner P, Pittet D, Pepey B, Nije-kinge T, Aukenthaler R. Etiological agents of infectious diarrhoea: implications for requests for microbial culture. J Clin Microbiol 1997;35:1427–1431.
3. Claassen E. Effects of Intestinal Flora on the Immune System. In: Intestinal Flora and Human Health. Yakult. An overview of scientific Literature. 2001.
4. Shanahan H. Recent advances in the understanding of inflammatory bowel disease – unravelling the complexity. Odyssey 6;2:32–36.
5. Bauer TM, Lalvani A, Fehrenbach J, Steffen I, Aponte JJ, Segovia R, Vila J, Philippczik G, Steinbrückner B, Frei R, Bowler I, Kist M. Derivation and validation of guidelines for stools cultures for enteropathogenic bacteria other than *Clostridium difficle* in hospitalised patients. JAMA 2001;285:313–319.
6. Vasa CV, Glatt MD. Effectiveness and appropriateness of empiric metronidazole for *Clostridium difficile*-associated diarrhoea. Am J Gastroenterol 2003;98:354–358.
7. Roffe C. Biotherapy for antibiotic associated and other diarrhoeas. J Infect 1995;32:1–10.
8. Bartlett J. Antibiotic associated diarrhoea. N Engl J Med 2002;346:334–339.
9. Kasper H. Development and Modification of the Intestinal Flora. In: Intestinal Flora and Human Health. Yakult. An overview of scientific Literature. 2001.
10. Meakins SM, Adak GK, Lopmann BA, O'Brien SJ. General outbreaks of infectious intestinal disease (IID) in hospitals, England and Wales, 1992–2000. J Hosp Infect 2003;53:1–5.
11. Khan R, Cheesbrough J. Impact of changes in antibiotic policy on *Clostridium difficile*-associated diarrhoea (CDAD) over a five-year period in a district hospital. J Hosp Infect 2003;54:104–108.

12. Wilcox MH, Smyth ETM. Incidence and impact of *Clostridium difficile* infection in the UK 1993–1996. J Hosp Infect 1998;39:181–187.

13. Hogenauer C, Hammer HF, Krejs GJ, Reisinger EC. Mechanisms and management of antibiotic-associated diarrhea. Clin Infect Dis 1998;27:702–710.

14. Boardman A. Diagnosis and management of pseudomembranous colitis and *Clostridium difficile*-associated disease. Primary Care Update OB/GYNS 1998;5:219–228.

15. Eckel F, Huber W, Weiss W, Lersch C. Recurrent pseudomembranous colitis as a cause of recurrent severe sepsis. Z Gastroenterol 2002;40:255–258.

16. Barbut F, Meynard JL. Managing antibiotic associated diarrhoea. BMJ 2002;324: 1345–1346.

17. Wilcox MH. Treatment of *Clostridium difficile* infection. J Antimicrob Chemother 1998; 41:41–46.

18. Modi N, Wilcox MH. Evidence for antibiotic induced *Clostridium perfringens* diarrhoea. J Clin Pathol 2001;54:748–751.

19. Wilcox MH, Cunniffe JG, Trundle C, Redpath C. Financial burden of hospital-acquired *Clostridium difficile* infection. J Hosp Infect 1996;34:23–30.

20. Sullivan A, Edlund C, Nord CE. Effect of antimicrobial agents on the ecological balance of human microflora. Lancet 2001;1:101–114.

21. Levy J. The effects of antibiotic use on gastrointestinal function. Am J Gastroenterol 2000;95:8–10.

22. Borriello SP, Barclay FE, Welsh AR, Stringer MF, Watson GN, Williams RK, Seal DV, Sullens K. Epidemiology of diarrhoea caused by enterotoxigenic *Clostridium perfringens*. J Med Microbiol 1985;20:363–372.

23. Schiller B, Chiorazzi N, Farber BF. Methicillin-resistant staphylococcal enterocolitis. Am J Med 1998;105:164–166.

24. McDonald M, Ward P, Harvey K. Antibiotic associated diarrhoea and methicillin-resistant *Staphylococcus aureus*. Med J Aust 1982;1:462–464.

25. Inamatsu T, Ooshima H, Masuda Y, Fukayama M, Adachi K, Takeshima H, Hashimoto H. Clinical spectrum of antibiotic associated enterocolitis due to methicillin resistant *Staphylococcus aureus*. Nippon Rinsho 1992;50:1087–1092.

26. Morita H, Tani M, Adachi H, Kawai S. Methicillin-resistant *Staphylococcus aureus* (MRSA) enteritis associated with prophylactic cephalosporin administration and hypochlorhydria after subtotal gastrectomy. Am J Gastroenterol 1991;86:791–792.

27. Hovius SE Rietra PJ. Salmonella colitis clinically presenting as a pseudomembranous colitis. Neth J Surg 1982;34:81–82.

28. Sun M. In search of Salmonella's smoking gun. Science 1984;226:30–32.

29. Olsen SJ, DeBess EE, McGivern TE, Marano N, Eby T, Mauvais S, Balan VK, Zirnstein G, Cieslak PR, Angulo FJ. A nosocomial outbreak of fluoroquinolone-resistant salmonella infection. N Engl J Med 2001;344;1572–1579.

30. Rokosz A,Sawicka-Grzelak A, Pituch H, uczak M. Cultivation of fungi from fecal specimens in cases of antibiotic associated diarrhea (AAD). Med Dosw Mikrobiol 2002;54(4):371–377.

31. Krause R, Haberl R, Strempfl C, Daxbock F, Krejs G, Reisinger EC, Wenisch C. Intestinal Candida phospholipase is not elevated in patients with antibiotic associated diarrhea. Scand J Infect Dis 2002;34:815–816.

32. Krause R, Krejs GJ, Wenisch C, Reisinger EC. Elevated fecal Candida counts in patients with antibiotic-associated diarrhoea: role of soluble fecal substances. Clin Diagn Lab Immunol 2003;10:167–168.

33. Cleau D, Humblot S, Jobard JM, Berger M. Acute right side hemorrhagic colitis with demonstration of *Klebsiella oxytoca* after treatment with amoxicillin. Presse Med 1994;23 (40):1879–1880.

34. Minami J, Katayama S, Matsushita O, Sakamoto H, Okabe A. Enterotoxic activity of *Klebsiella oxytoca* cytotoxin in rabbit intestinal loops. Infect Immun 1994;1:172–177.

35. Kim SW, Peck KR, Jung SI, Kim YS, Kim S, Lee NY, Song JH. *Pseudomonas aeruginosa* as a potential cause of antibiotic-associated diarrhea. J Korean Med Sci 2001;16:742–744.

36. Pituch H, Obuch-Woszczatylski P, Meisel-Mikolajczyk F, Luczak M. Prevalence of entero-toxigenic *Bacteroides fragilis* strains (ETBF) in the gut of children with clinical diagnosis of antibiotic associated diarrhoea (AAD). Med Dosw Mikrobiol 2002;54:357–363.

37. Hall IC, O'Toole E. Intestinal flora in newborn infants with a description of a new pathogenic anaerobe *Bacillus difficilis*. Am J Dis Child 1935;49:390–402.

38. Spencer R. Clinical impact and associated costs of *Clostridium difficile*-associated disease. J Antimicrob Chemother 1998;41:5–12.

39. Worsley MA. Infection control and prevention of *Clostridium difficile* infection. J Antimicrob Chemother 1998;41:59–66.

40. Brazier JS. The diagnosis of *Clostridium difficile*-associated disease. J Antimicrob Chemother 1998;41:29–40.

41. Snyder ML. Further studies on *Bacillus difficilis* (Hall and O'Toole). J Infect Dis 1937;60: 223–231.

42. Tedesco FJ, Barton RW, Alpers DH. Clindamycin-associated colitis. A prospective study. Ann Intern Med 1974;81(4):429–433.

43. Green RH. The association of viral activation with penicillin toxicity in guinea pigs and hamsters. Yale J Biol Med 1974;47(3):166–181.

44. Verity P, Wilcox MH, Fawley W, Parnell P. Prospective evaluation of environmental con-tamination by *Clostridium difficile* in isolation side rooms. J Hosp Infect 2001;49(3):204–209.

45. Wilcox MH, Fawley WN, Wigglesworth N, Parnell P, Verity P, Freeman J. Comparison of the effect of detergent versus hypochlorite cleaning on environmental contamination and inci-dence of *Clostridium difficile* infection. J Hosp Infect 2003;54(2):109–114.

46. Bolton RP, Tait SK, Dear PR, Lowsowsky MS. Asymptomatic neonatal colonisation by *Clostridium difficile*. Arch Dis Child 1984;56:466–472.

47. Larson HE, Barcley FE, Honour P, Hill ID. Epidemiology of *Clostridium difficle* in infants. J Infect Dis 1982;146:727–733.

48. Wongwanich S, Pongpech P, Dhiraputra C, Huttayananont S, Sawanpanyalert P. Character-istics of *Clostridium difficile* strains isolated from asymptomatic individuals and from diar-rheal patients. Clin Microbiol Infect 2001;7(8):438–441.

49. McFarland LV, Mulligan ME, Kwok RY, Stamm WE. Nosocomial acquisition of *Clostridium difficile* infection. N Engl J Med 1989;320:204–210.

50. Harmsen HJ, Wildeboer-Veloo AC, Raangs GC, Wagendorp AA, Klijn N, Bindels JG, Well-ing GW. Analysis of intestinal flora development in breast-fed and formula-fed infants by using molecular identification and detection methods. J Pediatr Gastroenterol Nutr 2000;30:61–67.

51. Donta ST, Myers MG. *Clostridium difficile* toxin in asymptomatic neonates. J Pediatr 1982;100(3):431–434.

52. Borriello SP, Wilcox MH. *Clostridium difficile* infections of the gut: the unanswered ques-tions. J Antimicrob Chemother 1998;41:67–69.

53. Magdesian KG, Madigan JE, Hirsh DC, Spenser SJ, Yajarayma JT, Carpenter TE, Hansen LM, Silva J Jr. *Clostridium difficile* and Horses: a review. Rev Med Microbiol 1997;8: S46–S48.

54. Nakamura S, Mikawa M, Nakashio S, Takabatake M, Okado I, Yamakawa K, Serikawa T, Okumura S, Nishida S. Isolation of *Clostridium difficile* from faeces and the antibody in sera of young and elderly adults. Microbiol Immunol 1981;25:345–351.

55. Riggs MM, Sethi AK, Zabarsky TF, Eckstein EC, Jump RL, Donskey CJ. Asymptomatic carriers are a potential source for transmission of epidemic and nonepidemic *Clostridium difficile* strains among long-term care facility residents. Clin Infect Dis 2007; 45(8):992–998.

56. Rivera EV, Woods S. Prevalence of asymptomatic *Clostridium difficile* colonization in a nursing home population: a cross-sectional study. J Gend Specif Med 2003;6(2):27–30.

57. Spencer R. The role of antimicrobial agents in the aetiology of *Clostridium difficile*-associted disease. J Antimicrob Chemother 1998;41:21–27.

58. Péchiné S, Janoir C, Collignon A. Variability of *Clostridium difficile* surface proteins and specific serum antibody response in patients with *Clostridium difficile*-associated disease. J Clin Microbiol 2005;43(10):5018–5025.
59. Eveillard M, Fourel V, Barc MC, Kernéis S, Coconnier MH, Karjalainen T, Bourlioux P, Servin AL. Identification and characterisation of adhesive factors of *Clostridium difficile* involved in adhesion to human colonic enterocyte-like Caco-2 and mucus secreting HT29 cells in cukture. Mol Microbiol 1993;7;371–381.
60. Karjalainen T, Barc MC, Collignon A, Trollé S, Boureau H, Cotte-Laffitte J, Bourlioux P. Cloning of a genetic determinant from *Clostridium difficile* involved in adherence to tissue culture cells and mucus. Infect Immun 1994;62:4347–4355.
61. Waligora AJ, Barc MC, Bourlioux P, Collignon A, Karjalainen T. *Clostridium difficile* cell attachment is modified by environmental factors. Appl Environ Microbiol 1999;65: 4234–4238.
62. Hennequin C, Collignon A, Karjalainen T. Analysis of expression of GroEL (Hsp60) of *Clostridium difficile* in response to stress. Microb Pathog 2001;31:255–260.
63. Borriello SP. *Clostridium difficile* and its toxin in the gastrointestinal tract in health and disease. Res Clin Forums 1979;1:33–35.
64. Calabi E, Fairweather N. Patterns of sequence conservation in the S-layer proteins and related sequences in *Clostridium difficile*. J Bacteriol 2002;184:3886–3897.
65. Calabi E, Calabi F, Phillips AD, Fairweather NF. Binding of *Clostridium difficile* surface layer proteins to gastrointestinal tissues. Infect Immun 2002;70:5770–5778.
66. Borriello SP, Bhatt R. Chemotaxis by *Clostridium difficile*. In Medical and Dental Aspects of Anaerobes (Duerden B, Wade JG, Brzier JG, Eley JS, Wren B, Hudson MJ. Eds). Sceintific Reviews Ltd Middlesex. 1995, p. 241.
67. Davies HA, Borriello SP. Detection of capsule in strains of *Clostridium difficile* of varying virulence and toxigenicity. Microb Pathog 1990;9:141–146.
68. Borriello SP, Davies HA, Kamiya S, Reed PJ. Virulence Factors of *Clostridium difficile*. Rev Infect Dis 1990;12:S185–S191.
69. Dhalluin A, Bourgeois I, Pestel-Caron M, Camiade E, Raux G, Courtin P, Chapot-Chartier MP, Pons JL. Acd, a peptidoglycan hydrolase of *Clostridium difficile* with *N*-acetylglucosaminidase activity. Microbiology 2005;151:2343–2351.
70. Steffen EK, Hentges DJ. Hydrolytic enzymes of anaerobic bacteria isolated from human infections. J Clin Microbiol 1981;14:153–156.
71. Bongaerts GP, Lyerly DM. Role of bacterial metabolism and physiology in the pathogenesis of *Clostridium difficile* disease. Microb Pathog 1997;22:253–256.
72. Stubbs S, Rupnik M, Gibert M, Brazier J, Duerden B, Popoff M. Production of actin-specific ADP-ribosyltransferase (binary toxin) by strains of *Clostridium difficile*. FEMS Microbiol Lett 2000;186:307–312.
73. Maciel AA, Oriá RB, Braga-Neto MB, Braga AB, Carvalho EB, Lucena HB, Brito GA, Guerrant RL, Lima AA. Role of retinol in protecting epithelial cell damage induced by *Clostridium difficile* toxin A. Toxicon 2007;50(8):1027–1040.
74. Hammond GA, Johnson JL. The toxigenic element of *Clostridium difficile* strain VPI 10463. Microb Pathog 1995;19:203–213.
75. Wren BW. Molecular characterisation of *Clostridium difficile* toxins A and B. Rev Med Microbiol 1992;3:21–27.
76. Samra Z, Talmor S, Bahar J. High prevalence of toxin-A negative toxin B-positive *Clostridium difficile* in hospitalized patients with gastrointestinal disease. Diagn Microbiol Infect Dis 2002;43:189–192.
77. Pothoulakis C, Castagliuolo I, Kelly C, LaMont T. *Clostridium difficile*-associated diarrhoea and colitis: pathogenisis and therapy. Int J Antimicrob Agents 1993;3:17–32.
78. Lyerly DM, Saum KE, MacDonald D, Wilkins TD. Effect of toxins A and B given intravenously to animals. Infect Immun 1985;47:349–352.

79. Lyerly DM, Johnson JL, Frey SM, Wilkins TD. Vaccination against lethal *Clostridium difficile* enterococcus with a nontoxic recombinant peptide of toxin A. Curr Microbiol 1990;21:29–33.
80. Barroso LA, Wang SZ, Phelps CJ, Johnson JL, Wilkins TD. Nucleotide sequence of *Clostridium difficile* toxin B gene. Nucleic Acids Res 1990;18:4004.
81. Hecht G, Pothoulakis JT, LaMont JT, Madara JL. *Clostridium difficile* toxin A perturbs cytoskeletal structure and tight junction permeability of cultured human epithelial monolayers. J Clin Invest 1988;82:1516–1524.
82. Grossmann EM, Longo WE, Kaminski DL, Smith GS, Murphy CE, Durham RL, Shapiro MJ, Norman JG, Mazuski JE. *Clostridium difficile* toxin: cytoskeletal changes and lactate dehydrogenase release in hepatocytes. J Surg Res 2000;88(2):165–172.
83. Pothoulakis C, Lamont JT. Microbes and microbial toxins: paradigms for microbial-mucosal interactions II. The integrated response of the intestine to *Clostridium* toxins. Am J Physiol Gastrointest Liver Physiol 2001;280:178–183.
84. Chen ML, Pothoulakis JT, LaMont JT. Protein kinase C signaling regulates ZO-1 translocation and increased paracellular flux of T84 colonocytes exposed to *Clostridium difficile* toxin A. J Biol Chem 2002;277:4247–4254.
85. Steiner TS, Flores CA, Pizarro T, Guerrant R. Fecal lactoferrin interleukin-1 beta and interleukin-8 are elevated in patients with sever *Clostridium difficile* colitis. Clin Diagn Lab Immun 1997;4:719–722.
86. Rocha MFG, Soares AM, Ribeiro RA, Lima AAM. Absence of intestinal secreation on supernatants from macrophages stimulated with *Clostridium difficile* toxin B on rabbit ileum. Toxicon 2001;39:335–340.
87. Wren BW, Heard SR, Tabaqchali S. Association between the production of toxins A and B and types of *Clostridium difficile*. J Clin Pathol 1987;40:1397–1401.
88. Rupnik M, Avesani V, Janc M, von Eichel-Streiber C, Delmee M. A novel toxinotyping scheme and correlation of toxinotypes with serogroups of *Clostridium difficile* isolates. J Clin Microbiol 1998;36:2240–2247.
89. Von Eichel-Streiber C, Meyer zu Heringdorf E, Habermann E, Sartingen S. Closing in on the toxic domain through analysis of a variant *Clostridium difficile* cytotoxin B. Mol Microbiol 1995;17:313–321.
90. Kuijper EJ, de Weerdt J, Kato H, Kato N, van Dam AP, van der Vorm ER, Weel J, van Rheenen C, Dankert J. Nosocomial outbreak of *Clostridium difficile*-associated diarrhoea due to a clindamycin-resistant enterotoxin A-negative strain. Eur J Clin Microbiol Infect Dis 2001;20:528–534.
91. Alfa MJ, Kabani A, Lyerly D, Moncrief S, Neville LM, Al-Barrak A, Harding GKH, Dyck B, Olekson K, Embil JM. J Clin Microbiol 2000;7:2706–2714.
92. Chaves-Olarte E, Freer E, Parra A, Guzman-Verri C, Moreno E, Thelestam M. R-Ras glucosylation and transient RhoA activation determine the cytopathic effect produced by toxin B variants from toxin A-negative strains of *Clostridium difficile*. J Biol Chem 2003;278:7956–7963.
93. Razavi B, Apisarnthanarak A, Mundy LM. *Clostridium difficile*: emergence of hypervirulence and fluoroquinolone resistance. Infection 2007;35(5):300–307.
94. Bartlett JG. *Clostridium difficile*: clinical considerations. Rev Infect Dis 1990;12:S243–S251.
95. Tedesco FJ, Corless JK, Brownstein RE. Rectal sparing in antibiotic associated pseudomembranous colitis; a prospective study. Gastroenterology 1983;83:1259–1260.
96. Skoutelis AT, Westenfelder GO, Beckerdite M, Phair JP. Hospital carpeting and epidemiology of *Clostridium difficile*. Am J Infect Control 1993;22:212–217.
97. Gravisse J, Barnaud G, Hanau-Berçot B, Raskine L, Riahi J, Gaillard JL, Sanson-Le-Pors MJ. *Clostridium difficile* brain empyema after prolonged intestinal carriage. J Clin Microbiol 2003;41(1):509–511.
98. Nakamur I, Kunihiro M, Kato H. Bacteremia due to *Clostridium difficile*. Kansenshogaku Zasshi 2004;78(12):1026–1030.

99. Qualman SJ, Petric M, Karmali MA, Smith CR, Hamilton SR. *Clostridium difficile* invasion and toxin circulation in fatal paediatric pseudomembranous colitis. Am J Clin Pathol 1990;94:410–416.

100. Bartlett JG. Management of *Clostridium difficile* infection and other antibiotic associated diarrhoeas. Eur J Gastroenterol Hepatol 1996;8:1054–1061.

101. Shek FW, Stacey BS, Rendell J, Hellier MD, Hanson PJ. The rise of *Clostridium difficile*: the effect of length of stay patient age and antibiotic use. J Hosp Infect 2000;45:235–237.

102. McFarland LV, Stamm WE. Review of *Closttridium difficile* associated diseases. Am J Infect Control 1986;14:99–109.

103. Spivack JG, Eppes SC, Klein JD. *Clostridium difficile*-associated diarrhea in a pediatric hospital. Clin Pediatr (Phila) 2003;42(4):347–352.

104. McGowan KL, Kader HA. *Clostridium difficile* infection in children. Clin Microbiol Newslett 1999;21:49–53.

105. Benson L, Song X, Campos J, Singh N. Changing epidemiology of *Clostridium difficile*-associated disease in children. Infect Control Hosp Epidemiol 2007;28(11):1233–1235.

106. Nash JQ, Chattopadhyay B, Honeycombe J, Tabaqchali S. *Clostridium difficile* and cytotoxin in routine faecal specimens. J Clin Pathol 1982;35(5):561–565.

107. Anand A, Glatt AE. *Clostridium difficile* infection associated with antineoplastic chemotherpay: a review. Clin Infect Dis 1993;17:109–113.

108. Andrews CN, Raboud J, Kassen BO, Enns R. *Clostridium difficile*-associated diarrhea: predictors of severity in patients presenting to the emergency department. Can J Gastroenterol 2003;17(6):369–373.

109. Olsen MM, Shanholtzer MT, Lee JT, Gerding DN. Ten years of prospective *Clostridium difficile*-associated disease surveillance and treatment at the minneapolis VA medical center 1982–1991. Infect Control Hosp Epidemiol 1994;15:371–381.

110. Wilcox MH. Respiratory antibiotic use and *Clostridium difficile* infection: is it the drugs or the doctors? Thorax 2000;55:633–634.

111. Settle CD, Wilcox MH, Fawley WN, Corrado OJ, Hawkey PM. Prospective study of the risk of *Clostridium difficile* diarrhoea in elderly patients following treatment with cefotaxime or piperacillin-tazobactam. Aliment Pharmacol Ther 1998;12:1217–1223.

112. Thomas C, Stevenson M, Riley TV. Antibiotics and hospital-acquired *Clostridum difficile*-associated diarrhoea: a systemic review. J Antimicrob Chemother 2003;51(6):1339–1350.

113. McFarland LV, Surawicz CM, Stamm WE. Risk factors for *Clostridium difficile* carriage and *C. difficile*-associated diarrhea in a cohort of hospitalized patients. J Infect Dis 1990;162 (3):678–684.

114. Thomas C, Riley TV. Restriction of third generation cephalosporin use reduces the incidence of *Clostridium difficile*-associated diarrhoea in hospitalised patients. Commun Dis Intell 2003;27:S28–S31.

115. Chang VT, Nelson K. The role of physical proximity in nosocomial diarrhea. Clin Infect Dis 2000;31(3):717–722.

116. Nanke Y, Kotake S, Akama H, Tomii M, Kamatani N. Pancytopenia and colitis with *Clostridium difficile* in a rheumatoid arthritis patient taking methotrexate, antibiotics and non-steroidal anti-inflammatory drugs. Clin Rheumatol 2001;20(1):73–75.

117. Periman P. Antibiotic associated Diarrhoea. Letter. N Engl J Med 2002;347:145.

118. Blot E, Escande MC, Besson D, Barbut F, Granpeix C, Asselain B, Falcou MC, Pouillart P. Outbreak of *Clostridium difficile*-related diarrhoea in an adult oncology unit: risk factors and microbiological characteristics. J Hosp Infect 2003;53:187–192.

119. Hussain A, Aptaker L, Spriggs DR, Barakat RR. Gastrointestinal toxicity and *Clostridium difficile* diarrhoea in patients treated with paclitaxel containing chemotherpay regimes. Gynecol Oncol 1998;71:104–107.

120. Bignardi GE. Risk Factors for *Clostridium difficile* infection. J Hosp Infect 1998;40:1–15.

121. Mastroianni OC, Nanetti A, Valentini R, et al. Nosocomial *Clostridium difficile* associated diarrhoea in patients with AIDS: a three-year survey and review. Clin Infect Dis 1997;25: S204–S205.

122. Mainardi JL, Lacassin F, Guilloy Y, Goldstein FW, Leport C, Acar JF, Vildé JL. Low rate of *Clostridium difficile* colonisation in ambulatory and hospitalized HIV-infected patients in a hospital unit: a prospective survey. J Infect 1998;37:108–111.
123. Anup R, Balasubramanian KA. Surgical stress and the gastrointestinal tract. J Surg Res 2000;92:291–300.
124. Issa M, Vijayapal A, Graham MB, Beaulieu DB, Otterson MF, Lundeen S, Skaros S, Weber LR, Komorowski RA, Knox JF, Emmons J, Bajaj JS, Binion DG. Impact of *Clostridium difficile* on inflammatory bowel disease. Clin Gastroenterol Hepatol 2007;5(3):345–351.
125. Freiler JF, Durning SJ, Ender PT. *Clostridium difficile* small bowel enteritis occurring after total colectomy. Clin Infect Dis 2001;33(8):1429–1431.
126. Kyne L, Sougioultzis S, McFarland LV, Kelly CP. Underlying disease severity as a major risk factor for nosocomial *Clostridium difficile* diarrhea. Infect Control Hosp Epidemiol 2002;23(11):653–659.
127. Sethi D, Wheeler JG, Cowden JM, Rodrigues LC, Sockett PN, Roberts JA, Cumberland P, Tompkins DS, Wall PG, Hudson MJ, Roderick PJ. A study of infectious intestinal disease in England: plan and methods of data collection. Commun Dis Pub Health 1999; 2:101–107.
128. Tompkins DS, Hudson MJ, Smith HR, Eglin RP, Wheeler JG, Brett MM, Owen RJ, Brazier JS, Cumberland P, King V, Cook PE. A study of infectious intestinal disease in England: microbiological findings in cases and controls. Commun Dis Pub Health 1999;2:108–113.
129. Beaugerie L, Flahault A, Barbut F, Atlan P, Lalande V, Cousin P, Cadilhac M, Petit JC; Study Group. Antibiotic-associated diarrhoea and *Clostridium difficile* in the community. Aliment Pharmacol Ther 2003;17(7):905–912.
130. Karlström O, Fryklund B, Tullus K, Burman LG. A prospective nationwide study of *Clostridium difficile*-associated diarrhoea in Sweden. Clin Infect Dis 1998;26:141–145.
131. Wistrom J, Norrby SR, Myhre E, et al. Frequency of antibiotic associated diarrhoea in 2462 antibiotic-treated hospitalized patients: a prospective study. J Antimicrob Chemother 2001; 47(1):43–50.
132. Gay TW. Hand hygiene and *Clostridium difficile*. Ann Intern Med 2007;3:69–70.
133. McFarland LV, Mulligan ME, Kwok RY, Stamm WE. Nosocomial acquisition of *Clostridium difficile* infection. N Engl J Med 1989;320(4):204–210.
134. Johnson S, Gerding DN. *Clostridium difficile*-associated diarrhoea. Clin Infect Dis 1998; 26:1027–1036.
135. Cheng SH, Lu JJ, Young TG, Perng CL, Chi WM. *Clostridium difficile* associated diseases: comparison of symptomatic infection versus carriage on the basis of risk factors toxin production and genotyping results. Clin Infect Dis 1997;25:157–158.
136. Shim JK, Johnson S, Samore MH, Bliss DZ, Gerding DN. Primary symptomless colonisation by *Clostridium difficle* and decreased risk of subsequent diarrhoea. Lancet 1998;351: 633–636.
137. Clabots CR, Johnson S, Olson MM, Peterson LR, Gerding DN. Acquisition of *Clostridium difficile* by Hospitalised patients: evidence for colonized new admissions as a source of infection. J Infect Dis 1992;166:561–567.
138. Bender BS, Bennett R, Laughon BE, Greenough WB III, Gaydos C, Sears SD, Forman MS, Bartlett JG. Is *Clostridium difficile* endemic in chronic care facilities? Lancet 1986;2:11–13.
139. Sparks SG, Carman RJ, Sarker MR, McClane BA. Genotyping of enterotoxigenic *Clostridium perfringens* fecal isolates associated with antibiotic-associated diarrhea and food poisoning in North America. J Clin Microbiol 2001;39(3):883–888.
140. Boone JH, Carman RJ. *Clostridium perfringens*: food poisoning and antibiotic-associated diarrhoea. Clin Microbiol Rev 1997;19(9):65–67.
141. Carman RJ. *Clostridia perfringens* in spontaneous and antibiotic-associated diarrhoea of man and other animals. Rev Med Microbiol 1997;8:S43–S45.
142. Borriello SP, Welch AR, Larson HE, Barclay F. Diarrhoea and simultaneous excretion of *Clostridium difficile* cytotoxin and *C. perfringens* enterotoxin. Lancet 1984;2(8413):1218.

143. Borriello SP, Williams RK. Treatment of *Clostridium perfringens* enterotoxin-associated diarrhoea with metronidazole. J Infect 1985;10(1):65–67.
144. Collee JG, Knowlden JA, Hobbs BC. Studies on the growth sporulation and carriage of *Clostridium welchii* with special reference to food poisoning strains. J Appl Bacteriol 1961;24:326.
145. Weese JS, Staempfli HR. Diarrhea associated with enterotoxigenic *Clostridium perfringens* in a red-footed tortoise (Geochelone carbonaria). J Zoo Wildl Med 2000;31(2):265–266.
146. Petit L, Gilbert M, Popoff MR. *Clostridium perfringens*: toxinotype and genotype. Trends Microbiol 1999;7(3):104–110.
147. Adams V, Lyras D, Farrow KA, Rood JI. The clostridial mobilisable transposons. Cell Mol Life Sci 2002;59(12):2033–2043.
148. Walker PD, Murrell TG, Nagy LK. Scanning electronmicroscopy of the jejunum in enteritis necroticans. J Med Microbiol 1980;13(3):445–450.
149. Cheng Q, Hwa V, Salyers A. A locus that contributes to colonization of the intestinal trqact by *Bacteroides thetaiotaomicron* contains a single regulatory gene (chuR) that links two polysaccharide utilization pathways. J Bacteriol 1992;174:7185–7193.
150. O'Brien DK, Melville SB. Multiple effects on *Clostridium perfringens* binding uptake and trafficking to lysosomes by inhibitors of macrophage phagocytosis receptors. Microbiology 2003;149(6):1377–1386.
151. Hatheway CL. Toxigenic clostridia. Clin Mirobiol Rev 1990;3:66–98.
152. Awad MM, Ellemor DM, Bryant AE, Matsushita O, Boyd RL, Stevens DL, Emmins JJ, Rood JI. Construction and virulence testing of a collagenase mutant of *Clostridium perfringens*. Microb Pathog 2000;28(2):107–117.
153. Alape-Giron A, Flores-Diaz M, Guillouard I, et al. Identification of residues critical for toxicity in *Clostridium perfringens* phospholipase C the key toxin in gas gangrene. Eur J Biochem 2000;267:5191–5197.
154. Mollby R, Holme T. Production of phospholipase C (alpha-toxin) haemolysins and lethal toxins by *Clostridium perfringens* types A to D. J Gen Microbiol 1976;96(1):137–144.
155. Rood JI. Virulence genes of *Clostridium perfringens*. Ann Rev Microbiol 1998;52:333–360.
156. Songer JG. Clostridial enteric diseases of domestic animals. Clin Microbiol Rev 1996;9:216–234.
157. Bullifent HL, Moir A, Awad MM, Scott PT, Rood JI, Titball RW. The level of expression of -toxin by different strains of *Clostridium perfringens* is dependent on differences in promoter structure and genetic background. Anaerobe 1996;2:365–371.
158. Ginter A, Williamson ED, Dessy F, Coppe P, Bullifent H, Howells A, Titball RW. Molecular variation between the alpha-toxins from the type strain (NCTC 8237) and clinical isolates of *Clostrium perfringens* associated with disease in man and animals. Microbiology 1996;142:191–198.
159. Lindsay JA. *Clostridium perfringnes* type A enterotoxin (CPE): more than just explosive diarrhoea. Crit Rev Microbiol 1996;22(44):257–277.
160. Hardy SP, Rirchie C, Allen MC, Ashley RH, Granum PE. *Clostridium perfringens* type A enterotoxin forms mepacrine-sensitive pores in pure phospholipid bilayers in the absence of putatibe receptor proteins. Biochm Biophys Acta 2001;1515:38–43.
161. Sarker MR, Shivers RP, Sparks SG, Juneja VK, McClane BA. Comparative experiments to examine the effects of heating on vegetative cells and spores of *Clostridium perfringens* isolates carrying plasmid genes versus chromosomal enterotoxin genes. Appl Environ Microbiol 2000;66(8):3234–3240.
162. Heredia NL, Labbe RG, Rodriguez MA, Garcia-Alvarado JS. Growth sporulation and enterotoxin production by *Clostridium perfringenes* type A in the presence of human bile salts. FEMS Microbiol Lett 1991;68:15–21.
163. Ohtani K, Kawsar HI, Okumura K, Hayashi H, Shimizu T. The VirR/VirS regulatory cascade affects transcription of plasmid-encoded putative virulence genes in *Clostridium perfringens* strain 13. FEMS Microbiol Lett 2003;222:137–141.

164. Brynestad S, Sarker MR, McClane BA, Granum PE, Rood JI. Enterotoxin plasmid from *Clostridium perfringens* is conjugative. Infect Immun 2001;69(5): 3483–3487.
165. Miyamoto K, Chakrabarti G, Morino Y, McClane BA. Organisation of the plasmid CPE locus in *Clostridium perfringens* type A isolates. Infect Immun 2003;71(3):1611.
166. McClane BA. New insights into the genetics and regulation of expression of *Clostridium perfringens* enterotoxin. Curr Top Microbiol Immunol 1998;225:37–55.
167. Katahira J, Sugiyama H, Inoue N, Horiguchi Y, Matsuda M, Sugimoto N. *Clostridium perfringnes* enterotoxin utilizes two structurally related membrane proteins as functional receptors *in vivo*. J Biol Chem 1997;272(42):26652–26658.
168. Long H, Crean CD, Lee WH, Cummings OW, Gabig TG. Expression of *Clostridium perfringens* enterotoxin receptors 3 and claudin-4 in prostate cancer epithelium. Cancer Res 2001;61(21):7878–7881.
169. Chakrabarti G, Xin Z, McClane BA. Death pathways activated in CaCo-2 cells by *Clostridium perfringens* enterotoxin. Infect Immun 2003;71:4260–4270.
170. Allen SD, Siders JA, Marler LM. Current issues and problems in dealing with anaerobes in the clinical laboratory. Clin Lab Med 1995;15(2):333–364.
171. Samuel SC, Hancock P, Leigh DA. An investigation into *Clostridium perfringens* enterotoxin-associated diarrhoea. J Hosp Infect 1991;18(3):219–230.
172. Hancock P. Antibiotic-associated diarrhoea: *Clostridium difficile* or *C. perfringens*? Rev Med Microbiol 1997;8:S66–S67.
173. Abrahao C, Carman RJ, Hahn H, Liesenfeld O. Similar frequency of detection of *Clostridium perfringens* enterotoxin and *Clostridium difficile* toxins in patients with antibiotic-associated diarrhea. Eur J Clin Microbiol Infect Dis 2001;20(9):676–677.
174. Asha NJ, Wilcox MH. Laboratory diagnosis of *Clostridium perfringens* antibiotic-associated diarrhoea. J Med Microbiol 2002;51(10):891–894.
175. Carney T, Perry JD, Ford M, Majumdar S, Gould FK. Evidence for antibiotic induced *Clostridium perfringens* diarrhoea. J Clin Pathol 2002;55(3):240.
176. Langhendries JP. Early bacterial colonisation of the intestine: why it matters? Arch Pediatr 2006;13(12):1526–1534.
177. Thompson-Chagoyan OC, Maldonado J, Gil A. Colonization and impact of disease and other factors on intestinal microbiota. Dig Dis Sci 2007;52(9):2069–2077.
178. Todd B. *Clostridium difficile*: familiar pathogen, changing epidemiology: a virulent strain has been appearing more often, even in patients not taking antibiotics. Am J Nurs 2006;106(5):33–36.
179. Flemming K, Ackermann G. Prevalence of enterotoxin producing *Staphylococcus aureus* in stools of patients with nosocomial diarrhea. Infection 2007;35:356–358.
180. Vaishnavi C, Kaur S. Is campylobacter involved in antibiotic associated diarrhoea? Indian J Pathol Microbiol 2005;48(4):526–529.
181. Hall J, Horsley M. Diagnosis and management of patients with *Clostridium difficile*-associated diarrhoea. Nurs Stand 2007;21(46):49–56; quiz 58.
182. Koh TH, Tan AL, Tan ML, Wang G, Song KP. Epidemiology of *Clostridium difficile* infection in a large teaching hospital in Singapore. Pathology 2007;39(4):438–442.
183. Crogan NL, Evans BC. *Clostridium difficile*: an emerging epidemic in nursing homes. Geriatr Nurs 2007;28(3):161–164.
184. Ricciardi R, Rothenberger DA, Madoff RD, Baxter NN. Increasing prevalence and severity of *Clostridium difficile* colitis in hospitalized patients in the United States. Arch Surg 2007;142(7):624–631; discussion 631.
185. Makris AT, Gelone S. *Clostridium difficile* in the long-term care setting. J Am Med Dir Assoc 2007;8(5):290–299.
186. Schroder O, Gerhard R, Stein J. Antibiotic-associated diarrhea. Z Gastroenterol 2006;44(2):193–204.

187. Samore MH, Vekataraman L, DeGirolami PC, Arbeit RD, Karchmer AW. Clinical and molecular epidemiology of sporadic and clustered cases of nosocomial *Clostridium difficile*. Am J Med 1996;100:32–40.
188. Loo VG, Poirier L, Miller MA, Oughton M, Libman MD, Michaud S, Bourgault AM, Nguyen T, Frenette C, Kelly M, Vibien A, Brassard P, Fenn S, Dewar K, Hudson TJ, Horn R, René P, Monczak Y, Dascal A. A predominantly clonal multi-institutional outbreak of *Clostridium difficile*-associated diarrhea with high morbidity and mortality. N Eng J Med 2005;353:2442–2449.
189. McDonald LC, Killgore GE, Thompson A, Owens RC Jr., Kazakova SV, Sambol SP, Johnson S, Gerding DN. An epidemic, toxin gene-variant strain of *Clostridium difficile*. N Engl J Med 2005;353:2433–2441.
190. Muto CA, Pokrywka M, Shutt K, Mendelsohn AB, Nouri K, Posey K, Roberts T, Croyle K, Krystofiak S, Patel-Brown S, Pasculle AW, Paterson DL, Saul M, Harrison LH. A large outbreak of *Clostridium difficile*-associated disease with an unexpected proportion of death and colectomies at a teaching hospital following increased fluoroquinolone use. Infect Control Hosp Epidemiol 2005;26:273–280.

Chapter 11
The Significance of *Helicobacter Pylori* Acquisition and the Hygiene Hypothesis

Steven L. Percival

Introduction

Helicobacter pylori is a micro-aerophilic, spiral-shaped bacterium that efficiently colonizes the human stomach mucosa of both the young and the elderly.[1] Warren was the first to successfully observe *H. pylori* from gastric biopsies in 1982.[2] However, as early as 1893, spiralic bacteria were described in the stomachs of autopsied rabbits, and the bacterium was first described in humans in 1906.[3] When *H. pylori* was first isolated, it was described as Campylobacter-like and was subsequently named as *Campylobacter pyloridis* which was later changed to the more grammatically correct *C. pylori*.[1] However, further studies showed that the organism differed sufficiently from true Campylobacters, justifying the need for the new genus Helicobacter. The name *Helicobacter pylori* is Latin for "spiral rod of the lower part of the stomach" and causes inflammation in the form of chronic active gastritis. It has been linked with a diverse spectrum of gastrointestinal disorders including peptic ulcer disease, gastric adenocarcinoma, and gastric mucosa-associated lymphoid tissue (MALT) lymphoma.[4] Although only a very small minority (1–2%) of infected individuals will develop a malignant disease, the public health relevance of this infection is high, with the World Health Organization International Agency for Research on Cancer classifying *H. pylori* as a class I carcinogen in humans.[5]

Humans are currently the only known reservoir for *H. pylori*, although a number of different animals have been shown to be easily infected with the bacteria. Its route (s) of transmission remains undefined but current thinking supports a direct person-to-person transmission by faecal–oral or oral–oral,[6] with increasing evidence suggesting that contaminated water is a potential route of transmission.[5] The faecal–oral route of transmission is thought to come indirectly from contaminated water or

S.L. Percival
West Virginia University Schools of Medicine and Dentistry Robert C, Byrd Health Sciences Center-North, Morgantown, WV, USA

S.L. Percival (ed.), *Microbiology and Aging.*
DOI: 10.1007/978-1-59745-327-1_11, © Springer Science + Business Media, LLC 2009

food. Positive cultures have also been obtained during air sampling after subjects infected with the bacteria have been induced to vomit. Although it is estimated that approximately 50% of the world's population is infected with *H. pylori*, prevalence varies widely by age as well as country, ethnic background, and socio-economic conditions.[7] The developing world carries the greatest burden, with over 70% of the children infected with *H. pylori* by age 15. In contrast, the developed world has, since the 1950s, experienced a decrease in prevalence with each successive generation, so that at present around only 20–30% of individuals harbour *H. pylori*.[3] This reduction has been attributed to improved socio-economic status, modernization, and personal hygiene but may equally have come about because of improvements in drinking water quality. Recently, population-based studies in Italy, the US, and Denmark have indicated that *H. pylori* infection in children can reduce the incidence of allergy and asthma manifestations forming an argument for the hygiene hypothesis theory. The hygiene hypothesis of asthma and atopy has been extensively studied, with the theory suggesting that naturally occurring infections and microbial exposure during childhood is necessary for the normal maturation of the immune response to achieve a balance between T-helper type 1 (protective immunity) and T-helper type 2 (allergic diseases) cytokine responses and thereby reduce the future risk of developing atopy.[8] If the hygiene hypothesis is correct, the reduction in childhood infections and subsequent immunotherapy in the past three decades may account for the rise in asthma and atopy rates associated with urbanization and Western lifestyle.[9]

Medical Significance

In contrast to infection with other mucosal pathogens, only a small percentage of individuals carrying *H. pylori* ever develop clinical sequelae; most people infected with *H. pylori* are asymptomatic.[10] If left untreated, *H. pylori* infection is lifelong.[7] *H. pylori* induce gastric inflammation in virtually all hosts, and although clinical disease typically occurs decades after initial infection acquisition, gastritis may progress over time from an initially superficial nonatrophic form to more severe atrophic gastritis with intestinal metaplasia leading to duodenal ulceration, gastric adenocarcinoma, and gastric MALT lymphoma.[4]

Gastric carcinogenesis is a multi-factorial process in which chronic inflammation plays a major role. *H. pylori* infection induces physiological changes and DNA adducts formation in the gastric microenvironment. Subsequent reduction in antioxidant levels increases the risk of carcinogenesis and damage to DNA from intragastric release of free radicals. Ingestion of dietary carcinogens, deficiencies in dietary antioxidants, smoking, and anti-secretory medications are also thought to be important co-factors in *H. pylori*-related cancer.[11] Development of atropy and metaplasia of the gastric mucosa is strongly associated with *H. pylori* infection, and despite a sharp worldwide decline in both the incidence and mortality of gastric cancer, the condition remains the world's second leading cause of cancer mortality behind lung cancer.[11] It has been estimated that there were more than 870,000 deaths from the disease in the year 2000, accounting for approximately 12% of all cancer deaths.[11] *H. pylori* has also been linked to other several diseases such as coronary heart disease[12] and sudden infant death syndrome.[13]

Pathogenicity/Virulence

As *H. pylori* infects approximately 50% of the world's population, the bacterium must have evolved highly effective mechanisms to enable efficient colonization and persistence for long periods in the gastric epithelium. After being ingested, the bacteria must evade the bactericidal activity of gastric luminal contents and then enter the mucous layer.[1] Also, both its spiral shape and high motility allow the bacterium to resist peristaltic flushing.[14] Urease production and motility are essential for the first step of infection. By breaking down urea present in the gastric juice and extracellular fluid, the bacterium is able to generate bicarbonate and ammonia in its pericellular environment so that hydrogen ions are effectively neutralized before damaging the cell. Essentially the *H. pylori* generates a neutral microenvironment that surrounds the bacterium. *H. pylori* is thereby able to survive in the gastric acid layer enough for it to colonize the gastric mucosa and induce gastritis with resistant neutrophil infiltration; *H. pylori* is particularly resistant to the oxidative inflammatory response of neutrophils, which can in turn damage the host gastric mucosa.[15]

Once attached to the gastric mucosa, *H. pylori* can damage host tissue by causing vacuolation in gastric epithelial cells. This vacuolation is caused by the production of a cytotoxin known as *vacuolating cytotoxin A* (*vac*A), a protein which is endocytosed by epithelial cells where it causes endosome–lysosome fusion.[16] Besides the diverse functions on epithelial cells (i.e. cellular vacuolation induction of apoptosis, loosening of cellular junctions, and the formation of urea channels), *vac*A also has immunomodulatory activity. It inhibits the processing of antigenic peptides in B cells and their presentation to human CD4+ T cells.[4] Recently *vac*A was also reported to alter T-cell function by inhibiting T-cell proliferation, suggesting a possible mechanism of how *H. pylori* might evade the adaptive immune response to establish a chronic infection.[17]

Approximately 60–70% of *H. pylori* strains in the industrialized world posses the cytotoxin-associated antigen (*cag*A) a 120–145-kDa protein localized at one end of the cag pathogenicity island a genomic fragment containing 31 putative genes.[4] Several of these genes encode components of a type IV secretion system that translocates *cag*A protein in the host cell.[11] After entering an epithelial cell, *cag*A is phosphorylated and binds to SHP-2 tyrosine phosphatase, leading to a cellular response and cytokine production by the host cell. The degradation of SHP-2 by *cag*A is an important mechanism by which *cag*A promotes gastric epithelial carcinogenesis by inducing DNA damage.[17] *Cag*A may also diminish anti-*H. pylori* immune response and play a role in the development of MALT lymphoma by impairing p53-dependent apoptosis.[4] The presence of *cag*A is generally always associated with increased inflammation and generally more severe infections.

A number of studies have indicated that genetic factors play a role in the clinical outcome of *H. pylori* infection. *H. pylori* inflammatory response induces a cascade of proinflammatory cytokines (i.e. IL-10, IFN, TNF, IL-β) and it has been proposed that cytokine imbalance is responsible for disease progression and dictates the disease outcome after *H. pylori* infection. Single nucleotide polymorphisms may affect overall cytokine production, and it has been suggested that variant cytokine alleles may contribute to individual differences in proinflammatory responses and account for heterogeneous outcomes following a *H. pylori* infection. Such a correlation has been reported in gastric carcinoma in which IL-β polymorphisms confer a twofold increase in risk for gastric adenocarcinoma after *H. pylori* infection.[4]

Transmission and Epidemiology of *H. Pylori*

The source of *H. pylori* is principally the human stomach; however, as mentioned previously, many animals have been shown to be easily infected with *H. pylori*. There have also been suggestions of a zoonotic transmission.[18] It is not really known whether *H. pylori* infections are acquired at home or in the community. In developing countries the patterns of *H. pylori* transmission suggest a common source of exposure rather than person-to-person spread,[19] and several community and environmental studies are consistent with water playing a role in transmission.[20–24] Viable *H. pylori* cells are possibly disseminated through faecal material[25] which may well provide a route for contaminating drinking water. Studies have shown that *H. pylori* may survive for prolonged periods in water over a range of physical variables.[26] However, *H. pylori* cells are readily inactivated by chlorine, suggesting that the organism would be controlled by disinfection regimes normally employed in the treatment of drinking water.[27] The absence of a proven analytical method or standard protocol for assessing cell viability has resulted in the publication of a variety of methods and survival times for *H. pylori* in the aquatic environment. Although evidence has been published that viable but non-culturable (VBNC) *H. pylori* cells are still alive,[20, 28, 29] no evidence has been published either on resuscitation of these cells or on their ability to cause infection.

In Chile, *H. pylori* prevalence rates correlated with socio-economic status, age, and the consumption of uncooked vegetables.[30] Although *H. pylori* was suggested to have been spread by a number of transmission routes, contamination of irrigation water by human faecal material and the subsequent contamination of vegetables (which were eaten raw) were suggested as a major risk factor for the acquisition of *H. pylori*.[30] This interpretation has been questioned, as the concentration of *H. pylori* cells present in faecal material is low compared to other faecal pathogens.[31] Furthermore, the prevalence of *H. pylori* IgG antibodies in sewage workers in Sweden compared to a control group matched for age and socio-economic status demonstrated no increased risk of infection as a result of an exposure to human faecal material.[32]

In Bangladeshi children, no significant correlation was found between quality of drinking water and *H. pylori* infection rates. Household crowding and behavioural differences between Hindu and Muslim families were suggested as the most significant risk factors for acquisition of *H. pylori*.[33] In Peru, *H. pylori* DNA was amplified by polymerase chain reaction (PCR) in 24 out of 48 samples tested, suggesting that waterborne transmission was an important risk factor.[23] A further study by Hulten et al.[34] used two PCR assays to examine municipal treated and well-water samples from all 25 counties of Sweden for the presence of Helicobacter DNA: 9 out of 24 wells, 3 out of 25 municipal sources, and 3 out of 25 wastewater samples were found to be positive for Helicobacter DNA. It is possible that the positive data were the result of other Helicobacter species and not specifically *H. pylori*. The use of PCR and other molecular methods for the detection of pathogens in environmental samples has limitations chiefly in the inability of these techniques to differentiate between naked DNA and dead and living cells. Furthermore, the natural environment contains many microorganisms that are not yet identified or cultured, and therefore there is a risk that positive results from PCR studies may be due to unknown organisms.

In Peruvian children from Lima, *H. pylori* prevalence (as determined by the ^{13}C-urea breath test) was found to have a high correlation with socio-economic status – children whose homes had external water sources were found to be three times more likely to be infected by *H. pylori* than those with internal water sources. No difference was found when those children from high- and low-income families with an internal water source were compared.[24] Children of high-income families supplied with municipal water were 12 times more likely to become colonized with *H. pylori* than those supplied from community wells, suggesting that municipal water was a strong risk factor in the acquisition of *H. pylori*; the unexpected finding was thought to be due to breaks in the municipal pipes allowing for surface contamination of water.[35] A report from Bolivia also indicated that contaminated water is a common source of infection with *H. pylori*. Children living in families using special water containers that prevented hands or objects from coming into direct contact with the family drinking water were significantly less likely to be infected with *H. pylori* than children whose family did not use the special water container. This suggests that hands contaminated with *H. pylori* rather than a contaminated water delivery system transfer the bacteria to the drinking water.[35] More recently, in rural China *H. pylori* DNA has been amplified from drinking water samples and its identity verified by sequence analysis.[36] In addition, a study in Leipzig, Germany, showed a positive correlation with the drinking of *H. pylori*-contaminated well water and the acquisition of a *H. pylori* infection.[20]

Evidence has been also been published suggesting the presence of *H. pylori* in both surface and ground waters in the US. The presence of *H. pylori* in both surface and ground waters showed a significant correlation with total coliforms but not with *E. coli*. In a small number of samples ($n = 7$), clinical data with respect to *H. pylori* prevalence was obtained demonstrating a significant correlation between *H. pylori* infection and presence of the bacterium in drinking water sources.[37]

An individual's age may also influence the route of transmission of *H. pylori*. In one study the key risk factor for acquisition of *H. pylori* in childhood was the water source compared to socio-economic status and education level in adults.[38] A study undertaken by MacKay et al.[39] of 65 infants in the rural village of Keneba found that the use of supplemental water was a strong risk factor for *H. pylori* colonization in these infants (OR 4.71; 95%CI 1.17–22.5). *H. pylori* DNA was also isolated from biofilms within water storage pots, suggesting that drinking water played an important role in the transmission of *H. pylori* in that community.[39]

Age and Acquisition of *H. Pylori*

H. pylori infection is acquired during childhood and *H. pylori* seroprevalence increases with age. Age has therefore been identified as a risk factor for infection.[40, 41] The child is the most venerable to infection from *H. pylori*,[12, 42] with infections in children documented at 10–80% worldwide. The conditions induced by *H. pylori* are more problematic in adults when compared to children; however, a large number of individuals are asymptomatic.

The prevalence of *H. pylori* varies in developing countries when compared to industrialized countries – the incidence of *H. pylori* infection is lower in developed countries when compared to developing countries. In most developed countries, between 10% and 20% of adults below the age of 30 are infected with *H. pylori*.[43] In Vietnam, for example, *H. pylori* was found on average in 34.5% of children sampled[44]; however, these levels did vary on location, as levels of *H. pylori* infection in urban areas were found to be 64% when compared to levels of 41.2% in rural areas.[45] In the Andes, a prevalence of *H. pylori* of 69% in 2–9 year olds has been documented.[18] The prevalence of *H. pylori* in young children in Netherlands is low[46] compared to Brazil.[47]

Research has shown that by the age of 10, over 50% of children worldwide are infected with *H. pylori* and acquisition has been shown to occur within the first 2 years of life,[48] with newly acquired *H. pylori* infections occurring before the age of 10.[49] However, the risk of infection with *H. pylori* decreases rapidly after the age of 5.[50] Levels of *H. pylori* infection in children living in Gambia have been found to be at a level of 19% at the age of 3 months. At the age of 30 months, this had been found to have increased to 85%.[51] Studies from the US have also shown age-specific differences in the prevalence of *H. pylori* infection in children, with black and hispanic children found to have the highest acquisition.[52, 53]

Despite mounting evidence, the age group at greatest risk from *H. pylori* is presently unknown and varied. In the early 1990s, a number of studies showed that the incidence of *H. pylori* in children was low. However, as mentioned previously, with more recent studies it has been suggested that the incidence of *H. pylori* infection in children is between 1.7 and 15%.[54] Further studies have shown that children who are of school age have a low risk of *H. pylori* infection and re-infection.[55] An increase in prevalence of *H. pylori* reflects a birth cohort effect rather than an increased rate of infection with age.

H. pylori seroconversion has been associated with the slowing weight gains in children aged 2 years or older,[56] suggesting *H. pylori* is capable of affecting growth in children.[57] Seroprevalence of *H. pylori* is found to be high in elderly people. In one study it was found that seroprevalence of *H. pylori* infection was between 82 and 86% in asymptomatic individuals.[58]

The Hygiene Hypothesis Theory

Atopy has been increasing in prevalence in the industrialized world for at least two decades, but the same increase has not been noted in the developing world.[59] Atopy characterized by the raised immunoglobulin (Ig) E levels underlies allergic diseases such as asthma, rhinoconjunctivitis, and eczema. The interaction of an environmental allergen with the innate immune system, its uptake by antigen-presenting cells, and the subsequent T-cell priming leads to the stimulation of cytokines such as interleukin (IL)-4, IL-5, and IL-13. These cytokines interact with their receptors to stimulate IgE production and increased numbers of eosinophils and mast cells; all these components are capable of precipitating inflammation in the respiratory tract.[60] Currently more than 130 million people suffer from asthma and the numbers are increasing.[60] Clear differences in the prevalence of allergies between rural and urban areas within one country are also evident: for example, in Ethiopia asthma is more prevalent in urban than in rural areas.[9]

Evidence suggests that exposure to food and orofaecal pathogens such as hepatitis A, *Toxoplasma gondii*, and *H. pylori* reduces the risk of atopy by >60%.[8] Such infections give rise to an increase in T helper 1 (Th1) cell production, which diverts the immune system away from T helper 2 (T2) cell production, and therefore reduces the prevalence of Th2 atopic diseases.[59] Furthermore, studies of gut commensals indicate differences in the rate of microbial colonization as well as the bacterial type involved in children with and without a pre-deposition to allergy.[60] On the basis of such data it has been postulated that the lack of intense infections in industrialized countries owing to improved hygiene vaccination and use of antibiotics may alter the immune system such that it responds inappropriately to innocuous substances.[61] The resulting hypothesis suggests that limited exposure to bacterial and viral pathogens during early childhood leads to an inefficient stimulation of Th1 cells, which in turn cannot counterbalance the expansion of Th2 cells and result in a predisposition to allergy.[60] Elsewhere it has been suggested that *H. pylori* infection may also be associated with increased production of IL-10, which possesses anti-allergic properties and has been shown to suppress lipopolysaccharide-activated eosinophils in allergic disease models.[62] However, the observation that parasites associated with a Th2 dominated immune response, e.g. hook worms, are also associated with a reduced prevalence of atopic diseases contradicts the hygiene hypothesis.[63] A common feature of worm infection *T. gondii* and *H. pylori* is their ability to produce a chronic persistent infection. This suggests that persistent exposure of gut commensal organisms is needed to stimulate the production of IL-10 and TGF-β, which are required for the maturity of inducible regulatory T cells needed to prevent the development of highly polarized T helper cells; failure of regulatory T-cell function has been linked to the development of allergic diseases.[64] Since it has been suggested that a *H. pylori* infection is likely to occur during the first 5 years of life, the bacterium may have a particularly marked effect on the developing immune system.[62]

Other predictors inversely related to atopic diseases are factors related to exposure to farm animals. Several studies have shown a protective effect of being raised on a farm or exposure to animal stables during childhood and of being a farmer on the prevalence of asthma and nasal allergies.[63] Additionally, consumption of unpasteurized milk is inversely related to atopic diseases.[64]

Conclusion

Current knowledge implies that acquisition of H. pylori seems to occur predominately in childhood and that once acquired, the infection persists lifelong in most infected individuals resulting in more infections manifesting in the adult population. Although still inconclusive, epidemiological studies strongly suggest person-to-person transmission, but recent experimental and epidemiological evidence suggests that H. pylori transmission may involve the consumption of contaminated drinking water. Although H. pylori is not classified as a food- or waterborne pathogen, it is recognized as an important pathogen. In the case of H. pylori its ability to survive in a coccoid VBNC form and its correlation with water and raw vegetables irrigated with such water represent a concern to epidemiologists and the like. In fact, it could be argued that survival of bacteria under a VBNC form allows for a hidden contamination from the environment.

The decline of orofecal infections and changes in the overall pattern of commensals and pathogens that stimulate the immune system may be strong determinants of the epidemic of allergic diseases observed in westernized societies. This has been as a consequence of improved sanitation and better hygiene practices and living conditions resulting in decreased risk of H. pylori acquisition in childhood.[3] However, recently H. pylori has been inversely associated with atopy and allergic manifestations data, which is consistent with the hygiene hypothesis theory. This suggests that H. pylori provides a stimulus essential for the adequate stimulation of the immune system to avoid allergic diseases. It has been postulated that H. pylori can direct the immune system toward a Th1 response that counterbalances proallergic responses of Th2 cells which are associated with allergic reactions.[60] Since epidemiological evidence suggests that exposure to H. pylori-contaminated drinking water is more common in developing countries, it could be argued that H. pylori may confer a protective effect and may account for the reduced prevalence of allergic diseases in developing countries. Several studies support this suggestion. In Russian Karelia where atopy and atopic diseases are uncommon, surface water bodies, lakes, and rivers are used as domestic water frequently without any chemical or other treatment.[64] Therefore, total elimination of H. pylori from the human host may not be favourable, as these data imply that carriage of H. pylori may have a beneficial effect. However, despite this, H. pylori infection in early childhood is postulated to induce a low-grade inflammatory condition which over time can develop into pre-malignant changes and eventually gastric carcinoma.[35] This is supported by the statistics that show that gastric carcinoma is more common in the developing world. Consequently, *H. pylori* remains a significant problem in the developing world and its importance is unlikely to diminish in the foreseeable future. It is imperative that we acquire a better understanding of the risk factors for acquiring the infection, yet at the same time should not overlook the potential for the bacterium to be transmitted via a waterborne pathway.[65,66] Acquisition in childhood of *H. pylori* has significance later on in life; however, the virulence of the bacterium and its role in the hygiene hypothesis are as yet inconclusive.

References

1. Owen RJ. Bacteriology of *Helicobacter pylori*. Bailliere's Clinical Gastroenterology 1995;9 (3):415–445.
2. Warren JR. Unidentified curved bacilli on gastric epithelium in active chronic gastritis. Lancet 1983;1:273.
3. Rothenbacher D, Brenner H. Burden of *Helicobacter pylori* and *H. pylori*–related diseases in developed countries: recent development and future implications. Microbes and Infection 2003;5:693–703.
4. Farinha P, Gascoyne RD. *Helicobacter pylori* and MALT Lymphoma. Gastroenterology 2005;128:1579–1605.
5. Sherman PM. Appropriate strategies for testing and treating *Helicobacter pylori* in children: when and how? The American Journal of Medicine 2004;117:30S–35S.
6. Park SR, Mackay WG, Reid DC. *Helicobacter sp* recovered from drinking water biofilm sampled from a water distribution system. Water Research 2001; 35:1624–1626.
7. Czinn SJ. *Helicobacter pylori* infection: detection investigation and management. The Journal of Pediatrics 2005;146:S21–S26.
8. McCune A, Lane A, Murray L, Harvey I, et al. Reduced risk of atopic disorders in adults with *Helicobacter pylori* infection. European Journal of Gastroenterology and Hepatology 2003;15:637–640.
9. Matricardi PM, Bonini S. High microbial turnover rate preventing atopy: a solution to inconsistencies impinging on the hygiene hypothesis? Clinical and Experimental Allergy 2000;30:1506–1510.
10. Peterson AM, Krogfelt KA. *Helicobacter pylori*: an invading micro-organism? A Review. FEMS Immunology and Medical Microbiology 2003;36:117–126.
11. Kelly JR, Duggan JM. Gastric cancer epidemiology and risk factors. Journal of Clinical Epidemiology 2003;56:1–9.
12. Kerr JR, Al-Khattaf A, Barson AJ, Burnie JP. An association between sudden infant death syndrome (SIDS) and *Helicobacter pylori* infection. Achieves of Disease in Children 2000;83 (5):429–434.
13. Go MF. Review article: natural history and epidemiology of *Helicobacter pylori* infection. Alimentary Pharmacology and Therapeutics 2002;16(1):3–15.
14. Velazquez M, Feirtag JM. *Helicobacter pylori*: characteristics pathogenicity detection methods and mode of transmission implicating foods and water. International Journal of Food Microbiology 1999;53:95–104.
15. Naito Y, Yoshikawa T. Molecular and cellular mechanisms involved in *Helicobacter pylori*-induced inflammation and oxidative stress. Free Radical Biology and Medicine 2002; 33:323–336.
16. Petersen AM, Krogfelt KA. *Helicobacter pylori*: an invading microorganism? A review. FEMS Immunology and Medical Microbiology 2003;36(3):117–126.

17. Rieder G, Fischer W, Haas R. Interaction of *Helicobacter pylori* with host cells: function of secreted and translocated molecules. Current Opinion in Microbiology 2005;8:67–73.
18. Goodman KJ, Correa P, Tenganá Aux HJ, Ramírez H, DeLany JP, Guerrero Pepinosa O, López Quiñones M, Collazos Parra T. *Helicobacter pylori* infection in the Colombian Andes: a population-based study of transmission pathways. American Journal of Epidemiology 1996;144(3):290–299.
19. Akcam Y, Ersan S, Alper M, Bicik Z, Aytug N. The transmission of *Helicobacter pylori* via exposure to common sources outweighs the person-to-person contact among spouses in developing countries. American Journal of Gastroenterology 2000;95:317–319.
20. Rolle-Kampczyk UE, Fritz GJ, Diez U, Lehmann I, et al. Well water – one source of *Helicobacter pylori* colonisation. International Journal of Hygiene and Environmental Health 2004;207:363–368.
21. Engstrand L. Helicobacter in water and waterborne routes of transmission. Journal of Applied Microbiology 2001;90:80S–84S.
22. Mackay WG, Gribbon LT, Barer MR, Reid DC. Biofilms in drinking water systems – a possible reservoir for *Helicobacter pylori*. Water Science and Technology 1998;38:181–185.
23. Hulten K, Han SW, Enroth H, Klein PD, Opekun AR, et al. *Helicobacter pylori* in the drinking water in Peru. Gastroenterology 1996;110:1031–1035.
24. Klein PD, Graham DY, Gaillour A, Opekun AR, Smith EO. Water source as a risk factor for *Helicobacter pylori* in Peruvian children. The Lancet 1991;337:1503–1506.
25. Thomas JE, Gibson BR, Darboe MK, Dale A, Weaver LT. *Helicobacter pylori* from human faeces. The Lancet 1992;340:1194–1195.
26. West AP, Millar MR, Tompkins DS. Effect of physical environment on survival of *Helicobacter pylori*. Journal of Clinical Pathology 1992;45:228–231.
27. Johnson CH, Rice EW, Reasoner DJ. Inactivation of *Helicobacter pylori* by chlorine. Applied and Environmental Microbiology 1997;63:4969–4970.
28. Rowan NJ. Viable but non-culturable forms of food and waterborne bacteria: Quo Vadis?. Trends in Food Science and Technology 2004;15:462–467.
29. Moreno Y, Ferrus MA, Alonso JL, Jimenez A, Herandez J. Use of fluorescent in situ hybridization to evidence the presence of *Helicobacter pylori* in water. Water Research 2003;37:2251–2256.
30. Hopkins RJ, Vial PA, Ferreccio C, Ovalle J, et al. Seroprevalence of *Helicobacter pylori* in Chile – vegetables serve as one route of transmission. Journal of Infectious Diseases 1993; 168:222–226.
31. Vincent P. Transmission and acquisition of *Helicobacter pylori* infection: evidences and hypothesis. Biomedicine and Pharmacotherapy 1995;49:11–18.
32. Friis L, Engstrand L, Edling C. Prevalence of *Helicobacter pylori* infection among sewage workers. Scandinavian Journal of Work and Environmental Health 1996;22:364–365.
33. Clemens J, Albert MJ, Rao M, Huda S, et al. Sociodemographic hygienic and nutritional correlates of *Helicobacter pylori* infection of young Bangladeshi children. Paediatric Infectious Disease Journal 1996;15:1113–1118.
34. Hulten K, Enroth H, Nyström T, Engstrand L. Presence of *Helicobacter* species DNA in Swedish well water. Journal of Applied Microbiology 1998;85:282–286
35. Frenck RW Jr, Clemens J. Helicobacter in the developing world. Microbes and Infection 2003;5(8):705–713.
36. Sazaki K, Tajiri Y, Sata M, Fujii Y, et al. *Helicobacter pylori* in the natural environment. Scandinavian Journal of Infectious Disease 2001;31:275–279.
37. Hegarty JP, Dowd MT, Baker KH. Occurrence of *Helicobacter pylori* in surface water in the United States. Journal of Applied Microbiology 1999;87:697–701.
38. Olmos JA, Rios H, Higa R. Prevalence of *Helicobacter pylori* infection in Argentina – results of a nationwide epidemiological study. Journal of Clinical Gastroenterology 2000; 31:33–37.

39. Mackay WG, Bunn JEG, Thomas JE, Reid DC, Weaver LT. Molecular evidence of *Helicobacter pylori* in biofilms of containers used for storing water. Archives of Disease in Childhood 2001;84(SS):A24–A27.

40. Braga AB, Fialho AM, Rodrigues MN, Queiroz DM, Rocha AM, Braga LL. *Helicobacter pylori* colonization among children up to 6 years: results of a community-based study from Northeastern Brazil. Journal of Tropical Pediatrics 2007;53(6):393–397.

41. Rodrigues MN, Queiroz DM, Rodrigues RT, Rocha AM, Braga Neto MB, Braga LL. *Helicobacter pylori* infection in adults from a poor urban community in northeastern Brazil: demographic, lifestyle and environmental factors. Brazilian Journal of Infectious Diseases 2005;9(5):405–410.

42. Tytgat GNJ, Lee A, Graham DY, Dixon MF, Rokkas T. The role of infectious agents in peptic ulcer disease. Gastroenterology International 1993;6:76–89.

43. Pounder RE, Ng D. The prevalance of *Helicobacter pylori* infection in different countries. Aliment Pharmacology and Therapeutics 1995;9:33–39.

44. Brenner H, Rothenbacher D, Bode G, Alder G. The individual and joint contributions of *Helicobacter pylri* infection and family history to the risk for peptic ulcer disease. Journal of Infection 1998;177:1124–1127.

45. Hoang TT, Bengtsson C, Phung DC, Sorberg M, granstrom M. Seroprevalence of *Helicobacter pylori* infection in urban and rural Vienam. Helicobacter 2003;8:481–482.

46. Mourad-Baars PE, Verspaget HW, Mertens BJ, Mearin ML. Low prevalence of *Helicobacter pylori* infection in young children in the Netherlands. European Journal of Gastroenterology and Hepatology 2007;19(3):213–216.

47. Rodrigues MN, Queiroz DM, Bezerra Filho JG, Pontes LK, Rodrigues RT, Braga LL. Prevalence of *Helicobacter pylori* infection in children from an urban community in northeast Brazil and risk factors for infection. European Journal of Gastroenterology and Hepatology 2004;16(2):201–205.

48. Rothenbacher D, Inceoglu J, Bode G, Brenner H. Acquisition of *Helicobacter pylori* infection in a high-risk population occurs within the first 2 years of life. Journal of Pediatrics 2000;136 (6):744–748.

49. Malaty HM, El-Kasabany A, Graham DY, Miller CC, Reddy SG, Srinivasan SR, Yamaoka Y, Berenson GS. Age at acquisition of *Helicobacter pylori* infection: a follow-up study from infancy to adulthood. Lancet 2002;16:931–935.

50. Rowland M, Daly L, Vaughan M, Higgins A, Bourke B, Drumm B. Age-specific incidence of *Helicobacter pylori*. Gastroenterology 2006;130:65–72.

51. Thomas JE, Dale A, Harding M, Coward WA, Cole TJ, Weaver LT. *Helicobacter pylori* colonization in early life. Pediatric Research 1999;45(2):218–223.

52. Malaty HM, Logan ND, Graham DY, Ramchatesingh JE. *Helicobacter pylori* infection in preschool and school-aged minority children: effect of socioeconomic indicators and breast-feeding practices. Clinical Infectious Diseases 2001;32(10):1387–1392.

53. Staat MA, Kruszon-Moran D, McQuillan GM, Kaslow RA. A population-based serologic survey of *Helicobacter pylori* infection in children and adolescents in the United States. Journal of Infectious Diseases 1996;174(5):1120–1123.

54. Pérez-Pérez GI, Sack RB, Reid R, Santosham M, Croll J, Blaser MJ. Transient and persistent *Helicobacter pylori* colonization in Native American children. Journal of Clinical Microbiology 2003;41(6):2401–2407.

55. Rowland M, Kumar D, Daly L, O'Connor P, Vaughan D, Drumm B. Low rates of *Helicobacter pylori* reinfection in children. Gastroenterology 1999;117(2):336–341.

56. Passaro DJ, Taylor DN, Gilman RH, Cabrera L, Parsonnet J. Growth slowing after acute *Helicobacter pylori* infection is age-dependent. Journal of Pediatric Gastroenterology and Nutrition 2002;35(4):522–526.

57. Richter T, Richter T, List S, Müller DM, Deutscher J, Uhlig HH, Krumbiegel P, Herbarth O, Gutsmuths FJ, Kiess WJ. Five- to 7-year-old children with *Helicobacter pylori* infection are

smaller than Helicobacter-negative children: a cross-sectional population-based study of 3,315 children. Pediatric Gastroenterology and Nutrition 2001;33(4):472–475.

58. Pilotto A, Fabrello R, Franceschi M, Scagnelli M, Soffiati G, Mario FD, Fortunato A, Valerio G. *Helicobacter pylori* infection in asymptomatic elderly subjects living at home or in a nursing home: effects on gastric function and nutritional status. Age and Ageing 1996; 25:245–249.

59. Elston D. The hygiene hypothesis and atopy: bring back the parasites? Journal of American Academy of Dermatology 2006;54:172–179.

60. Yazdanbakhsh M, Kremsner PG, Ree R. Allergy parasites and the hygiene hypothesis. Science 2002;296:490–494.

61. Bach JF. Six questions about the hygiene hypothesis. Cellular Immunology 2005; 233:158–161.

62. Cremonini F, Gasbarrini A. Atopy *Helicobacter pylori* and the hygiene hypothesis. European Journal of Gastroenterology and Hepatology 2003;15:635–636.

63. Radon K, Windstetter D, Eckart J, Dressel H, Leitritz L, et al. Farming exposure in childhood exposure to markers of infection and the development of atopy in rural subjects. Clinical and Experimental Allergy 2004;34:1178–1183.

64. Hertzen L, Haahtela T. Disconnection of man and the soil: reason for the asthma and atopic epidemic? J Allergy Clin Immunol 2006;117:334–344.

65. Percival SL, Chalmers RM, Embrey M, Hunter PR, et al. Microbiology of Waterborne Diseases. 2004. Elsevier Academic Press. London.

66. Gomes BG, De Martinis ECP. The significance of *Helicobacter pylori* in water food and environmental samples. Food Control 2004;15:397–403.

Chapter 12
Probiotics and the Ageing Gut

Steven L. Percival

Introduction

Probiotic food and supplements are very popular particularly in an ageing population. There usage has principally been confined to gastrointestinal (GI) related conditions. However, "live probiotics" are now being used to alleviate infection and diseases in many areas of the human body. It is well acknowledged that there is a growing body of evidence to support the fact that the complex and vast microflora inside our gastrointestinal tract (GIT) contributes to health and disease.[1] For this micoflora to function optimally in the adult gut, the "balance" of the microflora must be maintained and this appears to be increasingly difficult because of lifestyle changes and the problems associated with human ageing. Various factors (e.g. diet, antibiotic treatment, stress, age) may "shift" the balance of the gut microflora away from potentially beneficial or health-promoting bacteria (e.g. Lactobacilli and Bifidobacteria) towards a predominance of potentially harmful or pathogenic bacteria such as Clostridia, sulfate-reducers, and certain *Bacteroides* species.[2] Predominance of these latter populations are known to predispose an individual to a number of clinical conditions such as cancer and inflammatory disorders while making the host more susceptible to infections by transient enteropathogens such as Salmonella, *Escherichia coli*, and Listeria.[3] Consequently, people are seeking healthier lifestyles, and evidence is mounting that supports the idea that our health can be affected by the daily consumption of specific bacteria such as "probiotics." *Probiotic* is derived from Greek and means "for life." Fuller defined probiotics as "live microbial feed supplements which beneficially affect the host by improving the intestinal microbial balance."[4] However, a later definition by the Food and Agricultural Organization of the United Nations and the World Health Organization to provide health benefits[5] proposed probiotics as "live microorganisms which when administered in adequate amounts confer a health benefit on the host."[6] A probiotic is considered as a food or supplement containing viable microorganisms that on

S.L. Percival
West Virginia University Schools of Medicine and Dentistry Robert C, Byrd Health Sciences Center-North, Morgantown, WV, USA

S.L. Percival (ed.), *Microbiology and Aging.*   275
DOI: 10.1007/978-1-59745-327-1_12, © Springer Science + Business Media, LLC 2009

ingestion affect the host in a beneficial manner by modulating mucosal and systemic immunity as well as improving nutritional and microbial balance in the intestinal
tract.[7] Health benefits associated with the consumption of probiotic bacteria include
modulation of immune function, protection against enteric infections and immuno-
inflammatory disorders, anti-tumorigenic effects, alleviation of lactose intolerance,
and blood cholesterol reduction.[8,9]

Although there are many microbial strains that are claimed to have probiotic
activity, only a handful of species dominate the marketplace, with Lactobacilli and
Bifidobacteria being the most extensively studied.[10] With many probiotics it is
found that the most clinically significant strains are generally the most susceptible
to death. Consequently, many probiotics die before providing any benefit. In
addition, the mechanism by which probiotics act on the human host is poorly
understood, which can make the outcomes obtained from many trials difficult to
determine and expect. However, in the last decade probiotics have shown to provide
some benefit to help fight infections in an ageing population and also to help
modulate the humans immune system in both children and adults.

The scope of this chapter is to evaluate the scientific evidence in support of the
modest health claims in terms of efficacy of probiotics in GI disorders including the
mechanisms of action related to their therapeutic effect in children and adults.

History of Probiotics

Although the word "probiotic" by definition was not established until 1965, the
concept was worked upon by the Noble Prize winning Russian Scientist Elie
Metchnikoff much earlier. Metchnikoff believed that the microbial population in
the colon was having an adverse effect on the host through so called "autointox-
ination."[2] In the "Propagation of Life" Metchnikoff suggested that the long life of
Bulgarian peasants resulted from their consumption of fermented milk products
containing Lactobacilli.[11] As a result, Metchnikoff began to modify the colonic
flora through ingested soured milks. He used a Gram-positive rod which he called
Bulgarian bacillus and later *Bacillus bulgaricus*; it is probable that this organism
later became known as *Lactobacillus bulgaricus*, which together with *S. thermophilus* is responsible for the traditional fermentation of milk into yogurt.[2] Several
definitions of probiotics have since evolved, but a more modern definition has
proposed probiotics as "microbial cell preparations or components of microbial
cells that have a beneficial effect on health and wellbeing."[7]

Gut Physiology

Initial bacterial colonization of a previously germ-free human intestine begins at
birth and is an important component of the development of mucosal host
defences.[12,13] Diet and environmental factors may also influence this process.[14]
The GIT of the average human adult is colonized by approximately 10^{14} microbial

cells representing more than 500 different species, primarily consisting of Bacteroides, Lactobacillus, Clostridium, Fusobacterium, Bifidobacterium, Eubacterium, and Peptostreptococci species.[15] This indigenous microflora can be sometimes classified as potentially harmful or health promoting. The strains with beneficial properties include principally bifidobacteria and lactobacilli, as there is increasing evidence that these bacteria may antagonize pathogens directly through the production of antimicrobial compounds and exhibit powerful anti-inflammatory properties.[16] Moreover, the same genera have been attributed with other beneficial aspects such as stimulation of the immune response, competitive exclusion of pathogens, and production of lactase that aids digestion in lactose digestion.[17]

An important function of the intestinal microflora is to provide protection against incoming microorganisms. Studies have demonstrated that animals bred in a germ-free environment are highly susceptible to infections – therefore the intestinal microflora is considered an important constituent in the mucosal defence barrier; this is known as *colonization resistance*.[18] The role of intestinal microflora in oral tolerance induction also suggests that the gut microflora directs the regulation of systemic and local immune responses and provides strong stimuli for the maturation of gut lymphoid tissue; abrogation of oral tolerance is associated with lack of intestinal flora.[19] Recent investigation into the interaction between bacteria and the mucosal innate and adaptive immune system provides a basis for understanding the role of gut microflora in achieving a disease-free state in the host, despite the constant presence in the gut lumen of various antigens from food and microorganisms.[18]

Once established, the intestinal flora is beneficial to the host but also potentially pathogenic.[8] Consequently, disturbances in the intestinal microflora as a result of a number of factors (e.g. stress, antibiotic treatment, infection) can affect gut barrier function and induce GI disorders and gut-related inflammatory conditions, enhancing the predisposition to an increased risk of infectious disease as well as immuno-inflammatory or autoimmune diseases.[8]

Normalization of the properties of unbalanced intestinal microflora by specific strains of healthy gut microflora (e.g. Lactobacillus, Bifidobacterium) constitutes the rationale in probiotic therapy.

Therapeutic Effects of Probiotics

Probiotic Effects in Neonates and Children

The use of probiotics in children was reviewed extensively as a dietary supplement by the Committee on Nutrition of the European Society of Pediatric Gastroenterology, Hepatology and Nutrition, who published a report in 2001.[20] This report sparked off the use of probiotics in infants.

Probiotics in children has been used to help various conditions such as acute diarrhoeal disease, intestinal inflammation and infection, *Helicobacter pylori*, and constipation, and each of these will be highlighted in more detail later on in this chapter.

A newborn baby is very susceptible to infections and conditions such as diarrhoea are a common occurrence. In fact, if we consider the United States alone, there are generally between 21 and 37 million diarrhoeal episodes in 16.5 million children per year.[21] Today, this figure is very much higher, as actual numbers are often not reported. Necrotizing enterocolitis is a devastating disorder that affects neonates specifically in intensive care units. It is particularly prevalent in preterm infants ($<$1,500 g in weight).[21] The bacteria that are responsible for this condition include Clostridium, *Escherichia coli*, Klebsiella, Salmonella, *Staphylococcus aureus*, and Pseudomonas, to name but a few. It has been documented that if lactobacillus or Bifidobacteria colonize the gut first, the cases of necrotizing enterocolitis is significantly reduced.[22] Also, if neonates are administered antibiotics at birth, an abnormal microbiota is shown to remain 4 weeks later.[23] Human trials in children using *Lactobacillus acidophilus* and *Bifidobacterium infantis* was provided to 1,282 patients in Colombia. This treatment was shown to result in a 60% reduction in necrotizing enterocolitis.[24]

Strong evidence of the benefits of *L. rhamnosus* GG and *B. lactis* BB-12 and *L. reuteri* SD2222 against rotavirus in children have been found. In fact, there have been a number of clinical trails that have involved the use of probiotics and these have shown to reduce the duration of diarrhoea in children.[25–31] There is also growing evidence that probiotics can inhibit both the adherence and growth of many enteropathogens. *Lactobacillus* GG has been shown to have beneficial effects in reducing the incidence of eczema in infants.[32] In addition to this, infants that have been breast-fed have been found to have lower incidence of allergies. The role bifidobacteria play in this is considered to be significant.[33–38]

Probiotic Effects in Adults and Children

The use of probiotics in adults to help treat certain conditions and ailments is increasing. The clinical areas where these have been utilized, in both children and adults, have included lactose intolerance, gastritis due to *Helicobacter pylori*, small-bowel bacterial overgrowth, viral gastoenteritis, bacterial diarrhoea, antibiotic-associated and *C. difficile* induced diarrhoea, constipation, inflammatory bowel and irritable bowel syndromes, and nosocomial infections, to name but a few. Each of these areas will be considered in turn.

Lactose Intolerance

Approximately two-thirds of the world's adult population suffer from lactose malgestion.[15] Lactose malabsorption is characterized by the absence or decreased production of the lactose-cleaving enzyme β-galactosidase (lactase) in the mucosa of the small intestine, so that unsplit lactose reaches the colon.[39] This results in various degrees of abnormal discomfort (bloating, cramps, etc.). Lactase absorption has been shown to be improved by probiotic bacteria owing to bacterial β-galactosidase activity, changes in colonic microflora, and delayed transit time in the small bowel.[40] Studies have shown that milk containing *L. acidophilus* and Bifidobacteria improve the symptoms of lactose malabsorption in lactose-intolerant patients.[14] However, elsewhere, other studies have demonstrated that *L. acidophilus* does not improve lactose absorption.[3] Possible explanations include a low probiotic cell count[3] or that probiotic bacteria just pass through the small intestine without sufficient release of β-galactosidase and play more of a role in the colon.[11] Furthermore, numerous studies have shown that improved lactase digestion occurs in lactose malabsorbers who consumed yogurt rather than milk; this effect appears not to correspond to a replacement of endogenous lactase by bacterial β-galactosidase. Investigators have suggested that slower gastric emptying of yogurt and therefore the delayed passage of lactose allows the endogenous β-galactosidase more time to hydrolyse the lactose and is not attributed to microbial β-galactosidase.[11] To what extent probiotics contribute to relief of lactose intolerance symptoms is uncertain; some probiotics, for example, *L. rhamnosus* GG, are not able to ferment lactose.[10]

Helicobacter Pylori Infection

H. pylori is the major pathogen causing gastritis and peptic ulcers, and is a risk factor for gastric malignancies.[13] The organism can be found in 70–90% of the population in developing countries and 25–50% in developed countries.[41] Most intestinal bacteria cannot withstand the low pH environment of the stomach. However, in vivo studies have shown that Lactobacillus has the capacity to adhere and even transiently reside in the human upper GIT, and may even downregulate *H. pylori*.[42] In addition, a further in vivo study demonstrated how *H. pylori* colonization was inhibited with *L. salivarius*-fed mice when compared with lactobacillus-free mice.[9] A similar inhibition result was also observed in humans consuming *L. johnsonii*.[17] More recently, an intervention study involving administration of *L. casei* strain Shirota to 14 *H. pylori*-positive subjects indicated a slight trend towards a suppressive effect of *L. casei* on *H. pylori*.[9] Furthermore, investigators have suggested that inhibition by selected *L. reuteri* strains may help to prevent infection during early stage colonization by *H. pylori*.[13]

It has been postulated that Lactobacillus probiotic species colonize the intestine and exhibit several mechanisms of action against *H. pylori*. These include competing for nutrients, competitive pathogen exclusion, production of inhibitory compounds (e.g. lactate, hydrogen peroxide, short chain fatty acids, bacteriocins), and immunomodulatory stimuli.[41] More recently, the antimicrobial compounds secreted by Bifidobacterium were shown to inhibit the growth of clinical isolates of *H. pylori*, and their effects were promoted by organic acids resulting fermentation at an acid pH.

Finally, it has been proven that the effectiveness of antibiotic-based triple therapies can be improved by the addition of selected probiotic strains to *H. pylori* treatment protocols, in addition to alleviating any unwanted side effects.[40] The results of these studies alone indicate a supporting role for probiotics when used in combination with standard eradication therapy. However, despite promising evidence, attempts to improve *H. pylori* eradication rates through the use of probiotics alone have had mixed results.[7, 43] In children, *H. pylori* was eradicated when three probiotics were used in combination with the routinely used triple therapy for *H. pylori* treatment.[44]

Small-Bowel Bacterial Overgrowth

Overgrowth of bacteria in the small intestine can have many causes, including blind loops, stenosis of the intestine, diverticula, and motility disorders, with symptoms frequently chronic and relapsing.[45] *L. acidophilus* has been shown to reduce the symptoms of small-bowel bacterial overgrowth brought on by end-stage kidney disease.[17] A limited number of studies have also suggested that *L. plantarum* and *L. rhamnosus* GG may be beneficial in eliminating the symptoms associated with small-bowel bacterial overgrowth.[40]

Viral Diarrhoea

Acute Gastroenteritis

A major area of interest for the use of probiotics has been in patients who have acute diarrhoea caused by rotavirus infections, which is the most common cause of acute gastroenteritis in children.[15] Rotavirus can account for up to 60 and 50% of all diarrhoeal episodes in developing and developed countries, respectively, and an estimated 870,000 deaths in children every year.[46] In several placebo-controlled studies, a decrease of rotavirus associated diarrhoea in children has been reported after treatment with Lactobacillus GG, measured on reduction in duration of diarrhoea or decrease in numbers of bowel motions per day; it has consistently been shown to reduce the duration of diarrhoea by 50%.[18,47] Furthermore, a 15-month study on the effect of prophylactic use of a daily dose of *Lactobacillus* GG in 204 malnourished Peruvian children reported a decrease in the incidence of acute diarrhoea.[40] Elsewhere, several studies have also shown that *L. reuteri*, *L. casei* Shirota, and *B. lactis* Bb12 can shorten the duration of rotavirus by approximately 1 day.[10] As an example, in 1994[30] Saavedra and colleagues randomized 55 hospitalized infants to receive *B. bifidum* (later renamed as *B. lactis*) and *S. thermophilus* in a milk formula or placebo. Only 10% of the children in the probiotic group shed rotavirus in their stools compared with 39% of the control group; the overall rate of diarrhoea was also reduced in the treatment group.[17] These data support a role for probiotics in reducing the frequency of diarrhoeal illnesses possibly because of the stabilization of the indigenous microflora, reduction in the duration of rotavirus shedding, and reduction in the increased gut permeability caused by rotavirus infection together with a significant increase in IgA-secreting cells to the rotavirus.[18] A further suggestion offered by Penner et al.[7] indicated that probiotics are able to inhibit the adhesion of rotavirus by modifying the glycosylation state of the receptor in epithelial cells using soluble factors excreted by the probiotics. Consequently, certain strains of lactic acid bacteria, particularly *Lactobacillus* GG, may promote a systemic and local immune response to rotavirus, which may be of importance for protective immunity against re-infections.

A review of the literature suggests that the positive effects of *Lactobacillus* GG in acute diarrhoea cannot be extrapolated absolutely to other probiotic strains or to patients with other causes of acute diarrhoea of viral or bacterial origin. For example, comparing several probiotic strains, Majamaa et al.[29] found a beneficial effect of *Lactobacillus* GG but not of *L. rhamnosus*, *L. delbrueckii*, and *S. thermophilus* in the efficacy of rotavirus gastroenteritis. Furthermore, placebo-controlled trials in children with acute diarrhoea have not demonstrated any beneficial effect of *L. acidophilus*, and inconsistent results have been reported using *Enterococcus* SF68 in adults with acute diarrhoea.[18] This evidence suggests that different probiotic strains may have different potential benefits.

Bacterial Diarrhoea

Acute bacterial diarrhoeal infections continue to increase and are largely of waterborne and foodborne origin.[48] Several pathogens such as *Salmonella* species, enteroinvasive *E. coli* and enterohemorrhagic *E. coli* species, *Campylobacter* species, and *Shigella* species can cause invasive diarrhoea.[13] These pathogens have the capacity to invade the mucosa of the small intestine and colon, and stimulate local and systemic inflammatory responses, possibly causing haemorrhage and ulceration of the mucosa.[18] Probiotics have been shown to be effective in treatment of these conditions. For example, *L. acidophilus* was found to inhibit the damage in tight junctions.[1] Another study suggested that antimicrobial substances produced by *L. acidophilus* may neutralize entertoxins from *E. coli*.[13] Elsewhere, *L. rhamnosus* and *L. acidophilus* strains inhibited colonization of the intestinal cell monolayer by *E. coli* 0157:H7 and also reduced cell invasion by this enterovirulent strain.[8] Moreover, the antimicrobial activity of *B. breve* Yakult against *S. enterica* serovar *typhimurium* has been investigated using an antibiotic-induced murine infection model. Intestinal growth and subsequent intestinal translocation of the pathogen were inhibited by *B. breve* colonization; in contrast, *B. bifidum* strain had no effect.[16] *L. casei* Shirota strain has also been shown to significantly reduce the numbers of *Listeria monocytogenes* in the tissues of infected rats, possibly by increasing cell-mediated immunity.[48]

It is postulated that probiotics may exert their anti-infective effects by influencing the regulation of mucin gene expression, composition, and release of mucus.[8] An in vitro study involving the co-culture of *Lactobacillus* GG and *L. plantarum* 299v with colonic epithelial cells was shown to enhance the expression of mucin genes (MUC2 and MUC3); furthermore, *Lactobacillus* GG and *L. plantarum* inhibited the adherence of enteropathogenic and enterohaemorrhagic *E. coli* to intestinal epithelial cells but not to non-epithelial Hep 2 cells, suggesting a protective role for mucin.[8]

In contrast to reports showing substantial evidence of the benefits from Lactobacilli therapy in patients with viral gastroenteritis, data in support of the use of probiotic strains for the prevention of travellers' diarrhoea (TD) are more limited. In some studies, *L. casei rhamnosus* has been shown to reduce the incidence of TD,[49] but in contrast, a placebo-controlled study conducted in adults travelling on holiday showed an overall incidence of 46.5% of diarrhoea in the placebo group vs. an incidence of 41% in the group given *L. casei rhamnosus* GG.[16] Since TD is often caused by a diverse range of microbial pathogens (e.g. *E. coli*, Salmonella, Campylobacter, etc.) it is unlikely that a single probiotic strain would inhibit such a broad spectrum of pathogens in vivo and, as such may account for many probiotic strains that have failed to show a positive impact for TD. Finally, *Cryptosporidium parvum* is a waterborne protozoan parasite that also causes acute diarrhoea in humans. A recent study has demonstrated that the antimicrobial substances excreted by *L. reuteri* and *L. acidophilus* can prevent infection against the oocyst stage of *C. parvum*.[50]

Since diarrhoea is a major cause of infant death worldwide and can be incapacitating in adults, the widespread use of probiotics could be an important noninvasive means to prevent and treat such diseases, particularly in developing countries.

Antibiotic-associated and C. difficile-induced Diarrhoea

Diarrhoea can also occur as an adverse effect of antibiotic therapy, with clinical symptoms ranging from mild diarrhoea to pseudomembranous colitis; it is mainly caused by an overgrowth of *Clostridium diffcile* due to a disturbance in gut microbial ecology.[47] Despite adequate treatment with oral vancomycin or metronidazole, clostridia-related diarrhoea can relapse in up to 25% of cases.[45] Several placebo-controlled studies have demonstrated a decrease in the incidence of diarrhoea or change in stool frequency and consistency in patients treated with probiotics; probiotic strains frequently applied in these studies are lactobacillus GG, *L. acidophilus*, and *S. boulardi*.[40] A recent review also concluded that *L. rhamnosus* GG and *S. boulardi* in combination with antibiotics decreased recurrence of *C. difficile* infection,[51] and *S. boulardi* appeared to have a specific protective mechanism against *C. difficile*.[46] Elsewhere, the efficacy of *L. plantarum* 299v in combination with metronidazole treatment of *C. difficile* was determined, but it was concluded that the trial was inadequately powered to show significant benefit (recurrence in 4 out of 11 *L. plantarum*-treated vs. 6 of 9 placebo-treated patients).[7] Finally, a study enrolling 45 antibiotic-associated diarrhoea patients from 10 different centres found a resolution of diarrhoea within 1 week in 91% of the patients treated with *Enterococcus* SF68 vs. 73% in the placebo group.[40] These results show promise for several different probiotic agents in preventing antibiotic-associated and *C. difficile*-induced diarrhoea. However, most studies on probiotics and diarrhoea focus on outcome parameters such as the incidence of diarrhoea or stool frequency and therefore clinical applications of these studies are limited by the lack of proper comparative studies with available probiotics and dose–response studies.

Constipation

Constipation is a major digestive complaint and is traditionally defined in terms of bowel movement varying from three to once weekly or less.[52] Current evidence suggests that probiotics, specifically lactic acid bacteria, may improve intestinal mobility and relieve constipation, possibly through a reduction in gut pH.[10] One study showed that the consumption of bifidus milk improved intestinal mobility and bowel behaviour in a group of 18 constipated elderly persons.[17] However, a review of the literature does not substantiate this claim, and the causes of constipation may actually relate to physical inactivity, low-fibre diet, insufficient liquid intake, and certain drugs.[10]

In children the administering of *Lactobacillus* GG induced no significant benefit to chronic constipation.[53]

Irritable Bowel Syndrome and Inflammatory Bowel Disease

Irritable bowel syndrome (IBS) is a functional GI disorder with heterogeneous pathophysiology and affects 8–22% of the population.[15] Treatment focuses primarily on the relief of clinical symptoms (i.e. abdominal pain, diarrhoea, bloating). Recent, controlled studies have assessed the use of probiotics for IBS. The therapeutic effects of *L. acidophilus* were demonstrated in a cross-over trial with 18 IBS patients.[40] Symptomatic improvement was also found in 19 of 28 patients in an uncontrolled study after the administration of *Enterococcus faecium* PR88.[45] More recently, the effects of a probiotic formulation containing 8 different probiotic species (known as VSL3) on GI transit and symptoms of patients with diarrhoea and IBS were evaluated. The study concluded there was no significant difference in symptom relief between the placebo and the VSL3-treated group with the exception of abdominal bleeding which was decreased by VSL3 treatment.[7] Elsewhere, the administration of *L. plantarum* 299 vs. placebo for 4 weeks decreased pain and flatulence and showed overall clinical improvement in patients with IBS.[1] In contrast however, no clinical improvement was reported after consumption of *Lactobacillus* GG for 8 weeks in bloating-predominant IBS patients.[40] Consequently, the ability of probiotics to impact on IBS remains to be proven, and further invention studies are required using a range of probiotic strains.

Elderly patients with various conditions such as refractory pouchitis, ulcerative colitis, and Crohn's disease have utilized the use of probiotics.[54]

Other Areas

Within an ageing population, other conditions that may benefit from the use of probiotics have been documented. For example, incidences of urinary tract infections (UTIs) and bacterial vaginosis are thought to affect over one billion woman each year. Certain Lactobacilli are able to colonize the vagina and reduce the risk of urinary tract infection, yeast vaginitis, and bacterial vaginosis.[55,56] Long-term UTIs if left untreated can lead to conditions such as kidney damage or, worse still, death. The vaginal microflora changes on a daily basis and during the menstrual cycle.[57] It is documented that the lactobacillus in most woman is continually being disrupted, which increases the chances for infections from pathogens.

As both lactobacilli and bifidobacteria are able to modify the microbiota of the gut, there is evidence that these bacteria have the ability to reduce β-glucuronidase and carcinogenic levels of harmful chemicals in the gut.[58] The use of probiotics to prevent allergic reactions has also been demonstrated.[32] Skin care has also been considered as another potential area for probiotic applications.[59]

Ongoing Research into Probiotics

The effect of probiotics on the immune system is an active area of interest and hence has been comprehensively reviewed. Most of the evidence from in vitro investigations, animal models, and human studies suggest that probiotics can enhance both specific and non-specific immune responses.[60] These effects are believed to be mediated through activating macrophages, increasing levels of cytokines, increasing natural killer cell activity, and/or increasing levels of immunoglobulins.[8] For example, a study involving the consumption of *L. johnsonni* La1 or *B. lactis* Bb12 for 3 weeks enhanced the phagocytic activity of the peripheral blood leukocytes (PMN cells and monocytes) in human volunteers.[8]

Other areas of research include the use of probiotics in inflammatory bowel disease (IBD), pouchitis, and ulcerative colitis. Studies have shown improvement in symptoms of these disorders with consumption of certain strains of Lactobacilli. A recent trial in 60 patients with IBD indicated that daily administration of a 400-ml drink containing 5×10^7 cfu/ml *L. plantarum* reduced pain and flatulence over the

4-week study period.[17] Suppression of growth and function of enteric pathogenic bacteria via production of short-chain fatty acids, secretion of bactericidal proteins, and prevention of epithelial adherence are thought to be some of the mechanisms of probiotic action.[54]

Hypercholesterolemia is a leading cause of atherosclerosis and cardiovascular disease.[13] A wide variety of probiotics have been used in clinical trials involving their usage in serum lipid modulation. A recent, well-controlled study has shown that consumption of milk containing *Enterococcus faecium* and *S. thermophilus* by 29 healthy males for 6 weeks resulted in a 10% reduction in low density lipoprotein (LDL) cholesterol.[47] Elsewhere, one study in hypercholesterolemic mice showed that administration of low levels of *L. reuteri* for 7 days decreased total cholesterol and triglyceride levels by 38 and 40% respectively, and increased the HDL:LDL ratio by 20%.[17] There is also evidence that probiotic bacteria may also play a role in blood pressure control, with animal and clinical studies documenting anti-hypertensive effects of probiotic ingestion.[10] Consequently, there is a need for long-term, well-controlled human studies to evaluate the benefit of probiotic consumption on heart disease and blood lipid levels.

Probiotics have been suggested to prevent the recurrence of certain cancers by inhibiting various carcinogens. Examples include nitrosamines. Certain bacteria are able to produce enzymes that transform precarcinogens into active carcinogens such as glycosidase, β-glucuronidase, azoreductase, and nitroreductase[45]; Bifidobacteria and Lactobacilli do not produce toxic or carcinogenic metabolites.[15] In fact, many probiotics have been shown to reduce the level of these detrimental enzyme activities. Probiotic strains (e.g. *L. acidophilus*, *B. longum*, and *L. rhamnosus* GG) have reduced the incidence of colonic tumours in rats dosed with colonic carcinogens or cooked food mutagens.[40] O'Mahony has shown that *Lactobacillus salivarius* UCC118 strain was able to reduce the prevalence of colon cancer in mice.[61] Elsewhere, human epidemiological studies suggest that probiotics delivered as fermented dairy products may reduce the risks of large adenomas in the colon.[15] Also *L. casei* has been shown to prevent bladder cancer.[62]

Some studies have also reported that probiotics can play a role in both the prevention and management of atopic dermatitis.[13] Furthermore, the immuno-inflammatory responses to dietary antigens in allergic individuals are shown to be alleviated by probiotics, this being attributable to enhanced production of the anti-inflammatory cytokines, IL-10 and TGF-β, and partly by the control of allergic inflammation of the gut.[18] Also, current research suggests that an altered gut microflora may play a role in autistic pathology, and studies have shown that probiotics may relieve GI symptoms associated with autism.[15]

Finally, since some probiotics have demonstrated immune-potentiating activities during the course of rotavirus infection, it has been suggested that they could enhance oral vaccine administration. Studies have been conducted with live polio vaccine and typhoid vaccine, administrating probiotics for an immunoadjunct effect – in these trials, levels of protective antibody were enhanced and overall vaccine efficiency was increased.[10] Also, an additional area of research is the use of a probiotic in combination with a prebiotic to form what is called a *symbiotic approach.* This combination is thought to benefit the host by improving the survival and implantation of live microbial dietary supplements into the GIT and by improving the microbial balance of the GIT.[15] Furthermore, the effectiveness of combining probiotics and prebiotics may be additive and synergistic, especially in lowering serum cholesterol levels and reducing colorectal cancer.[13]

Conclusion

Initial bacterial colonization of a human intestine begins at birth and is an important component for the development of mucosal host defences and also aids in the development of a beneficial microflora for adult life.[12,13,63] Data from studies on the effects of probiotics in GIT, both in children and also adults, tend to be encouraging and evidence is accumulating which confirms that probiotics can benefit the host by improving intestinal wellbeing, skin complaints, and atopic disease.[64,65] Research is also suggesting that some probiotic bacteria have anti-carcinogenic properties and may be able to reduce tumours, while others are able to modulate the immune system. The most conclusive evidence to date exists for the prevention and treatment of diarrhoea by *Lactobacillus* GG, *L. reuteri*, and *S. boulardi*. Two meta-analyses concluded that probiotics can reduce the risk of developing antibiotic-associated diarrhoea, and significant benefits have also been shown in rotavirus diarrhoea.[40] Elsewhere, many proposed beneficial health effects of probiotics still require further investigation. These include IBD, pouchitis, and ulcerative colitis. In conclusion, the probiotic approach involving the regular consumption of beneficial bacteria such as Lactobacilli and Bifidobacteria holds great promise for the prevention and treatment of clinical conditions associated with improved gut mucosal barrier function and sustained inflammatory responses. This may have important implications on reducing infections and as such have a role to play in the ageing process.

References

1. Saxelin M, Tynkkynen S, Mattila-Sandholm T, De Vos WM. Probiotics and other functional microbes: from markets to mechanisms. Curr Opin Biotechnol 2005;16:204–211.
2. Fooks LJ, Fuller R, Gibson GR. Prebiotics, probiotics and human gut microbiology. Int Dairy J 1999;9:53S–61S.
3. Sanders ME. Considerations for use of probiotic bacteria to modulate human health. J Nutr 2000;130:384–390.
4. Fuller R. Probiotics in man and animals. J Appl Bacteriol 1989;66:365–378.
5. Anon. Regulatory and clinical aspects of dairy probiotics. Food and agricultural organization of the united nations and world health organisation. Expert consultation report. Food and agriculture organization of the united nations and world health organisation working group report (online). 2001.

6. McFarland LV, Elmer GW Bioterapeutic agents: past, present and future. Microecol Ther 1995;23:46–73.
7. Penner R, Fedorak RN, Madsen KL. Probiotics and nutraceuticals: non-medical treatments of gastrointestinal diseases. Curr Opin Pharmacol 2005;5:596–603.
8. Gill HS. Probiotics to enhance anti-infective defences in the gastrointestinal tract. Best Pract Res Clin Gastroenterol 2003;17(5):755–773.
9. Sgouras D, Maragkoudakis P, Petraki K, Martinez-Gonzalez B, Eriotou E, Michopoulos S, Kalantzopoulos G, Tsakalidou E, Mentis A. *In vitro* and in vivo inhibition of *Helicobacter pylori* by *Lactobacillus casei* strain Shirota. Appl Environ Microbiol 2004;70(1):518–526.
10. Ouwehand AC, Salminen S, Isolauri E. Probiotics: an overview of beneficial effects. Antonie Van Leeuwenhoek 2002;82:279–289.
11. Fioramonti J, Theodorou V, Bueno L. Probiotics: what are they? What are their effects on gut physiology? Best Pract Res Clin Gastroenterol 2003;17(5):711–724.
12. Rinne M, Kalliomäki M, Salminen S, Isolauri E. Probiotic intervention in the first months of life: short-term effects on gastrointestinal symptoms and long-term effects on gut microbiota. J Pediatr Gastroenterol Nutr 2006;43(2):200–205.
13. Chen CC, Walker WA. Probiotics and prebiotics: role in clinical disease states. Adv Paediatr 2005;52:77–113.
14. Walker WA, Duffy LC. Diet and bacterial colonization: role of probiotics and prebiotics. J Nutr Biochem 1998;9:668–675.
15. Tuohy KM, Probert HM, Smejkal CW, Gibson GR. Using probiotics and probiotics to improve gut health. Drug Discov Today 2003;15:692–701.
16. Servin AL. Antagonistic activities of lactobacilli and bifidobacteria against microbial pathogens. FEMS Microbiol Rev 2004;28:405–440.
17. Kopp-Hoolihan L. Prophylactic and therapeutic uses of probiotics: A review. J Am Diet Assoc 2001;101:229–241.
18. Isolauri E, Salminen S, Ouwehand AC. Probiotics. Best Pract Res Clin Gastroenterol 2004; 18:299–313.
19. Isolauri E, Kirjavainen PV, Salminen S. Probiotics: a role in the treatment of intestinal infection and inflammation? Gut 2002;50(suppl III):iii54–iii59.
20. Agostoni C, Axelsson I, Braegger C, Goulet O, Koletzko B, Michaelsen KF, Rigo J, Shamir R, Szajewska H, Turck D, Weaver LT; ESPGHAN Committee on Nutrition. Probiotic bacteria in dietetic products for infants: a commentary by the ESPGHAN Committee on nutrition. J Pediatr Gastroenterol Nutr 2004;38:365–374.
21. Glass RI, Lew JF, Gangarosa RE, LeBaron CW, Ho MS. Estimates of morbidity and mortality rates for diarrheal diseases in American children. J Pediatr 1991;118:S27–S33.
22. Lucas A, Cole TJ. Breast milk and neonatal necrotising enterocolitis. Lancet 1990;336 (8730):1519–1523.
23. Gewolb IH, Schwalbe RS, Taciak VL, Harrison TS, Panigrahi P. Stool microflora in extremely low birthweight infants. Arch Dis Child Fetal Neonatal Ed 1999;80(3):F167–F173.
24. Hoyos AB. Reduced incidence of necrotizing enterocolitis associated with enteral administration of *Lactobacillus acidophilus* and *Bifidobacterium infantis* to neonates in an intensive care unit. Int J Infect Dis 1999;3(4):197–202.
25. Szajewska H, Kotowska M, Mrukowicz JZ, Armańska M, Mikołajczyk W. Efficacy of *Lactobacillus* GG in prevention of nosocomial diarrhea in infants. J Pediatr 2001;138 (3):361–365
26. Guandalini S, Pensabene L, Zikri MA, Dias JA, Casali LG, Hoekstra H, Kolacek S, Massar K, Micetic-Turk D, Papadopoulou A, de Sousa JS, Sandhu B, Szajewska H, Weizman Z. *Lactobacillus* GG administered in oral rehydration solution to children with acute diarrhea: a multicenter European trial. J Pediatr Gastroenterol Nutr 2000;30(1):54–60.
27. Guarino A, Canani RB, Spagnuolo MI, Albano F, Di Benedetto L. Oral bacterial therapy reduces the duration of symptoms and of viral excretion in children with mild diarrhea. J Pediatr Gastroenterol Nutr 1997;25(5):516–519.

28. Isolauri E, Juntunen M, Rautanen T, Sillanaukee P, Koivula T. A human Lactobacillus strain (*Lactobacillus casei* sp strain GG) promotes recovery from acute diarrhea in children. Pediatrics 1991;88(1):90–97.
29. Majamaa H, Isolauri E, Saxelin M, Vesikari T. Lactic acid bacteria in the treatment of acute rotavirus gastroenteritis. J Pediatr Gastroenterol Nutr 1995;20(3):333–338.
30. Saavedra JM, Bauman NA, Oung I, Perman JA, Yolken RH. Feeding of *Bifidobacterium bifidum* and *Streptococcus thermophilus* to infants in hospital for prevention of diarrhoea and shedding of rotavirus. Lancet 1994;344(8929):1046–1049.
31. Shornikova AV, Casas IA, Isolauri E, Mykkänen H, Vesikari T. *Lactobacillus reuteri* as a therapeutic agent in acute diarrhea in young children. J Pediatr Gastroenterol Nutr 1997;24 (4):399–404.
32. Isolauri E, Arvola T, Sütas Y, Moilanen E, Salminen S. Probiotics in the management of atopic eczema. Clin Exp Allergy 2000;30(11):1604–1610.
33. Gill HS, Guarner F. Probiotics and human health: a clinical perspective. Postgrad Med J 2004;80(947):516–526.
34. Kalliomäki M, Salminen S, Poussa T, Isolauri E. Probiotics during the first 7 years of life: a cumulative risk reduction of eczema in a randomized, placebo-controlled trial. J Allergy Clin Immunol 2007;119(4):1019–1021.
35. Kalliomäki M, Isolauri E. Role of intestinal flora in the development of allergy. Curr Opin Allergy Clin Immunol 2003;3(1):15–20.
36. Kalliomäki M, Salminen S, Poussa T, Arvilommi H, Isolauri E. Probiotics and prevention of atopic disease: 4-year follow-up of a randomised placebo-controlled trial. Lancet 2003;361 (9372):1869–1871.
37. Kalliomäki MA, Isolauri E. Probiotics and down-regulation of the allergic response. Immunol Allergy Clin North Am 2004;24(4):739–752.
38. Gueimonde M, Sakata S, Kalliomäki M, Isolauri E, Benno Y, Salminen S. Effect of maternal consumption of lactobacillus GG on transfer and establishment of fecal bifidobacterial microbiota in neonates. J Pediatr Gastroenterol Nutr 2006;42(2):166–170.
39. Kailasapathy K, Chin J. Survival and therapeutic potential of probiotic organisms with reference to *Lactobacillus acidophilus* and *Bifidobacterium* spp. Immunol Cell Biol 2000;78:80–88.
40. Goossens D, Jonkers D, Stobberingh E, van den Bogaard A, Russel M, Stockbrugger R. Probiotics in gastroenterology: indications and future perspectives. Scand J Gastroenterol 2003;239:15–23.
41. Hamilton-Miller JMT. The role of probiotics in the treatment and prevention of *Helicobacter pylori* infection. Int J Antimicrob Agents 2003;22:360–366.
42. Servin AL, Coconnier MH. Adhesion of probiotic strains to the intestinal mucosa and interaction with pathogens. Best Pract Res Clin Gastroenterol 2003;17:741–754.
43. Franceschi F, Cazzato A, Nista EC, Scarpellini E, Roccarina D, Gigante G, Gasbarrini G, Gasbarrini A. Role of probiotics in patients with *Helicobacter pylori* infection. Helicobacter 2007;12(2):59–63.
44. Sýkora J, Valecková K, Amlerová J, Siala K, Dedek P, Watkins S, Varvarovská J, Stozický F, Pazdiora P, Schwarz J. Effects of a specially designed fermented milk product containing probiotic *Lactobacillus casei* DN-114 001 and the eradication of *H. pylori* in children: a prospective randomized double-blind study. J Clin Gastroenterol 2005;39(8):692–698.
45. Rolfe RD. The role of probiotic cultures in the control of gastrointestinal health. Am Soc Nutr Sci 2000;130:396S–402S.
46. Thapar N, Sanderson IR. Diarrhoea in children: an interface between developing and developed countries. Lancet 2004;363:641–653.
47. McNaught CE, MacFie J. Probiotics in clinical practice: a critical review of the evidence. Nutr Res 2001;21:343–353.
48. Reid G, Burton J. Use of Lactobacillus to prevent infection by pathogenic bacteria. Microbes Infect 2002;4:319–324.

49. Saavedra JM. Clinical applications of probiotic agents. Am J Clin Nutr 2001;73:1147S–51S.
50. Foster JC, Glass MD, Polly D, Ward LA. Effect of *Lactobacillus* and *Bifidobacterium* on *Cryptosporidium parvum* oocyst viability. Food Microbiol 2005;20(3):351–357.
51. Sartor R. Probiotic therapy of intestinal inflammation and infections. Curr Opin Gastroenterol 2005;21:44–50.
52. Holzapfel WH, Schillinger U. Introduction to pre-and probiotics. Food Res Int 2002; 35:109–116.
53. Banaszkiewicz A, Szajewska H. Ineffectiveness of *Lactobacillus* GG as an adjunct to lactulose for the treatment of constipation in children: a double-blind, placebo-controlled randomized trial. J Pediatr 2005;146(3):364–369
54. Sartor R. Therapeutic manipulation of the enteric microflora in inflammatory bowel diseases: antibiotics, probiotics, and prebiotics. Gastroenterology 2004;126:1620–1633.
55. Reid G, Beuerman D, Heinemann C, Bruce AW. Effect of oral probiotic Lactobacillus therapy on the vaginal flora and susceptibility to urogenital infections. FEMS Immunol Med Microbiol 2001;32:37–41.
56. Velraeda MC, van der Belt B, van der Mei HC, Reid G, Busscher HJ. Interference in initial adhesion of uropathogenic bacteria and yeasts silicone rubber by a *Lactobacillus acidophilus* biosurfactant. J Med Microbiol 1998;49:790–794.
57. Eschenbach DA, Thwin SS, Patton DL, Hooton TM, Stapleton AE, Agnew K, Winter C, Meier A, Stamm WE. Influence of the normal menstrual cycle on vaginal tissue, discharge and microflora. Clin Infect Dis 2000;30:901–907.
58. Hosoda M, Hashimoto H, He F, Morita H, Hosono A. Effect of administration of milk fermented with *Lactobacillus acidophilus* LA-2 on fecal mutagenicity and microflora in the human intestine. J Dairy Sci 1996;79(5):745–749.
59. Ouwehand AC, Batsman A, Salminen S. Probiotics for the skin: a new area of potential application. Lett Appl Microbiol 2003;36:327–331.
60. Di Giacinto C, Marinaro M, Sanchez M, Strober W, Boirivant M. Probiotics ameliorate recurrent Th1-mediated murine colitis by inducing IL-10 and IL-10-dependent TGF-beta-bearing regulatory cells. J Immunol 2005;174(6):3237–3246.
61. O'Mahony L, Feeney M, O'Halloran S, Murphy L, Kiely B, Fitzgibbon J, Lee G, O'Sullivan G, Shanahan F, Collins JK. Probiotic impact on microbial flora, inflammation and tumour development in IL-10 knockout mice. Aliment Pharmacol Ther 2001;15:1219–1225.
62. Ohashi Y, Nakai S, Tsukamoto T, Masumori N, Akaza H, Miyanaga N, Kitamura T, Kawabe K, Kotake T, Kuroda M, Naito S, Koga H, Saito Y, Nomata K, Kitagawa M, Aso Y. Habitual intake of lactic acid bacteria and risk reduction of bladder cancer. Urol Int 2002;68(4): 273–280.
63. Gueimonde M, Kalliomäki M, Isolauri E, Salminen S. Probiotic intervention in neonates – will permanent colonization ensue? J Pediatr Gastroenterol Nutr 2006;42(5):604–606.
64. Chapat L, Chemin K, Dubois B, Bourdet-Sicard R, Kaiserlian D. *Lactobacillus casei* reduces CD8+ T cell-mediated skin inflammation. Eur J Immunol 2004;34(9):2520–2528.
65. Kalliomäki M, Salminen S, Arvilommi H, Kero P, Koskinen P, Isolauri E. Probiotics in primary prevention of atopic disease: a randomised placebo-controlled trial. Lancet 2001;357 (9262):1076–1079.

Chapter 13
Microbiological Theory of Autism in Childhood

Steven L. Percival

Introduction

Kanner first described the symptoms of autism in 1943. He defined autism as a "biological inability for social relatedness".[1] To date, autism is considered to be part of the term Autism spectrum disorders (ASD), which includes autism, attention deficit disorder (ADD), attention deficit hyperactivity disorder (ADHD), and other associated disorders. These disorders are composed of a complex and heterogeneous group of conditions.

Autism is a severely disabling disorder resulting in profound behavioural and emotional problems and is typified by defects in communication and repetitive patterns of behaviour.[2] It is a syndrome characterized by impairments in social relatedness and communication, repetitive behaviour, abnormal movements, and sensory dysfunction. ASD clinically is present at 3 years of age. Studies have, however, shown that abnormalities in social and communication skills may represent early indicators of autism. These can sometimes be detected as early as 14 months of age.[3] Because of the heterogeneity and clinical variability of autism, many researchers are now calling autism, *autisms*.[4]

The severity of disability of a person with "autism" varies widely. The less severe forms of autism have considerable co-morbidity with other neurodevelopmental disorders such as dyspraxia attention-deficit/hyperactivity disorder and dyslexia.[2,5] Surveys that have been conducted in the US have indicated an apparent 210% increase in the cases of profound autism in children diagnosed over the last 10 years. Recent estimates indicate that the frequency of mild to severe autism may be as high as 1:150.[6] In the UK there has been a sevenfold increase in newly diagnosed cases of autism between 1988 and 1999,[7] but it is unknown whether this is a true increase in new cases of autism[8] or merely the result of altered diagnostic criteria or increased awareness of the condition.[9] Boys are four times more likely to have autistic spectrum disorders than girls.

S.L. Percival
West Virginia University Schools of Medicine and Dentistry Robert C, Byrd Health Sciences
Center-North, Morgantown, WV, USA

S.L. Percival (ed.), *Microbiology and Aging.*
DOI: 10.1007/978-1-59745-327-1_13, © Springer Science + Business Media, LLC 2009

A study by Comi and Zimmerman[10] showed that the mean number of autoimmune disorders was greater in families with autism, and that 46% of ASD patient's families had two or more members with autoimmune disorders. As the number of family members with autoimmune disorders increased from 1 to 3, the risk of autism was greater, with an odds ratio that increased from 1.9 to 5.5. The most common autoimmune disorders observed were type 1 diabetes, adult rheumatoid arthritis, hypothyroidism, and systemic lupus erythematosus.

In the literature there are many varied theories about the causes of autism. But it is accepted that genetic and also environmental factors are involved in the pathogenesis of autism.[11–13] The majority of autistic cases seem likely to arise from a multiplicity of yet unidentified genetic and environmental factors. Consequently, causes associated with autism include genetic predisposition, alterations in catecholamine and serotonin metabolism, gastrointestinal (GI) abnormalities, bioactive peptides, autoimmunity, vaccination, fatty acid metabolism, and in utero factors, to name but a few. There is also growing concern from parents and health professionals that prenatal and postnatal exposure to xenobiotics (e.g. pesticides) and biotic (e.g., antigens) factors may act synergistically with unidentified susceptibility factors to produce autistic spectrum disorders. It is thought that this may be brought about by direct or indirect effects on the immune system and/or the developing central nervous system (CNS). Some research has been placed on environmental exposures to agents such as thimerosal.[14] Also, the effects of heavy metals (lead and mercury) on the immune system and autism continue.[15] Essentially, it is thought that any alteration to the immune function may have long lasting effects resulting in an increased likelihood of development and/or progression of autoimmune and/or allergic diseases.

While several mechanisms seem to be implicated in autism, there seems to be no common factor to link them together. Although there have been extensive analyses of autistic patients' blood and urine, to date no constant factors have been found.

While genetics has a role to play in autism, genetics alone is not able to determine the entire ASD phenotype. Therefore, as mentioned previously, nongenetic factors, such as environmental factors, must play roles as modifiers of processes determined by genetic susceptibility. This is because environmental factors may interact with the neuroimmune system. This will ultimately have a significant effect in disrupting neurodevelopmental pathways leading to alterations of neurobehaviour.[2,16] Over the last few years there has been a lot of interest regarding the role of immunity and immunological dysfunction in the pathogenesis of ASD.[17,18] Some studies suggest that up to 60% of patients with ASD have various types of systemic immune dysfunction.[19–21] Also, oxidative stress, which occurs when the levels of reactive oxygen species exceed the antioxidant capacities of a cell, has effects on the brain. The brain is considered to be vulnerable to oxidative stress. In addition to these, the microbiology of the host may have a role to play in relation to allergic effects on the developing host.[22]

It is the aim of this chapter to highlight some of the available literature on the possible causative agents of autism in children and provide an alternative theory implicating bacteria as an environmental factor causing or predisposing an individual to autism.

Current Theories on Autism

As mentioned previously, there are a number of factors that can be causative of autism in children. Each of these will be considered in turn, with each section linked to a microbiological association.

Genetic Predisposition

Autism affects between 2 and 5 children per 10,000. A genetic contribution has been proven by family and twin studies,[23–27] which show that concordance for autism is 60% for monozygotic twins and 3% for dizygotic twins of unlike sex. Lauristen and colleagues[28] in 2005 found that the highest risk of autism was in families with a history of autism. This study supports the commonly accepted knowledge that genetic factors are involved in the aetiology of autism. However, the concordance figure for monozygotic twins never reaches 100%, which indicates an important environmental role in the aetiology of autism. Genetic loci on 15 separate human chromosomes have been implicated in autism, many of which may have a role in fatty acid metabolism. From a study undertaken in 2001,[29] it was established that the most interesting chromosome regions concerning the aetiology of autism were chromosomes 7q31–35, 5q11–13, and 16p13.3 as suggested by different lines of genetic research. A more recent study by Gilling et al.[30] has shown that a 3.2-Mb deletion encompassing 17 genes at the 18q break point and an additional deletion of 1.27 Mb containing two genes on chromosome 4q35 may be significant. Quantitative Polymerase Chain Reaction (Q-PCR) analysis of 14 of the 17 genes deleted on chromosome 18 showed that 11 of these genes were expressed in the brain, suggesting that haplo insufficiency of one or more genes may have contributed to the childhood autism phenotype of the patient. Identification of multiple genetic changes in this patient with childhood autism agrees with the frequently suggested genetic model of ASDs as complex, polygenic disorders. There are other publications relating to the genetics of autism and these can be located elsewhere.[31–34]

Serotonin and Catecholamines

Serotonin

Over 30% of autistic individuals have been shown to have an increase in whole blood serotonin (5-hydroxytryptamine, 5-HT) levels.[35–37] Symptoms of autism such as sleep disturbance and emotional disturbance are also associated with delirium,[38] which could be caused by increased or decreased serotonin levels. The presence of a tripeptide that stimulates the uptake of serotonin into platelets (pyro-Glu-Tyr-Gly-NH$_2$) has been identified in urine of 67% of autistic cases compared with 18% controls.[39] Serotonin manufacture and release into the brain depends upon the availability of tryptophan, which is metabolized to form indole acrylic acid (IAA). IAA is complexed with glycine to form indole acroyl glycine (IAG), and it is this compound that is commonly found excreted in urine in higher concentrations from people who have neurodevelopmental disorders.[40]

Prenatal stress in pregnant rats significantly increases the levels of brain 5-HT, and its breakdown product 5-hydroxyindoleacetic acid (5-HIAA) accumulates in the offspring with concomitant behavioural deficits during infancy.[41] It has been suggested that similar mechanisms could operate in humans leading to abnormal development of specific monoamine-containing neurons in the fetus.[41]

The possible role of serotonin in autism has been explored using a number of different approaches.[42] In fact, there is documented research that has shown that elevated levels of serotonin occurs in the platelets of patients with autism.[43–45]

Some genetic studies that have been undertaken have also shown that people with autism have abnormalities in serotonin-related genes. Another area of research supporting serotonin as a neurobiological factor in ASD comes from pharmacological interventions.[46] Research has also shown that alterations in the serotonin system have caused behavioural improvements in autistic patients.[47,48]

Catecholamines

A significant increase in the levels of dopamine and epinephrine has been demonstrated in whole blood samples from autistic individuals; however, there is no significant alteration in norepinephrine concentration in these individuals.[49] Analysis of urine samples from autistic individuals often shows a significant increase in the concentration of total homovanillic acid (HVA) (a breakdown product of dopamine).[49,50] Urinary concentration of a metabolic product of norepinephrine (3-methoxy-4-hydroxy-phenylethylene-glycol (MHPG)) is often reduced in autistic individuals.[9]

Although there often appears to be a link between catecholamines and/or their breakdown products and autism, this link has not been explained by genetic analyses which have shown that there is no association between autistic disorders and loci for genes encoding enzymes involved in their biosynthesis (e.g., tyrosine hydroxylase, dopamine hydroxylase, and the dopamine receptor D3 (DRD3)).[49]

Microbiological Link

Bacterial endotoxin (lipopolysaccharide (LPS)) has been shown to activate cerebral catecholamine and serotonin metabolism[51,52] and to increase tryptophan within the brain.[53] Bacterial (*Salmonella typhimurium*) translocation has been shown to increase brain catecholamine metabolism,[54] and injection with the bacterium *Nocardia asteroides* has been shown to significantly increase the dopamine turnover in the neostriatum and increase the serotonin turnover in the cerebellum of mice.[55]

Hence bacteria may be responsible for the differences in catecholamine and 5-HT metabolism described in some autistic individuals.

In most bacteria that have been examined to date, it is found that catecholamines result in a dramatic increase in cell numbers and also the enhanced production of some virulence factors. Norepinephrine seems to act as an autoinducer on Gram-negative bacteria which acts as a bacterial signalling molecule.

Changes in the GI Tract

Over the past decade, a significant number of research papers have been published that have examined the biological basis of autism. Recent clinical studies have revealed a high prevalence of GI symptoms, inflammation, and dysfunction in children with autism. Mild and moderate degrees of inflammation were found in both the upper and lower intestinal tract. In addition, decreased sulphation capacity of the liver, pathologic intestinal permeability, increased secretary response to intravelenous secretin injection, and decreased digestive enzyme activities have been reported in many children with autism. Treatment of digestive problems appears to have a positive effect on autistic behaviour. This suggests that more research into the brain–gut connection is needed.

Sulphation Deficit

Studies of IgA to casein gluten and gliadin (the main protein constituent of wheat protein) in certain autistic individuals[56,57] have led to the suggestion that there may be increased permeability of the GI tract leading to increased transmucosal passage of casein and gluten.[56] (In these autistic individuals there were no gross GI changes that could potentially have explained the increased permeability.)

Sulphated proteins in the gut wall help to provide a protective mucosal layer within the GI tract. Insufficient sulphation results in protein aggregation which increases gut wall permeability; this could lead to an increase in the uptake of dietary peptides from the GI tract.

It has been suggested that the genetic component of autism could be a sulphation deficit caused by a loss or reduction of activity of phenyl sulphur-transferases (PST).[58]

Sulphation potential can be measured using a paracetamol substrate because this drug is sulphated prior to excretion. Measurement of the ratio of sulphated paracetamol/paracetamol-glucuronide (PS/PG) is used to indicate the sulphation capacity of an individual. It has been shown that a significant number of autistic individuals had a reduced capacity to sulphate paracetamol compared with age-matched control subjects.[58] Therefore the GI tract of these individuals is likely to have increased permeability to dietary peptides. Importantly, neurotoxic substances that are normally sulphated prior to excretion may persist in these individuals and cause or exacerbate neurological damage.[58]

Peptides

An increase in the peptide component of urine in many autistic individuals has been demonstrated.[59-61] with common patterns of peptides being observed in many young autistic individuals. Few of these peptides have been characterized. It has been suggested that there may be an underlying genetic peptidase deficit which could result in the inappropriate metabolism of casein and gluten, leading to the production of bioactive peptides possessing opiate qualities.[62-64] These could leach across the blood–brain barrier (BBB), causing neurological dysfunction or permanent damage by interfering with synapse pruning during childhood.[65] Bovine casomorphine 1–8 (a breakdown product of cows' milk) has been identified in urine of autistic individuals,[66] demonstrating that biologically active dietary peptides can enter the systemic circulation and be subsequently identified in urine.[67]

Autistic Enterocolitis

Recently, a new form of inflammatory bowel disease (IBD) has been described and termed "autistic enterocolitis"[68] (IBD includes conditions such as Crohn's disease (CD) and ulcerative colitis (UC)). The investigation of patients (both autistic and non-autistic) with bowel disorders led to the identification of autistic enterocolitis in 93% of autistic patients compared with 16% in non-autistic patients.[68] Inflammation of the oesophagus, stomach, and duodenum has also been shown in many of autistic individuals.[69] The cause of the inflammation is unknown, but it has been suggested that gut pathogen(s) or persistent infection by measles may be responsible.

Microbiological Link

The GI immune system must maintain an adequate immune response toward microbial pathogens while adopting tolerance toward dietary antigens. The gut-associated lymphoreticular tissue (GALT) ensures that an appropriate immune response is mounted when required while maintaining the integrity of the protective intestinal mucosa.[70] In cases of IBD, an exaggerated immune response is mounted toward dietary or bacterial antigens, leading to inflammation and damage to the protective intestinal mucosa.[71]

Several pathogenic bacteria have been implicated in IBD including *Vibrio cholerae*, *Escherichia coli*, *Helicobacter pylori*, *Campylobacter* spp., *Salmonella* spp., *Yersinia* spp., *Listeria monocytogenes*, *Mycobacteria* spp., and *Streptococcus pheumoniae*.[72] However, there is evidence to suggest that non-pathogenic bacteria may also play a role in inflammation within the GI tract.[73] This has been shown in a study where IL-10-deficient mice, maintained in pathogen-free conditions, were found to be more susceptible to colonic inflammation, possibly resulting in an altered mucosal permeability or increased cytokine production leading to an inappropriate inflammatory response toward non-pathogenic luminal bacteria.[73]

Chemokine production may be regulated by butyrate (an intestinal bacterial metabolite) in response to bacterial endotoxin (LPS) stimulation.[74] LPS has been detected in the plasma of many, though not all, IBD patients.[75] This may be a result of an increased permeability of the GI tract or an alteration in the normal gut flora.[76,77] Lactobacilli (the principal Gram-positive bacteria in the GI tract) prevent Gram-negative bacterial translocation. It has been shown that there are fewer Lactobacilli in colonic biopsy specimens in patients with UC and faeces of CD patients[78,79] and that Lactobacillus is beneficial to patients with IBD[80,81] and can prevent colitis in IL-10-deficient mice described above.

It has also been reported that there is an increase in nitric oxide (NO) synthase activity in response to bacterial LPS[82] (endotoxaemia is accompanied by vasodilation and GI haemorrhage due to vascular damage). The vascular permeability and mucosal damage seen in UC has been associated with enhanced NO synthase activity found in these patients[83] and corroborated by reports of increased NO in the inflamed regions of the gut in human and animal IBD.[84] Patients with UC have been shown to overproduce hydrogen sulphide, which is toxic for the intestinal mucosa. The increase in H_2S is thought to be caused by the increase in sulphate-reducing bacteria (*Desulfibrio desulfuricans*) found in faecal samples from patients with UC.[85,86] Counts and carriage rates of SRB in faeces of patients with UC are not significantly different from those in controls. SRB metabolism is not uniform between strains, and alternative sources of hydrogen sulphide production exist in the colonic lumen which may be similarly inhibited by 5-ASA. The evidence for hydrogen sulphide as a metabolic toxin in UC remains circumstantial.[87]

After birth, the bacterial flora has not evolved to adult levels, and it is known that newborn and young infants have an immature intestinal mucosal barrier and increased GI mucosal permeability.[88] Hence, during this period there is an increased likelihood that bacteria and/or their products could cause an inflammatory response in the GI tract and pass through the gut epithelium. The initial symptoms in many cases of late-onset autism have appeared, or symptoms have worsened following a course of antimicrobial therapy for a variety of infections. It is probable that certain antimicrobials may have changed the balance of bacteria normally found in the gut and that this contributes to the picture of autism. It is likely that a toxin or other compounds produced by bacteria, particularly *Clostridium* spp., may be involved. The reason for this is particularly in relation to species of Clostridium because studies have shown that when two antimicrobials, vancomycin and metronidazole, are given orally, a significant improvement in autistic symptoms is observed. Also, clostridia produce many toxins that cause both GI disorders similar to those seen in autistic children and potent neurotoxic effects.

Overall, the GI features associated with autism could be caused by a combination of genetic reduction in PST activity, peptidase deficiency, enterocolitis inflammation, and altered GI permeability exacerbated by pathogenic or non-pathogenic bacteria and/or the increased production of NO or H_2S.

Autoimmunity

The Autoimmunity Theory of Autism

Investigations into the prevalence of autism in families that also suffer from autoimmune disease led to the identification of a positive correlation between the titre of measles-virus antibody and the presence of brain autoantibodies[89] suggestive of a viral-induced autoimmune response. Brain autoantibodies directed against myelin basic protein (MBP) and neuron axon filament protein (NAFP) were found in at least 70% of autistic individuals who also possessed antibodies to measles virus or to Herpes virus.[89] Antibodies to neither MBP nor NAFP were detected in developmentally normal control children who also possessed antibodies to measles virus or to Herpes virus.[89] Proteins of Herpes simplex type 1 and measles virus have been shown to cross-react with an intermediate filament protein of human cells,[90] which could explain the appearance of autoantibodies during viral infections. These results suggest that there may be a link between autism and measles or Herpes antigens; however, this area of research has not progressed and remains controversial.

A number of epidemiological studies suggest that a family history of autoimmune disorders is more common among children with autism than healthy control children.[91,92] Suggestions that autoimmunity may be etiologically important in autism was first reported in 1971.[93] It is thought that common genes found in a number of families may be associated with autoimmune states in families.[94] A number of studies have found that autistic individuals have an increased frequency of autoantibody production specifically anti-brain autoantibodies.[95–97] The pathophysiological significance of autoantibodies reported in autistic children is presently not known. However, autoimmunity in families suggests autoantibodies that target the CNS may be a factor thought to possibly affect neuronal development in autistic children. However, we also have to take into account that anti-brain autoantibodies are also found in patients with neurological disorders other than autism, as well as in normal individuals. Observation have also shown that the risk of having a child with autism was highest among women with allergies recorded during the second trimester,[98] possibly indicating autoimmunity as a risk factor associated with autism.

Microbiological Link

Bacteria have been implicated as the causative agents in several autoimmune disorders such as acute rheumatic fever, which known to be caused by streptococcal infection (streptococcus-induced carditis), and Guillain–Barré syndrome (GBS) which is a post infectious syndrome of *Campylobacter jejuni*[99,100] this occurs via epitope mimicry between the human ganglioside GM1 and lipopolysaccharide of *C*.

jejuni. Proteus mirabilis and *Mycobacterium tuberculosis* have been implicated as causative factors in rheumatoid arthritis[101] and *Klebsiella pneumoniae* and *Yersinia enterocolitica* have been implicated with the onset of ankylosing spondylitis[102,103] a rheumatic disease affecting joints in the spine, hips, and shoulders.

There have been suggestions that vaccination may cause the onset of autoimmune diseases such as arthritis (rubella as a component of the measles, mumps, and rubella (MMR) vaccination), rheumatoid arthritis (tetanus and hepatitis B vaccinations) and diabetes mellitus (*Haemophilus influenzae* type B vaccination).[104] The epitope mimicry theory attempts to explain how vaccination could cause autoimmune disease: epitopes within the vaccine (either the bacterial/viral antigenic component of the vaccine), or the adjuvant itself, may resemble host antigens and induce an autoimmune response.[104]

It has also been suggested that bacterial superantigens (SAg) (particularly those of *Staphylococcus aureus* and *Streptococcus pyogenes*) are involved with the onset of rheumatoid arthritis.[105] There is a strong possibility that superantigens may compromise the ability of the host's immune system to clear bacterial antigens, leading to a perpetuation of inflammatory and immune responses. Hence it is not unreasonable to suggest that bacteria may be associated with an autoimmune component of autism.

Vaccination

Some illnesses have been shown to be directly attributable to vaccination such as Guillain–Barré syndrome (GBS) which results in motor paralysis and mild sensory disturbances. Prior viral infections such as Herpes virus, Epstein–Barr virus (EBV), cytomegalovirus (CMV), and measles are thought to be risk factors for the onset of GBS after vaccination. A putative link between MMR vaccination and autism was proposed by Wakefield et al.[106] However, MMR vaccination prevalence has remained constant over the last 10 years, in a period showing a sevenfold increase in the prevalence of autism. Therefore, Kaye et al.[7] have proposed that there was no correlation between MMR vaccination and the incidence of autism. Many papers have now suggested it is time to look beyond MMR in autism research.[107] However, it is interesting to note the presence of brain autoantibodies in at least 70% of autistic individuals (but absent in non-autistic individuals) also possessed antibodies to measles virus or to Herpes virus.

Microbiological Link

The "Hygiene Hypothesis" was first proposed in 1989 by David Strachan on the basis of the observation that hay fever skin prick positivity and specific IgE in children correlated inversely with family size. He stated that higher standards of personal cleanliness over recent years have reduced opportunities for cross-infection in young families and that this may have resulted in more widespread clinical expression of aptopic disease. He also indicated that the development of allergic diseases could be prevented by infections during early childhood transmitted by unhygienic contact with other siblings or acquired prenatally. This therefore would possibly aid in providing a tolerance of the host to potentially problematic bacteria.

A state of tolerance to bacterial products leading to their persistence within the body can be induced via the bacterial component of the vaccine adjuvant. Adjuvant prolongs the presentation of the vaccination antigen to the immune system, prevents its degradation, and stimulates the immune system's cells. Many adjuvants contain cell wall components from *Mycobacterium tuberculosis*, such as Freund's complete adjuvant (FCA) and Ribi Adjuvant System (RAS). *M. tuberculosis* cell wall components include lipoarabinomannan (LAM). Riedel and Kaufmann[108] conducted in vitro experiments to show that a state of tolerance could be induced in human macrophages by using arabinosylated lipoarabinomannan (ARA-LAM).

The persistence of bacterial products (toxins) within the body causes neurological dysfunction (e.g., hepatic encephalopathy where coma is associated with an increase in bacterially derived gamma-aminobutyric acid (GABA). This could potentially lead to an induction or exacerbation of autistic behaviour. Is it possible that vaccination could lead to tolerance of bacterial antigens leading to their persistence in the body?

Gamma-Aminobutyric Acid

GABA is the principal inhibitory neurotransmitter in the brain and any alteration in the GABAergic system will cause neurological changes. The genetic locus 15q11–q13 has been implicated with autism susceptibility: a region known to contain the GABA(A) receptor gene complex and the GABA(B3) subunit receptor gene.[109] Analysis of families with a history of autism has produced evidence that this genetic locus is linked with autism.[109]

The Blood–Brain Barrier

BBB is physical and biochemical. The biochemical barrier consists of peptidases that destroy exogenous peptides and prevents bacterial peptides entering the brain. The circumventricular organs within the brain are not protected by the BBB and there is a 10- to 1,000-fold increase in the uptake rates for small solutes in these areas when compared with the rest of the brain. During fetal development, the BBB and blood–cerebrospinal fluid (CSF) barriers are more permeable to low molecular weight lipid-insoluble compounds[110] and therefore there may also be increased permeability to smaller compounds such as GABA or other neuromodulators/neurotransmitters.

In hepatic encephalopathy (HE), where there are large quantities of circulating bacterial products, there was found to be an abnormally permeable BBB prior to the onset of HE[111] allowing GABA to pass easily into the brain. The liver normally removes the gut-derived GABA from the portal venous blood. However, during liver failure many neuroactive nitrogenous products of gut bacteria enter the systemic circulation and pass to the brain via the more permeable BBB.

Certain viruses (measles, parainfluenza virus type 3, Herpes simplex virus type 1, and cytomegalovirus (CMV)) are able to infect endothelial cells and in so doing may cause vessel wall injury.[111,112] Hence, viral infection causing inflammation within the capillaries of the brain may increase the permeability of the BBB in this region, allowing easier diffusion of neuroactive substances, which are normally carefully regulated with neurological consequences.

Microbiology Link

GABA-releasing bacteria are known and include *H. influenzae, E. coli, B. fragilis, P. mirabilis, P. enterococcus, S. aureus, P. aeruginosa* and *K. pneumoniae*.[113] Bacterial lipopolysaccharide (LPS) can stimulate an increase in GABA and taurine output in adult rats,[114] and, interestingly, autistic urine fractions have been found to stimulate the release of GABA and taurine. It has been suggested that intestinal bacteria could be a major source of a substance present in plasma that can bind to GABA receptors[110] to impair neurological transmission. Therefore, an increase in GI tract permeability, as described in a previous section, coupled with an increasingly permeable BBB could lead to severe neurological dysfunction.

Fatty Acid Metabolism

Clinical and biochemical research have indicated changes in the metabolism of fatty acids in several psychiatric disorders. It has therefore been suggested that fatty acids may have a role to play in autism.[115] Loci on 15 different human chromosomes have been implicated in autism and many of these could potentially play a role in fatty acid metabolism.[116] It has been suggested that the genetic component of autism may be an over-activity of the enzyme cytosolic (type IV) phospholipase A2 (cPLA2), which is responsible for removing arachidonic acid (AA) from membrane phospholipids.[117]

The essential fatty acid (EFA), linoleic acid, is the precursor for the formation of the highly unsaturated fatty acids (HUFAs), arachidonic acid (AA) and dihomo-gamma linolenic acid (DGLA). Alpha-linolenic acid is the precursor for the eicosapentanoic acid (EPA) and docosahexanoic acid (DHA), both HUFAs. DHA is the major constituent of synaptic end sites, and AA is present in the growth cone region and synaptosomes. The eicosanoids are derived from AA and include prostaglandins, thromboxanes, and leukotrienes, which regulate a wide range of physiological processes including the normal functioning of neural synapses, with high concentrations leading to pathological conditions.

AA and DHA are found in lower concentrations in many neurodevelopmental diseases[118,119] compared to controls. Reduced amounts of HUFA have been found in the red blood cell membranes of one patient with autistic spectrum disorder and in a significant number of schizophrenic individuals. There are reports that supplements of fatty acids can help to alleviate symptoms of dyslexia, ADHD, and dyspraxia in some cases,[120] suggesting that autism may be a fatty acid metabolism disorder.

Infants require more HUFA during the last trimester of pregnancy and in the first few months of post-natal development compared with later in development. Therefore, if the intake of EFA is insufficient, this could seriously affect the brain development of the fetus. Thus the environmental factor of autism may be attributable to the dietary intake of EFA from which the HUFA are produced. In rats there is a higher requirement of HUFA in males than in females,[121,122] and if this is also true of humans, a deficiency in HUFA would affect more males than females as observed in autism.

Microbiological Link

Bacterial endotoxin (LPS) has been shown to alter the lipid and fatty acid metabolism in peroxisomes, decrease cholesterol and fatty acid content, and alter the cholesterol/fatty acid ratio.[123] CPLA2 activity and release of AA is known to be upregulated by bacteria.[123] A novel phospholipid diacylglycerol pyrophosphate (DGPP) present in bacteria is capable of activating macrophages to release arachidonic acid metabolites such as protaglandins,[124] and it has been suggested that bacterial constituents may be responsible for enhanced cyclooxygenase 2 (COX-2) expression in vivo[125] (COX is required in the formation of prostaglandins from AA). Hence the co-morbidity seen in neurodevelopmental disorders may be attributable to bacteria-induced cPLA2 DGPP or COX-2 expression.

In Utero Factors

Prenatal stress and an increased HUFA requirement during pregnancy have been linked with fetal characteristics of autism. Morphological abnormalities within the limbic system and cerebellum regions of the brain have frequently been reported at post mortem examination of autistic individuals with approximately 10–20% having macrocephalia, which is most noticeable in the occipital and parietal lobes. The pre-frontal cortex (PFC affected in schizophrenia) has been proposed as a potential site of toxicant-induced damage which may lead to autistic behaviour since lesions in this region are known to lead to distractibility and an impairment of the ability to inhibit inappropriate behaviour: both features of autism. Specific regions of the brain have differing "windows of vulnerability" during development[126] and it is thought that maturity of the PFC may even continue beyond puberty. Thus the PFC is a potentially promising site of toxicant-induced damage leading to ASD.

Microbiological Link

Bacterial products and toxins entering the systemic circulation (via increased GI tract permeability and/or altered BBB permeability) could cause damage to the developing brain from the period including fetal development to puberty.

Neurotransmission and Bacteria

There are many reasons to suspect an underlying bacterial cause of autism. Having described some of the major theories of autism and indicated how bacteria may be playing a role, in this final section what will be highlighted will be the possibility that bacterial products may also interfere with normal neurotransmission by the production of neuropeptide-processing enzymes.

A Basic Local Alignment *Search* Tool (BLAST) search against finished and unfinished microbial genomes (http://www.ncbi.nlm.nih.gov) has indicated several predicted bacterial proteins that could affect neurotransmission. Certain predicted bacterial proteins show strong similarity and identity with neprilysin, endothelin-eonverting Enzyme (ECE), carboxypeptidase E proprotein, and prohormone convertases, often having a conserved active site. Many of these enzymes are required for correct processing of neuropeptides. Bacterial homologues could cause inappropriate processing of neuropeptides to alter peptidergic transmission. Neprilysins inactivate peptide neurotransmitters in the synaptic cleft, and therefore the bacterial neprilysins could reduce peptidergic neurotransmission.

The homology between the bacterial and human proteins is especially good in some cases so that it is possible that epitope mimicry could elicit an autoimmune response and affect neurotransmission in that way.

Conclusions

On the basis of the literature to date, there is no single underlying cause of ASD. There is growing awareness that ASD can have an infectious nature that may be a co-factor for the illness or appear as an opportunistic infection(s) that can aggravate patient morbidity.[127–132] There are several plausible genetic defects that could result in autistic behaviour in children such as alterations in GABAergic transmission, fatty acid metabolism, PST defects, or peptidase deficiencies, among others. However, it is known that there must be an environmental role in the aetiology of autism. It is proposed here in this chapter that bacteria may be responsible for exacerbation of an existing genetic predisposition for autism and that the many diverse, apparently unrelated data recorded from autistic individuals may be unified by this bacterial hypothesis. In fact, there is growing evidence that bacteria and viruses are significant to autism.[133] ASD patients generally have a high prevalence of one or more *Mycoplasma* spp. and sometimes show evidence of infections with *Chlamydia pneumoniae*. The significance of these infections in ASD is discussed in by Nicolson and collegues.[133] Many autistic children experience severe dietary and/or GI problems (including abdominal pain, constipation, diarrhoea, and bloating). Such symptoms may be due to a disruption of the indigenous gut flora promoting the overgrowth of potentially pathogenic (toxin-producing) microorganisms.[134] Typically, parents claim that GI problems and behaviour symptoms manifest in parallel. The first true link towards bacteria and autism transpired in 1998 when Bolte published a hypothesis that *Clostridium tetani* (or other bacteria in the gut) might play a role in late-onset autism.[134]

There are many reasons to consider that intestinal bacteria may be involved in autism, but on the basis of the literature to date it is generally appreciated that onset of autism is known to occur often following antimicrobial therapy. Also, the GI symptoms associated with autism are very common at the onset and these often persist. Additionally, antimicrobials are known to have a significant effect in both the relapse and continuation of the autistic condition. Because of this, the bacteria that have been most considered to be associated with autism have been clostridium. The reasons for this are highlighted in this chapter, but just to reiterate, the antimicrobials that most commonly predisposes to late-onset autism are trimethoprim/sulphamethoxazole, a drug that is not very effective against gut clostridia. Also, a number of autistic patients have been shown to respond to vancomycin and oral metronidazole. As these antibiotics are geared towards anaerobic Gram-positive bacteria, an association of autism with clostridium has been suggested. Also, high tetanus antitoxin titres have been recorded in a number of patients with late-onset autism. In addition to this, Clostridium and other intestinal flora are known to produce enterotoxins and neurotoxins as well as a number of detrimental metabolites.[135] Recent studies[136–138] have demonstrated that certain clostridial species were specific to autistic samples and not seen in faecal samples from healthy subjects. Also, bacteria such as *Clostridium bolteae* and *Cetobacterium somerae* have been observed in stools of children with autism, and it is probable that there are interactions between intestinal microflora.[139] To date, however, there is a very limited amount of work that has investigated the clostridial populations and other gut flora in ASD individuals.

The gut microbiology and the acquisition of certain bacteria during the ageing process may have a significant part to play in autism. However, because there is a lack of detailed comparisons of the composition of the gut flora of people with ASD compared with healthy controls, this has significantly hindered this line of investigation. While a number of authors have researched and hypothesized about the likely role of clostridia in autism, this area still needs to be substantiated with further studies. To date, by far the best evidence available suggesting a role for gut bacteria in autism has transpired from the results generated in a study undertaken by Parracho et al. in 2005.[140] In this study, 40 boys and 10 girls (aged between 3 and 16), all of whom had been diagnosed with ASDs, had their intestinal flora compared with that of control individuals. Results generated in this study showed that there was a significantly higher incidence of *Clostridium histolyticum* in the faecal flora of ASD patients when compared to healthy children. The predominant bacterial population in samples from ASD patients was *C. histolyticum* (*Clostridium* clusters 1 and 11). This study clearly provides further evidence of an association between clostridia and the development of certain autistic characteristics. The degree of association is presently unknown. As we are now within an era of bacterial communities and sociomicrobiology (biofilmology), any possible association between bacteria and autism may be more complex than a "one bug one disease" hypothesis! It is hoped that research in this direction may provide further clues concerning the cause(s) of this distressing condition.

References

1. Kanner L. Autistic disturbances of affective contact. Nervous child 1943;2:217–250.
2. Lord C, Cook EH, Leventhal BL, Amaral DG. Autism spectrum disorders. Neuron 2000;28:355–363.
3. Landa RJ, Holman KC, Garrett-Mayer E. Social and communication development in toddlers with early and later diagnosis of autism spectrum disorders. Arch Gen Psychiatry 2007; 64:853–864.
4. Geschwind DH, Levitt P. Autism spectrum disorders: developmental disconnection syndromes. Curr Opin Neurobiol 2007;17:103–111.
5. Richardson AJ, Ross MA. Fatty acid metabolism in neurodevelopmental disorder: a new perspective on associations between attention-deficit/hyperactivitiy disorder dyslexia dyspraxia and the autistic spectrum. Prostaglandins, leukotrienes and essential fatty acids. Prostaglandins Leukot Essent Fatty Acids 2000;63:1–10.
6. Rice CE, Baio J, Van Naarden Braun K, Doernberg N, Meaney FJ, Kirby RS. ADDM Network. A public health collaboration for the surveillance of autism spectrum disorders. Paediatr Perinat Epidemiol 2007;21:179–190.
7. Kaye JA, Melero-Montes MM, Jick H. Mumps measles and rubella vaccine and the incidence of autism recorded by general practitioners: a time trend analysis. BMJ 2001;322:460–463.
8. Little J. Epidemiology of neurodevelopmental disorders in children. Prostaglandins Leukot Essent Fatty Acids 2000;63(1/2):11–20.
9. Fombonne E. The prevalence of autism. JAMA 2003;289(1):87–89.
10. Comi AM, Zimmerman AW, Frye VH, Law PA, Peeden JN. Familial clustering of autoimmune disorders and evaluation of medical risk factors in autism. J Child Neurol 1999;14: 388–394.
11. Herbert MR, Russo JP, Yang S, Roohi J, Blaxill M, Kahler SG, Cremer L, Hatchwell E. Autism and environmental genomics. Neurotoxicology 2006;27:671–684.

12. Minshew NJ, Williams DL. The new neurobiology of autism: cortex, connectivity, and neuronal organization. Arch Neurol 2007;64:945–950.
13. Pardo CA, Vargas DL, Zimmerman AW. Immunity, neuroglia and neuroinflammation in autism. Int Rev Psychiatry 2005;17:485–495.
14. Hornig M, Chian D, Lipkin WI. Neurotoxic effects of postnatal thimerosal are mouse strain dependent. Mol Psychiatry 2004;9:833–845.
15. Bigazzi PE. Autoimmunity and heavy metals. Lupus 1994;3:449–453.
16. Landa RJ, Holman KC, Garrett-Mayer E. Social and communication development in toddlers with early and later diagnosis of autism spectrum disorders. Arch Gen Psychiatry 2007; 64:853–864.
17. Pardo CA, Vargas DL, Zimmerman AW. Immunity, neuroglia and neuroinflammation in autism. Int Rev Psychiatry 2005;17:485–495.
18. Ashwood P, Wills S, Van de WJ. The immune response in autism: a new frontier for autism research. J Leukoc Biol 2006;80:1–15.
19. Korvatska E, Van de WJ, Anders TF, Gershwin ME. Genetic and immunologic considerations in autism. Neurobiol Dis 2002;9:107–125.
20. Licinio J, Alvarado I, Wong ML. Autoimmunity in autism. Mol Psychiatry 2002;7:329.
21. Torrente F, Ashwood P, Day R, Machado N, Furlano RI, Anthony A, Davies SE, Wakefield AJ, Thomson MA, Walker-Smith JA, Murch SH. Small intestinal enteropathy with epithelial IgG and complement deposition in children with regressive autism. Mol Psychiatry 2002;7:375–382, 334.
22. Everest P. Stress and bacteria: microbial endocrinology. Gut 2007;56(8):1037–1038.
23. Buitelaar JK, Willemsen-Swinkels SHN. Autism: current theories regarding its pathogenesis and implications for rational pharmacotherapy. Pediatr Drugs 2000;2:67–81.
24. Fombonne E, Mazaubrun C. Prevalence of infantile autism in four French regions. Soc Psychiatry Psychiatr Epidemiol 1992;27:203–210.
25. Folstein S, Rutter M. Infantile autism: a genetic study of 21 twin pairs. J Child Psychol Psychiatry 1977;18:297–321.
26. Ritvo ER, Freeman BJ, Mason-Brothers A, Mo A, Ritvo AM. Concordance for the syndrome of autism in 40 pairs of afflicted twins. Am J Psychiatry 1985;142:74–77.
27. Steffenburg S, Gillberg C, Hellgren L, Anderson L, Gillberg IC, Jakobsson G, Bohman M. A twin study of autism in Denmark Finland Iceland Norway and Sweden. J Child Psychol Psychiatry 1989;3:405–416.
28. Lauritsen MB, Pedersen CB, Mortensen PB. Effects of familial risk factors and place of birth on the risk of autism: a nationwide register-based study. J Child Psychol Psychiatry 2005;46 (9):963–971.
29. Lauritsen M, Ewald H. The genetics of autism. Acta Psychiatr Scand 2001;103:411–427.
30. Gilling M, Lauritsen MB, Møller M, Henriksen KF, Vicente A, Oliveira G, Cintin C, Eiberg H, Andersen PS, Mors O, Rosenberg T, Brøndum-Nielsen K, Cotterill RM, Lundsteen C, Ropers HH, Ullmann R, Bache I, Tümer Z, Tommerup N. A 3.2 Mb deletion on 18q12 in a patient with childhood autism and high-grade myopia. Eur J Hum Genet 2008;16(3):312–319.
31. Muhle R, Trentacoste SV, Rapin I. The genetics of autism. Pediatrics 2004;113(5):e472–e486.
32. Spence SJ. The genetics of autism. Semin Pediatr Neurol 2004;11(3):196–204.
33. Sebat J, Lakshmi B, Malhotra D, Troge J, Lese-Martin C, Walsh T, Yamrom B, Yoon S, Krasnitz A, Kendall J, Leotta A, Pai D, Zhang R, Lee YH, Hicks J, Spence SJ, Lee AT, Puura K, Lehtimäki T, Ledbetter D, Gregersen PK, Bregman J, Sutcliffe JS, Jobanputra V, Chung W, Warburton D, King MC, Skuse D, Geschwind DH, Gilliam TC, Ye K, Wigler M. Strong association of de novo copy number mutations with autism. Science 2007;316(5823):445–449.
34. Lopez-Rangel E, Lewis ME. Further evidence for epigenetic influence of MECP2 in Rett, autism and Angelman's syndromes. Clin Genet 2006;69(1):23–25.
35. Israngkun PP, Newman HAI, Patel ST. Potential biochemical markers for infantile autism. Neurochem Pathol 1986;5:51–70.

36. Minderaa RB, Anderson GM, Volkmar FR, Harcherick D, Akkerhuis GW, Cohen DJ. Whole blood serotonin and tryptophan in autism: temporal stability and the effects of medication. J Autism Dev Disord 1989;19:129–136.
37. Anderson GM, Horne WC, Chatterjee D, Cohen DJ. The hyperserotonemia of autism. Ann N Y Acad Sci 1990;600:331–342.
38. van der Mast RC, Fekkes D. Serotonin and amino acids: partners in delerium pathophysiology. Semin Clin Neuropsychiatry 2000;5(2):125–131.
39. Pedersen OS, Lui Y, Reichelt KL. Serotonin-uptake stimulating peptide found in plasma of normal individuals and in some autistic urines. J Peptide Res 1999;53:633–640.
40. Bell JG, Satgent DR, Tocher DR, Dick JR. Red blood cell fatty acid compositions in a patient with autistic spectrum disorder: a characteristic abnormality in neurodevelopmental disorders? Prostaglandins Leukot Essent Fatty Acids 2000;63(1/2):21–25.
41. Peters DA. Prenatal stress: effects on brain biogenic amine and plasma corticosterone levels. Pharamacol Biochem Behav 1982;17(4):721–725.
42. Scott MM, Deneris ES. Making and breaking serotonin neurons and autism. Int J Dev Neurosci 2005;23:277–285.
43. Burgess NK, Sweeten TL, McMahon WM, Fujinami RS. Hyperserotoninemia and altered immunity in autism. J Autism Dev Disord 2006;36:697–704.
44. Cook EH. Autism: review of neurochemical investigation. Synapse 1990;6:292–308.
45. Lam KS, Aman MG, Arnold LE. Neurochemical correlates of autistic disorder: a review of the literature. Res Dev Disabil 2006;27:254–289.
46. McDougle CJ, Scahill L, McCracken JT, Aman MG, Tierney E, Arnold LE, Freeman BJ, Martin A, McGough JJ, Cronin P, Posey DJ, Riddle MA, Ritz L, Swiezy NB, Vitiello B, Volkmar FR, Votolato NA, Walson P. Research Units on Pediatric Psychopharmacology (RUPP) Autism Network. Background and rationale for an initial controlled study of risperidone. Child Adolesc Psychiatr Clin N Am 2000;9:201–224.
47. Moore ML, Eichner SF, Jones JR. Treating functional impairment of autism with selective serotonin-reuptake inhibitors. Ann Pharmacother 2004;38:1515–1519.
48. Posey DJ, Erickson CA, Stigler KA, McDougle CJ. The use of selective serotonin reuptake inhibitors in autism and related disorders. J Child Adolesc Psychopharmacol 2006;16:181–186.
49. Martineau J, Perrot A, Hérault J, Mallet J, Petit E, Sauvage D, Guérin P, Lelord G, Hameury L, Müh J-P. Catecholaminergic metabolism and autism. Dev Med Child Neurol 1994;36:688–697.
50. Garreau B, Barthélémy C, Jouve J, Bruneau N, Müh JP, Lelord G. Urinary homovanillic acid levels of autistic children. Dev Med Child Neurol 1988;30:93–98.
51. Dunn AJ. Endotoxin-induced activation of cerebral catecholamine and serotonin metabolism: comparison with interleukin-1. J Pharmacol Exp Ther 1992;261(3):964–969.
52. Dunn AJ, Welch J. Stress- and endotoxin-induced increases in brain tryptophan and serotonin metabolism depend on sympathetic nervous system activity. J Neurochem 1991;57(5):1615–1622.
53. Dunn AJ. Effects of cytokines and infections on brain neurochemistry. Clin Neurosci Res 2006;6(1–2):52–68.
54. Ando T, Brown RF, Berg RD, Dunn AJ. Bacterial translocation can increase plasma corticosterone and brain catecholamine and indoleamine metabolism. Am J Physiol Regul Integr Comp Physiol 2000;279(6):R2164–2172.
55. Hyland K, Beaman BL, LeWitt PA, DeMaggio AJ. Monoamine changes in the brain of BALB/c mice following sub-lethal infection with *Nocardia asteroides* (GUH-2). Neurochem Res 2000;25(4):443–448.
56. D'Eufemia P, Celli M, Finocchiaro R, Pacifico L, Viozzi L, Zaccagnini M, Cardi E, Giardini O. Abnormal intestinal permeability in children with autism. Acta Paediatr 1996;85:1076–1079.

57. Reichelt K-L, Ekrem J, Scott H. Gluten milk proteins and autism: dietary intervention effects on behaviour and peptide secretion. J Appl Nutr 1990;42(1):1–11.
58. Alberti A, Pirrone P, Elia M, Waring RH, Romano C. Sulphation deficit in 'low functioning' autistic children: a pilot study. Biol Psychiatry 1999;46(3):420–424.
59. Le Couteur A, Trygstad O, Evered C, Gillberg C, Rutter M. Infantile autism and urinary excretion of peptides and protein-associated peptide complexes. J Autism Dev Disord 1988;18:181–190.
60. Gilberg C, Trygstad O, Foss I. Childhood psychosis and urinary excretion of peptides and protein-associated complexes. J Autism Dev Disord 1982;12 (3):229–241.
61. Trygstad OE, Reichelt KL, Foss I, Edminson PD, Saelid G, Bremer J, Hole K, Ørbeck H, Johansen JH, Bøler JB, Titlestad K, Opstad PK. Patterns of peptides and protein-associated-peptide complexes in psychiatric disorders. Br J Psychiatry 1980;136:59–72.
62. Zioudrou C, Streaty RA, Klee WA. Opioid peptides derived from food proteins. J Biol Chem 1979;254:2446–2449.
63. Huebner FR, Lieberman KW, Rubino RP, Wall JS. Demonstration of high opioid-like activity in isolated peptides from wheat gluten hydrolysates. Peptides 1984;5:1139–1147.
64. Lottspeich F, Henschen A, Brantl V, Teschemacher H. Novel opioid peptides derived from casein (beta-casomorphins) III Synthetic peptides corresponding to components from bovine casein peptone. Hoppe Seyler's Z Physiol Chem 1990;361:1835–1839.
65. Reichelt WH, Knivsberg A-M, Nodland M, Stensrud M, Reichelt KL. Urinary peptide levels and patterns in autistic children from seven countries and the effect of dietary intervention after 4 years. Dev Brain Dysfunct 1997;10:44–55.
66. Reichelt KL, Knivsberg A-M, Lind G, Nodland M. Brain Dysfunct 1991;4:308–319.
67. Reichelt KL, Hole K, Hamberger A, Saelid G, Edminsson PD, Braestrup C, Lingjaerde O, Orbeck H. Biologically active peptide-containing fractions in schizophrenia and childhood autism. Adv Biochem Psychopharmacol 1986;28:627–643.
68. Wakefield AJ, Anthony A, Murch SH, Thomson M, Montgomery DSM, Davies S, O'Leary JJ, Berelowitz M, Walker-Smith JA. Enterocolitis in children with developmental disorders. Am J Gastroenterol 2000;95(9):2285–2295.
69. Horvath K, Papadimitriou JC, Rabsztyn A, Drachenberg C, Tildon JT. Gastrointestinal abnormalities in children with autistic disorder. J Pediatr 1999;135:559–563.
70. Brandtzaeg P, Baekkevold ES, Farstad IN, Jahnsen FL, Johansen FE, Nilsen EM, Yamanaka T. Regional specialization in the mucosal immune system: what happens in the microcompartments? Immunol Today 1999;20:141–151.
71. MacDermott RP. Immunology of inflammatory bowel disease. Curr Opin Gastroenterol 1999;14:54–67.
72. Caradonna L, Amati L, Magrone T, Pellegrino NM, Jirillo E, Caccavo D. Enteric bacteria lipopolysaccharides and related cyotokines in inflammatory bowel disease: biological and clinical significance. J Endotoxin Res 2000;6(3):205–214.
73. Sellon RK, Tonkonogy S, Schultz M, Dieleman LA, Grenther W, Balish E, Rennick DM, Sartor RB. Resident enteric bacteria are necessary for the development of spontaneous colitis and immune system activation in interleukin-10-deficient mice. Infect Immunol 1998; 66:5524–5231.
74. Ohno Y, Lee J, Fusunyan RD, MacDermott RP, Sanderson IR. Macrophage inflammatory protein-2: chromosomal regulation in rat small intestinal epithelial cells. Proc Natl Acad Sci USA 1997;94:10279–10284.
75. Caradonna L, Amati L, Lella P, Jirillo E, Caccavo D. Phagocytosis killing lymphocyte-mediated antibacterial activity serum autoantibodies and plasma endotoxin in inflammatory bowel disease. Am J Gastroenterol 2000;95:1495–1502.
76. Wellmann W, Fink PC, Benner F, Schmidt FW. Endotoxaemia in active Crohn's disease treatment with whole gut irrigation and 5-aminosalicylic acid. Gut 1986;27:814–820.
77. Wyatt J, Vogelsang H, Hub LW, Waldhoe T, Lochs H. Intestinal permeability and the prediction of relapse in Crohn's disease. Lancet 1993;341:1437–1439.

78. Fabia R, Ar'Rajab A, Johansson ML, Andersson R, Willén R, Jeppsson B, Molin G, Bengmark S. Impairment of bacterial flora in human ulcerative colitis and experimental colitis in the rat. Digestion 1993;54:248–255.

79. Favier C, Neut C, Milon C, Cortot A, Colombel JF, Milon J. Fecal (-D-galactosidase production and bifidobacteria are decreased in Crohn's disease. Dig Dis Sci 1997;42:817–822.

80. De Simone C, Ciardi A, Grassi A, Lambert Gardini S, Tzantzoglou S, Trinchieri V, Moretti S, Jirillo E. Effect of *Bifidobacterium bifidium* and *Lactobacillus acidophilus* on gut mucosa and peripheral blood B lymphocytes. Immunopharmacol Immunotoxicol 1992;14:331–340.

81. Gionchetti P, Rizzello F, Venturi A, et al. Maintenance treatment of chronic pouchitis: a randomized placebo-controled double-blind trial with a new probiotic preparation. Gastroenterology 1998;114:G4037 p A985.

82. Coffey MJ, Phare SM, Peters-Golden M. Prolonged exposure to lipopolysaccharide inhibits macrophage 5-lipoxygenase metabolism via induction of nitric oxide synthesis. J Immunol 2000;165(7):3592–3598.

83. Middleton SJ, Shorthouse M, Hunter JO. Increased nitric oxide synthesis in ulcerative colitis. Lancet 1993;341:465–466.

84. Jourd'heuil D, Morise Z, Conner EM, Grisham MB. Oxidants transcription factors and intestinal inflammation. J Clin Gastroenterol 1997;25:561–572.

85. Pitcher MC, Beatty ER, Gibson GR, et al. Incidence and activities of sulphate-reducing bacteria in patients with ulcerative colitis. Gut 1995;36:A63.

86. Pitcher MC, Cummings JH. Hydrogen sulphide: a bacterial toxin in ulcerative colitis? Gut 1996;39:1–4.

87. Pitcher MC, Beatty ER, Cummings JH. The contribution of sulphate reducing bacteria and 5-aminosalicylic acid to faecal sulphide in patients with ulcerative colitis. Gut 2000; 46(1):64–72.

88. Gotteland M, Cruchet Muñoz S, Araya Quezada M, Espinoza Madariaga J, Brunser Tesarschü O. Intestinal permeability in the first year of life. The effect of diarrhea. An Esp Pediatr 1998;49(2):125–128.

89. Cohly HH, Panja A. Immunological findings in autism. Int Rev Neurobiol 2005;71:317–341.

90. Fujinami RS, Oldstone MB, Wroblewska Z, Frankel ME, Koprowski H. Molecular mimicry in virus infections: cross reaction of measles virus phosphoprotein or of herpes simplex viral protein with human intermediate filaments. Proc Natl Acad Sci USA 1983;80(8):2346–2350.

91. Comi AM, Zimmerman AW, Frye VH, Law PA, Peeden JN. Familial clustering of autoimmune disorders and evaluation of medical risk factors in autism. J Child Neurol 1999; 14:388–394.

92. Sweeten TL, Bowyer SL, Posey DJ, Halberstadt GM, McDougle CJ. Increased prevalence of familial autoimmunity in probands with pervasive developmental disorders. Pediatrics 2003;112:e420.

93. Money J, Bobrow NA, Clarke FC. Autism and autoimmune disease: a family study. J Autism Child Schizophr 1971;1:146–160.

94. Ginn LR, Lin JP, Plotz PH, Bale SJ, Wilder RL, Mbauya A. Familial autoimmunity in pedigrees of idiopathic inflammatory myopathy patients suggests common genetic risk factors for many autoimmune diseases. Arthritis Rheum 1998;41:400–405.

95. Kozlovskaia GV, Kliushnik TP, Goriunova AV, Turkova IL, Kalinina MA, Sergienko NS. Nerve growth factor auto-antibodies in children with various forms of mental dysontogenesis and in schizophrenia high risk group. Zh Nevropatol Psihiatr S S Korsakova 2000;100:50–52.

96. Singh VK, Rivas WH. Prevalence of serum antibodies to caudate nucleus in autistic children. Neurosci Lett 2004;355:53–56.

97. Silva SC, Correia C, Fesel C, Barreto M, Coutinho AM, Marques C. Autoantibody repertoires to brain tissue in autism nuclear families. J Neuroimmunol 2004;152:176–182.

98. Croen LA, Grether JK, Yoshida CK, Odouli R, Van de Water J. Maternal autoimmune diseases, asthma and allergies, and childhood autism spectrum disorders: a case-control study. Arch Pediatr Adolesc Med 2005;159(2):151–157.

99. Yuki N. Current cases in which epitope mimicry is considered a component cause of autoimmune disease: Guillain–Barré syndrome. Cell Mol Life Sci 2000;57:527–533.

100. Cunningham MW, McCormack JM, Talaber LR, Harley JB, Ayoub EM, Muneer RS, Chun LT, Reddy DV. Human monoclonal antibodies reactive with antigens of the group A Streptococcus and human heart. J Immunol 1988;141:2706–2760.

101. Jones DB, Coulson AF, Duff GW. Sequence homologies between hsp60 and autoantigens. Immunol Today 1993;14:115–118.

102. Rose NR, Mackay IR. Molecular mimicry: a critical look at exemplary instances in human diseases. Cell Mol Life Sci 2000;57:542–551.

103. Ebringer RW, Cawdell DR, Cowling P, Ebringer A. Sequential studies in ankylosing spondylitis: association of *Klebsiella pneumoniae* with active disease. Ann Rheum Dis 1978;37:146–151.

104. Shoenfeld Y, Aron-Maor A. Vaccination and autoimmunity – 'vaccinosis': a dangerous liaison? J Autoimmun 2000;14:1–10.

105. Goodacre JA, Brownlie CED, Ross DA. Bacterial superantigens in autoimmune arthritis Br J Rheumatol 1994;33:413–419.

106. Wakefield AJ, Murch SH, Anthony A, Linnell J, Casson DM, Malik M, Berelowitz M, Dhillon AP, Thomson MA, Harvey P, Valentine A, Davies SE, Walker-Smith JA. Ileal-lymphoid-nodular-hyperplasia non-specific colitis and pervasive developmental disorder in children. Lancet 1998;351:637–641.

107. Chen W, Landau S, Sham P, Fombonne E. No evidence for links between autism, MMR and measles virus. Psychol Med 2004;34(3):543–553.

108. Riedel DD, Kaufmann SH. Differential tolerance induction by lipoarabinomannan and lipopolysaccharide in human macrophages. Microbes Infect 2000;2(5):463–471.

109. Bass MP, Menold MM, Wolpert CM, Donnelly SL, Ravan SA, Hauser ER, Maddox LO, Vance JM, Abramson RK, Wright HH, Gilbert JR, Cuccaro ML, DeLong GR, Pericak-Vance MA. Genetic studies in autistic disorder and chromosome 15. Neurogenetics 2000;2(4):219–226.

110. Saunders NR, Knott GW, Dziegielewska KM. Barriers in the immature brain. Cell Mol Neurobiol 2000;20(1):29–40.

111. Jones EA, Schafer DF, Ferenci P, Pappas SC. The GABA hypothesis of hepatic encephalopathy: current status. Yale J Biol Med 1984;57:301–316.

112. Friedman HM, Macarak EJ, MacGregor RR, Wolfe J, Kefalides NA. Virus infection of endothelial cells. J Infect Dis 1981;143(2):266–273.

113. Minuk GY. Gamma-aminobutyric acid (GABA) production by eight common bacterial pathogens. Scand J Infect Dis 1986;18:465–467.

114. Feleder C, Arias P, Refojo S, Nacht S, Moguilevsky JA. Age-related differences in the effects of bacterial endotoxin (LPS) upon the release of LHRH gonadotropins and hypothalamic inhibitory amino acid neurotransmitters measured in tissues explanted form intact male rats. Exp Clin Endocrinol Diab 2000;108:220–227.

115. Vancassel S, Durand G, Barthélémy C, Lejeune B, Martineau J, Guilloteau D, Andrès C, Chalon S. Plasma fatty acid levels in autistic children. Prostaglandins Leukot Essent Fatty Acids 2001;65(1):1–7.

116. Bennett CN, Horrobin DF. Gene targets related to phospholipid and fatty acid metabolism in schizophrenia and other psychiatric disorders: an update. Prostaglandins Leukot Essent Fatty Acids 2000;63(1/2):47–59.

117. Bell JG, MacKinlay EE, Dick JR, MacDonald DJ, Boyle RM, Glen AC. Essential fatty acids and phospholipase A2 in autistic spectrum disorders. Prostaglandins Leukot Essent Fatty Acids 2004;71(4):201–204.

118. Piven J, Tsai G, Nehme E, Coyle JT, Chase GA, Folstein SE. Platelet serotonin a possible marker for familial autism J Autism Dev Disord 1991;21:51–59.

119. Ross MA. Could oxidative stress be a factor in neurodevelopmental disorders? Prostaglandins Leukot Essent Fatty Acids 2000;63(1/2):61–63.

120. Stordy BJ. Dyslexia attention deficit disorder dyspraxia: do fatty acid supplements help? Dyslexia Rev 1997;9:5–7.
121. Archelos JJ, Hartung H-P. Pathogenic role of autoantibodies in neurological diseases. Trends Neurosci 2000;23:317–327.
122. Pudelkewicz C, Seufert J, Holman RT. Requirements of the female rat for linoleic and linolenic acids. J Nutr 1968;94:138–146.
123. Khan M, Contreras M, Singh I. Endotoxin-induced alterations of lipid and fatty acid compositions in rat liver peroxisomes. J Endotoxin Res 2000;6(1):41–50.
124. Balsinde J, Balboa MA, Dennis EA. Group IV cytosolic phospholipase A2 activation by diacylglycerol pyrophosphate in murine P388D1 macrophages. Ann NY Acad Sci 2000;905:11–15.
125. Morton RS, Dongari-Bagtzoglou AI. Cyclooxygenase-2 is upregulated in inflamed gingival tissues. J Periodontol 2001;72(4):461–469.
126. Rice D, Barone S. Critical periods of vulnerability for the developing nervous system: evidence from humans and animal models. Environ Health Perspect 2000;108:511–533.
127. Takahashi H, Arai S, Tanaka-Taya K, Okabe N. Autism and infection/immunization episodes in Japan. Jpn J Infect Dis 2001;54:78–79.
128. Yamashita Y, Fujimoto C, Nakajima E, Isagai T, Matsuishi T. Possible association between congenital cytomegalovirus infection and autistic disorder. J Autism Dev Disord 2003;33:355–459.
129. Libbey JE, Coon HH, Kirkman NJ, Sweeten TL, Miller JN, Lainhart JE, McMahon WM, Fujinami RS. Are there altered antibody responses to measles, mumps, or rubella viruses in autism? J Neurovirol 2007;13(3):252–259.
130. Libbey JE, Coon HH, Kirkman NJ, Sweeten TL, Miller JN, Stevenson EK, Lainhart JE, McMahon WM, Fujinami RS. Are there enhanced MBP autoantibodies in autism? J Autism Dev Disord 2008;38(2):324–332.
131. Libbey JE, Sweeten TL, McMahon WM, Fujinami RS. Autistic disorder and viral infections. J Neurovirol 2005;11(1):1–10.
132. Singh VK, Lin SX, Yang VC. Serological association of measles virus and human herpesvirus-6 with brain autoantibodies in autism. Clin Immunol Immunopathol 1998;89(1):105–108.
133. Nicolson GL, Gan R, Nicolson NL, Haier J. Evidence for *Mycoplasma* sp, *Chlamydia pneunomiae*, and human herpes virus-6 coinfections in the blood of patients with autistic spectrum disorders. J Neurosci Res 2007;85(5):1143–1148.
134. Bolte ER. Autism and *Clostridium tetani*. Med Hypotheses 1998;51:133–144.
135. Brook I. Clostridial infection in children. J Med Microbiol 1995;42:78–82.
136. Finegold SM, Molitoris D, Song Y, Liu C, Vaisanen ML, Bolte E, McTeague M, Sandler R, Wexler H, Marlowe EM, Collins MD, Lawson PA, Summanen P, Baysallar M, Tomzynski TJ, Read E, Johnson E, Rolfe R, Nasir P, Shah H, Haake DA, Manning P, Kaul A. Gastrointestinal microflora studies in late-onset autism. Clin Infect Dis 2002;35:S6–S16.
137. Song Y, Liu C, Finegold SY. Real-time PCR quantification of clostridia in feces of autistic children. Appl Environ Micobiol 2004;70:6459–6465.
138. Finegold SM. Therapy and epidemiology of autism-clostridial spores as key elements. Med Hypotheses 2008;70(3):508–511.
139. Martirosian G. Anaerobic intestinal microflora in pathogenesis of autism? Postepy Hig Med Dosw 2004;58:349–351.
140. Parracho HM, Bingham MO, Gibson GR, McCartney AL. Differences between the gut microflora of children with autistic spectrum disorders and that of healthy children. J Med Microbiol 2005;54:987–991.

Chapter 14
Decomposition of Human Remains

Robert C. Janaway, Steven L. Percival, and Andrew S. Wilson

Introduction

Early scientific research into "putrefaction" by eighteenth century physicians was driven by a need to understand and treat living patients who were suffering from "putrid diseases" (presumably conditions such as treponemal disease, non-specific osteomyelitus, bacterial skin infections, abscesses, and the like, which could result in the formation of necrotic tissue, but which today can be treated by modern medicine).[1,2] But these works clearly recognized and tried to seek explanation to some of the fundamental microbially induced changes in the human body, in particular, to soft tissue that occur during different stages in the decomposition process and which result in pH change, and the evolution of volatile compounds. As such, these works are an early precursor to the discipline that today we know as "taphonomy". This term, originally coined by the Russian palaeontologist Ivan Efremov to describe the "transformations from the biosphere to the lithosphere"[3] in explaining the formation of fossils, today has much broader meaning. The term has been widely adopted in archaeology and forensic science and is concerned with the decomposition of the body and associated death scene materials. As such, the disciplines of archaeological taphonomy/diagenesis[4–7] and forensic taphonomy[8–11] cover the location of buried or disturbed human remains[12] and time since death/burial estimation, and explain the survival/differential decomposition of physical remains and macromolecules such as proteins, lipids, and DNA.

Death may be defined under two categories: somatic and cellular death.[13] In somatic death, while the person has lost sentient personality, reflex nervous activity often persists. In cellular death, the cells of the body no longer function, cease to exhibit metabolic activity, and cannot function by means of aerobic respiration.[13] Understanding the distinction between somatic and cellular death is important when considering physiological changes that occur immediately after death, when, for

R.C. Janaway, S.L. Percival, and A.S. Wilson
School of Life Sciences, University of Bradford, Bradford, West Yorkshire, UK

S.L. Percival (ed.), *Microbiology and Aging*.
DOI: 10.1007/978-1-59745-327-1_14, © Springer Science + Business Media, LLC 2009

instance, the corpse still exhibits muscular contractions, but has less relevance to much more destructive, longer term decomposition.

After the cessation of heart function, the body becomes flaccid and blood ceases to circulate. The body goes through some well-documented changes, known as the "classic triad" of livor, rigor and algor mortis. That is, the blood drains to the lower areas, and the body stiffens and cools until it approaches ambient temperature. The rate at which these changes occur is largely governed by environmental conditions, especially temperature together with microbial load and diversity.

Post Mortem Hypostasis (Lividity, Livor Mortis)

One of the earliest effects of the heart ceasing to function is that blood will drain to the lower parts of the body under the influence of gravity, and this causes a characteristic discolouration of the dependant areas termed *post mortem hypostasis*. Depletion of oxygen from the blood results in a colour change from bright red to deep purple. The collection of this deep colouring in the lower parts of the body is apparent 1–2 h after death and becomes fully developed within about 6 h and firmly fixed after 12 h.

Rigor Mortis

Except in the cases that exhibit cadaveric spasm, the first effect of death in most cases is a general relaxation of muscular tone. The lower jaw drops, the eyelids lose their tension, the muscles are soft and flabby, and the joints are flexible. Within a few hours after death, and generally while the body is cooling, the muscles of the eyelids and the jaw begin to stiffen and contract followed by similar changes in the muscles of the trunk and limbs so that the whole body becomes rigid.[13] The muscular tissue passes through three phases after death:

1. It is flaccid but contractile, still possessing cellular life
2. It becomes rigid and incapable of contraction, being dead and
3. It once more relaxes but never regaining its power of contractility

Rigor mortis is caused by the breakdown of adenosine triphosphate (ATP) and the build-up of lactic acid to about 0.3% in the muscle tissues. At this point the muscles go into an irreversible state of contraction. In temperate climates this condition usually commences within 2–4 h of death, reaching a peak at 12 h, and starts to disappear at 24 h, with the cadaver becoming limp within 36 h. The flaccidity that follows stiffening is due to the action of alkaline liquids produced by putrefaction. In contrast to rigor mortis, cadaveric spasm is a rare phenomenon of the instantaneous stiffening of specific muscle groups occurring at time of death, e.g. the hand clutching a weapon. It is usually associated with sudden, violent death.[14]

Cooling (Algor Mortis)

After death the body starts to cool, because of loss of living body heat to the external environment. The rectal temperature of a healthy adult at rest is approximately 99°F with daily variations up to 1–1.5°F. The temperature varies throughout the day, being at its lowest between 2 A.M. and 6 A.M. and highest between 4 P.M. and 6 P.M. The rate of cooling is determined by the difference in temperature between the body and its environment. For instance, in temperate climates it has been suggested that for an average adult the heat loss in air will be 1.5°F/h, while in tropical climates it is 0.75°F/h.[14,15]

Under most environmental conditions body decomposition will eventually result in the loss of soft tissue, leaving the skeletal elements. However, the study of archaeological bone has indicated that there may be residual organic material, e.g., bone collagen, surviving even after hundreds of years of burial.[16,17] In addition, there has been considerable interest in the survival of DNA from heavily degraded remains both from the point of victim identification during the investigation of mass graves, natural disasters,[18] and the recovery of ancient DNA in archaeological studies.[19,20] In addition, research has been ongoing to document the body decomposition products that are left in transit graves, where a body has been temporarily buried, or on a surface where a body has lain for time since death estimation.[21] Thus, a detailed understanding of not only the gross loss of soft tissue but also the chemistry of surviving organic molecules in bone and the soil is of importance to both forensic and archaeological scientists.

As a body decomposes, soft tissues will progressively liquefy. There are a number of processes that cause this: the body's own enzymes will self-digest material at a cellular level in a process known as *autolysis*, while the usually much more destructive process of *putrefaction* is driven by bacterial enzymes. The bulk of these putrefactive microorganisms are anaerobic and are derived from the body's own gastrointestinal (GI) tract, and their activity during the major phase of tissue breakdown keeps the tissue mass anoxic. At later stages of decomposition, extracorporeal microorganisms such as soil fungi[22] may be involved, but these can only be associated with the exterior of the body mass or after the major phase of decomposition when the remaining material is better oxygenated.

Despite the possible actions of insects or scavenging animals, it is microorganisms that consistently play a fundamental role in the decomposition of human remains. While there are recognizable changes that a body may proceed through (e.g., from putrefactive decomposition towards skeletalization), there are key variables that influence the advancement or retardation of this process. Of greatest note are the environmental constraints of temperature, moisture content, and their influence on tissue. At one extreme is the process of desiccation (natural mummification) that can retard decomposition because of the drying of tissue below a critical threshold for bacterial action. This, of course, does not preclude superficial mould growth on the outside of partially desiccated remains.

Cadaveric Decay

Decay of the body is dominated by the two destructive processes of autolysis and putrefaction. Autolysis occurs independently from any bacterial action, while putrefaction, the reduction and liquefaction of tissue, is a microbiologically dominated process.

Autolysis is a process of postmortem self destruction due to intrinsic enzymes at a cellular level. It is not apparent at a macroscopic level but can be documented histologically. Importantly, it operates without the participation of bacteria.[23–25] The postmortem release of intra- and extracellular hydrolytic enzymes denature molecules and cell membranes. Cells become detached and the cell contents are broken down.[23] The partial destruction of cellular structures will greatly facilitate further bacterially driven putrefactive change. The breakdown results from the action of bacteria and enzymes that are already present in the tissues, or enzymes, which are otherwise derived from soil microorganisms and fungi.[26,27]

The tissues of a corpse are considered to be free of microorganisms within the first 24 h following death. It is likely that a lot of the microorganisms that are circulating through out the body are continually being deactivated, as the immune responses of the body are still active over 48 h after death. After death, the microorganisms present in the body (e.g., in the GI tract) initially invade the local tissues and gain access to the rest of the body (including bone which has a good blood supply) via the vascular and lymphatic systems. As the redox potential of tissues is known to fall very quickly flowing death, the growth of obligate aerobes is substantially reduced so that bacteria such as Micrococci, *Pseudomonas* and *Acinetobacter* spp. are the only remaining viable bacteria that are found at the outer surfaces of the decaying tissue. Anaerobic bacteria become generally more prevalent.[28] While the human GI tract is composed of a very complex microbiology, only a small number of bacteria, i.e. *Clostridium* spp., Streptococci, and the Enterobacteria during the first days of death, are involved in the putrefaction process.

Putrefactive change is usually first visible on the abdominal wall, owing to the conversion of haemoglobin by anaerobic bacteria. Initial activity is usually documented in the region of the right iliac fossa where the caecum is relatively superficial.[13] Putrefaction results in widespread decomposition of the body caused largely by action of bacterial enzymes, mostly anaerobic organisms from the bowel. The process of putrefaction commences immediately after death and is visible under normal conditions from 48 to 72 h afterwards.[27] Initial signs of putrefaction are green or greenish-red discolouration of the skin of the anterior abdominal wall due to the formation of sulph-haemoglobin. This spreads to the whole of the abdominal wall, chest, and thighs, and eventually to the skin of the whole body (marbling). This usually takes about 7 days. Over time, the corpse's skin begins to go greenish owing to the formation of sulph-haemoglobin in settled blood. The gases that are generated during this decomposition process include hydrogen sulphide, carbon dioxide, methane, ammonia, sulphur dioxide, and hydrogen. These gases increase to high levels in the large bowel and around tissues that are being broken down by natural autolysis and bacterial lysis.[29] Further anaerobic fermentation in the corpse results in the development of more by-products, specifically volatile fatty acids. Over time, the natural process of putrefaction of hydrocarbons, ammonia compounds, and biogenic amines begin to accumulate in the corpse.

Because of the changes that begin to occur in the body, the indigenous micro-biota that still exists, particularly the GI flora, increase their proliferation, accelerating the whole decomposition process. It has been documented that 90% of microorganisms isolated from tissue from human corpses are strict anaerobes. The highest concentrations of bacteria isolated include mainly Gram-positive non-sporulating anaerobes such as bifidobacteria. Lower numbers of Lactobacillus, *Streptococcus* spp., and bacteria belonging to the Enterobacteriaceae group have been observed. Other bacteria that have been isolated from decomposing tissues, but in lower numbers than the bacteria mentioned above, have included *Bacillus* sp., yeasts, *Staphylococcus* spp., and *Pseudomonas* sp.[30,31]

In the early stages of decomposition, bacteria isolated from human corpses have included, among others, *Staphylococcus* sp., *Candida* sp., *Malasseria* sp., *Bacillus* sp., and *Streptococcus* spp. While a number of non-fastidious bacteria have been identified from decaying human matter, because of the very high abundance of microorganisms associated with the host a major overgrowth of bacteria both culturable and non-culturable would be inevitable because of the availability of a food source. These include, among others, micrococci, coliforms, diptheroids, and *Clostridium* spp. Also, organisms such as *Serratia* spp., *Klebsiella* spp., *Proteus* spp., *Salmonella* spp., and bacteria such as Cytophaga and Pseudomonads and flavobacteria have been documented to be evident. Also, the host's "normal" microbiota will become mixed with environmental microorganisms such as Agrobacterium, amoeba, and many fungi, which are also significant to human decomposition.

From a microbiological point of view it is plausible to suggest that every microorganism, both endogenous and exogenous, of the host is involved in some aspect of the human decomposition process. Ultimately, the decomposition of human remains would not progress without these normal microbiota and external exogenous microorganisms developing a community in the form of different biofilms. The formation of the biofilm will enhance the continual survival of the host microbiology, but this time the community will become more detrimental to the host rather than beneficial. As has been outlined, the role of microbiology in human decomposition is significant. This role is more apparent when we consider bodies that have open wounds (e.g., death due to stabbing), as these undergo faster decomposition than bodies without wounds. This is principally due to the prevalence of high levels of bacteria within the wounds.[30] In addition to this, if a person dies as a result of bacterial or viral infection, postmortem alterations are accelerated.[32]

Intrinsic Microorganisms and the Chemistry of Death

The human body is composed of approximately 64% water, 20% protein, 10% fat, 1% carbohydrate, and 5% minerals.[33] Adipose tissue is on average 5–30% water, 2–3% protein, and 60–85% lipids, of which 90–99% are triglycerides,[34] while muscle largely consists of protein. Soft tissue decomposition is characterized by the progressive breakdown of these proteins, carbohydrates, and fats. The soft tissues eventually liquefy and disintegrate, leaving skeletalized remains articulated by ligaments.[24,27,35]

Protein Decomposition (Proteolysis)

Protein is broken down by enzyme action, but this does not proceed at a uniform rate throughout the body. The rate is determined by the amount of moisture, bacterial action, and temperature. Moisture favours decay, and proteolysis is slowed by cooling and increased by warming.

Soft tissue proteins such as those forming neuronal and epithelial tissues are destroyed first during decomposition, i.e., the lining membranes of the GI tract and pancreatic epithelium.[25] At an early stage of decomposition, proteins forming the brain, liver, and kidneys are also subject to putrefactive change, while proteins such as epidermis reticulin and muscle proteins are more resistant to breakdown.[23] The most resistant proteins are those associated with connective tissue and cartilage.

Within the hard tissues, proteins such as type I collagen (comprising 90–95% bone protein, alongside other proteins such as osteocalcin, osteopontin, and osteonectin) and amelogenin within tooth enamel are protected by their association with biological apatite. While these are subject to biological or chemical attack under many conditions, they exhibit resilience and as such persist into the archaeological record. These biomolecules have been the subject of considerable interest and utility within the archaeological science community.[36–38]

Keratin, which is an insoluble protein found in hair, nail, and skin can only be exploited as a nutrient source in the first instance by specialized keratinolytic microorganisms.[39,40] Given that the hair shaft is a complex heterogeneous structure, it is hardly surprising that microbially induced changes occur selectively on the basis of the relative resistance of these morphological structures to chemical enzymatic attack.[41] Where the depositional conditions are favourable, hair and nail can persist over considerable timescales, on naturally mummified and even on otherwise skeletal remains.[42]

Common bacteria that are very proteolytic and therefore are involved in protein breakdown include *Pseudomonas*, *Bacillus*, and *Micrococcus* spp. As well as these bacteria, sulphate-reducing bacteria found in the GI tract have a vast array of enzymes and have the ability to utilize sulphates and sulphur-containing compounds and as such are important bacteria in human decomposition.

In general, proteins break down into peptones, polypeptides, and amino acids, a process known as *proteolysis*. Proteolysis leads to the production of phenolic substances, and gases such as carbon dioxide, hydrogen sulphide, ammonia, and methane. The sulphur-containing amino acids of the proteins such as cysteine, cystine, and methionine undergo desulfhydralation and decomposition by bacteria, yielding hydrogen sulphide gas, sulphides, ammonia, thiols, and pyruvic acid. Thiols or mercaptans are decomposition gases containing the –SH (sulfhydryl group), and these are responsible for the very bad odours generated during human decomposition.

Protein decomposition also results in the production of a range of organic acids and other substances that become bacterial metabolites. These are generally of low or moderate molecular weight, anionic or non-ionic, and are susceptible to rapid breakdown by bacteria.[43]

Decomposition of Fat

Human body-derived lipids comprise 90–99% triglycerides, which contain numerous fatty acids attached to the glycerol molecule. The body's adipose tissue consists of approximately 60–85% lipids, with most of the remainder being water.[25] Of those fatty acids making up the composition of adipose tissue, mono-unsaturated $C_{18:1}$ oleic acid is the most widespread, followed then by polyunsaturated $C_{18:2}$ linoleic acid and monounsaturated $C_{16:1}$ palmitoleic acid and the corresponding saturated $C_{16:0}$ palmitic acid.[25]

For the most part, hydrolysis rather than oxidation dominates the fat degradation system, largely because of the fact that bacterial action will have driven the tissues into an anaerobic condition. Palmitic acid increases and the oleic acid becomes increasingly reduced in amount through hydrolyzation. Neutral fat undergoes hydrolysis during decomposition, resulting in the formation of fatty acids hydrolyzed by lipases. This proceeds slowly and the activity of this enzyme system soon diminishes. Analyses of postmortem fat exhibit the presence of oleic, palmitic, and stearic acids as soon as 8 h after death. These are the first phase of neutral fat breakdown. Neutral fats that have been hydrolyzed produce a large concentration of unsaturated fatty acids resulting in the production of aldehydes and ketones. Hydrolysis of triglycerides results in the formation of glycerine and free fatty acids. Bacterial enzymes lead to the transformation of unsaturated into saturated fatty acids. Fatty acids, the products of hydrolysis, will be quickly oxidized into aldehydes and ketones; this, however, can only take place in the presence of oxygen.

More effective than the intrinsic lipases are the lipolytic enzymes produced by bacteria, particularly those of Clostridia (especially *Cl. perfringens*), which derive from the GI tract[44] and are able to grow at relatively high redox potentials.[45] These lipolytic enzymes significantly aid the anaerobic hydrolysis and hydrogenation of fat under warm conditions.[27] Water is necessary for both the intrinsic and bacterial enzymes to work, though there is usually sufficient moisture in the fat tissue itself. If the process continues, the neutral fat is totally converted to hydroxy fatty acids, which are deposited in its place.[46] If no further chemical changes take place, these fatty acids remain as adipocere (*adipo* = fat, *cere* = wax).

If the burial circumstances keep the oxygen levels low, then the fat degradation products will remain as adipocere.[47] Adipocere is a waxy substance that sometimes forms from the adipose tissue of dead bodies and has generally been considered to result from bacterial action, commonly in warm, damp, anaerobic environments.[48] The presence of bacteria and water is crucial for adipocere to form.[49] Adipocere is formed by the alteration of the soft tissue of the corpse into a greyish-white, soft, cream-like substance, over time becoming a solid and resistant compound. Adipocere is a soft, greasy material which may be white or stained reddish brown when recent. When adipocere is analyzed, in addition to stearic, palmitic, and oleic acids, there is a fraction of calcium soaps.[27] Old adipocere is white or grey, and depending on its age and condition it has been likened to suet or cheese.[27]

Extensive adipocere formation will be found on a body when conditions will allow only partial degeneration of fatty tissue, i.e., by hydrolysis and hydrogenation but not oxidative reactions. Adipocere in corpses has been found after as little as 30–90 days following death.[15]

Varieties of aerobic or facultatively anaerobic microorganisms from the surface of the adipocere have been identified. In culture, a number of Gram-positive bacteria, associated with the indigenous human microbiota, are able to degrade the adipocere. The role of bacteria in adipocere formation and degradation must be understood before we can use the presence of adipocere to extrapolate information about the post-death interval.[50]

Apart from corpse-specific characteristics (e.g., sex, age, physique, cause of death), method of burial (e.g., material of the coffin, depth of grave, individual or mass grave, clothing) and time of burial, the conditions of the resting place (geology, topography, soil properties and frequency of use, air, water, and heat budget) can have a special impact on adipocere formation.[51] It is a traditional belief that adipocere forms in damp environments – such as after submersion or interment in damp or waterlogged ground. Adipocere will also form in bodies buried in dry vaults, and in some cases distal elements (e.g., limbs and hands) have shown signs of mummification while adipocere is present in others. It is suggested that coffins will retard the rate at which adipocere forms but clothing enhances its formation.[52] Gas-chromatography-mass spectrometry was used to characterize the fatty acids from soils and associated tissues excavated from a 1967 Foot and Mouth burial pit. Subcutaneous fats were mainly composed of 55–75% palmitic acid, 17–22% stearic acid, and 3–16% oleic acid as well as 5–7% myristic acid. The distribution of fatty acids confirmed that the tissues had decayed to adipocere.[53]

There is little known about which specific microorganisms bring about lipid break-down in soil, although it has been suggested that Gram-positive bacteria such as *Bacillus* spp., *Cellulomonas* spp., and *Nocardia* spp. are involved in the decomposition of adipocere.[50] In Brazilian cemetery studies, the presence of significant numbers but unspecified types of lipolytic bacteria (possibly *Clostridia* spp.) was reported for the groundwaters examined[54]; these were said to be directly related to the decom-position of the interred remains. Hydrogenation of fats under the influence of bacterial enzymes results in the partial conversion of unsaturated fatty acids into saturated fatty acids. As the fatty acids clearly have a bactericidal effect, further bacterial decomposition is stopped at this early adipocere stage. Additional micro-organisms from outside can no longer penetrate when this hermetic seal is in place.[55]

Within the archaeological record, lipids are considered to be robust molecules and have been recovered extensively from human remains, soils, and in association with artefactual material such as ceramics.[56,57]

Decomposition of Carbohydrates

The utilization of carbohydrates present in the soft tissue of corpses occurs in the early stages of decomposition.[26] For example glycogen, a complex polysaccharide, will break down into sugars (glucose) by the action of microorganisms. Most sugars are completely oxidized to carbon dioxide and water, while some are incompletely decomposed. For example, *Clostridium* spp. breakdown carbohydrates to form a number of organic acids and alcohols, and fungi decompose the sugars to form organic acids including glucuronic acid, citric acid, and oxalic acid.[58] Postmortem production of alcohol by anaerobic fermentation occurs during conversion of body sugar to ethanol by bacteria, and this can begin within 6–12 h under hot, humid conditions.[10] In the presence of oxygen, the glucose monomer is broken down through the pyruvic acid, lactic acid, and acetaldehyde stages to form carbon dioxide and water.[58] Other gases produced through bacterial carbohydrate fermentation include methane, hydrogen, and hydrogen sulphide.

Decomposition of Bone

The loss of soft tissue from the corpse is referred to as *skeletonization*. The rate of skeletonization will depend on many factors such as whether the body is buried or not, depth of burial, temperature, moisture, and access by insects and larger scavengers.[30] Under anaerobic burial conditions or where the tissues have significantly desiccated, the rate of skeletonization will be low.[29] In these circumstances, the degree of soft tissue survival is often scored according to the region of the body, and survival of organs using indices such as the Aufderheide's soft tissue index.[42]

In addition to the loss of tissue from bone, the bone itself is subject to decompositional change.[29,59] Bone is a composite tissue having three main components: a protein fraction, collagen acting as a supportive scaffold; a mineral component, biological apatite to stiffen the protein structure; and a ground substance of other organic compounds such as mucopolysaccharides and glycoproteins.[60,61] Bone collagen and biological apatite are strongly held together by protein–mineral bonds, which give bone its strength and contribute to its preservation.[62]

The loss of protein and/or partial loss of bone mineral result in weakening/embrittlement, which is associated with bone buried over archaeological timescales when compared to fresh bone. The physical condition of excavated bone will depend on the integrity of the bone mineral bond due to collagen survival and the depositional environment. It is usual for archaeological bone recovered from aerobic, non-acidic environments to be stained but otherwise appear to be in good condition. However, cracking and flaking may occur on drying. In coarser, calcareous sand or loam where it is damp and more oxygenated, the bone surface will be rougher and may warp, crack, or laminate on drying, while material from coarse calcareous gravels will lose much collagen and have the consistency of powdery chalk and be coated in a white encrustation of insoluble salts. Bone from acidic peat deposits appears as interwoven fibres, is pliable, and hardens on drying.[63] Acid in soil is the most common agent of bone destruction and works by dissolving the inorganic matrix of hydroxyapatite which produces an organic material susceptible to leaching by water. The collagen fibres are sometimes preserved by natural tannins.[63]

Bone collagen is attacked by bacterial collagenases that hydrolyse the proteins to peptides; these are then broken down to form amino acids.[64] It has been suggested that collagen degradation is affected by the activity of the gas-gangrene bacterium *Clostridium histolyctium* which operates in a pH range from 7 to 8.[65,66] Alternative claims implicate bacterial collagenases as largely responsible for degrading bone collagen by reducing them to peptides that leach away in groundwater.[67] Regardless of the mechanism, once the protein mineral bond has been broken, the bone mineral is vulnerable to partial dissolution via chemical weathering.[68,69] Bones are generally better preserved in soils with a neutral or slightly alkaline pH than in acidic soils, which will result in the dissolution of biological apatite. Over short timescales, dry sand is an aid to preservation (although sandy soils are often acidic), as it retards bacterial decomposition, while in fine-grained soil and dense clay aerobic bacteria cannot live.

In archaeology there has been a lot of recent attention concerning the degradation of bone in the soil (diagenesis). The impetus for this work has been both an attempt to explain the differential survival of different elements of the skeleton as well as differential preservation between individual burials and to underpin more detailed biochemical analysis of archaeological bone based on the survival of organic matter such as bone collagen and DNA in teeth and bone.[19,20,37]

Extrinsic Organisms Involved in Human Decomposition

Colonization of the corpse by extrinsic organisms may begin within hours of death. Of particular significance are insects that are used as important forensic indicators to calculate time-since-death estimations and are discussed in greater detail elsewhere.[70–72] The attractiveness of a cadaver will depend on odour and fly oviposition, defined by temperature. Blow flies (Calliphoridae) may be attracted to the body within minutes of exposure, and gravid female blowflies will detect the presence of a body on the basis of a scent plume from some considerable distance. In laboratory experiments with caged *Callophora vicina* presented with baits that were fresh and partly decomposed, the flies ignored the fresh bait. Eggs are laid in natural body openings (mouth, nose, eyes, ears, anus, and open wounds) and up to 180 eggs can be laid at one time. Eggs take 1–2 days to hatch depending on temperature and humidity (low temperature retards insect activity, and 4°C or below is the lower threshold for hatching in *Callophora vicina*). The formation of maggot masses by these hatched larvae can cause massive soft tissue damage that will open tissue up to further putrefactive decay.

Burial will often pose a barrier to blow flies – although, if there is an opportunity for eggs to be laid prior to burial, then they can subsequently hatch and the larvae will feed. Sealed post-medieval coffins have yielded evidence of blowfly activity (pupal cases), which suggests that eggs were laid prior to closure of the coffin.[73] Over longer timescales, different insects will colonize the corpse. Although the desiccation of mummified tissue will inhibit normal putrefactive changes, they remain susceptible to insect attack by the larvae of the brown house moth or beetles such as *Dermestes lardarius* or *Necrobia rufipes*.

Larger animals such as domestic cats and dogs as well as foxes, badgers, and rats will scavenge meat from corpses. Whether they scavenge or not will be determined by ease of access as well as individual feeding preferences and the abundance of available food. Larger animals will dig up and disinter parts of corpses from shallow burials, and scatter skeletal elements from both buried and surface-deposited remains.[74,75] Importantly, in the case of buried remains, during the early putrefactive stages of decomposition such digging will disturb the grave and the resultant aeration of the grave will accelerate putrefactive change. This has been documented in experimental studies using pig burials as human body analogues.[76] The action of these larger scavengers is outside the scope of this chapter.

During the later stages of decomposition, microorganisms may be derived from the soil; here soil history is an important factor and will influence the size and nature of the population of dormant microorganisms. At the microscopic level, biological agents of decay include bacteria and fungi which can mimic pathological changes in bone.[77] Microscopic focal destruction of bone (tunnels) was first noted during the last century[78] and it is now understood to be caused by invading soil microorganisms,[79] possibly an unidentified mycelium-forming fungus.[80] Beginning at the surface of the cortex, the organisms proceed along the vascular channels and osteons, creating tunnels that expand until only separated by thin bars of hypermineralized bone. In the burial environment, it is believed that soil water content and temperature are important factors in focal destruction, which does not occur in wet, water-logged, or dry soils but is favoured in soils with moderate moisture in summer weather. Histological and physical (mercury intrusion porosimetry) analyses of bone from 41 archaeological sites across five countries revealed that the majority (68%) had suffered microbial attack.[81]

Most fungi that are found on decomposing remains are aerobic, and consequently their growth is restricted to the surface of the cadaver and little deep penetration of the tissues takes place. Fungi are commonly found on the skin and exposed surfaces of decomposing remains. In some cases they can also be found growing in the intestines and other body cavities. In addition, fungi may also be found growing in soil that is infused with decomposition products from the body.[82] Microorganisms may have complex inter-relationships and many synthesize antibiotic compounds. For example, griseofulvin is an anti-mycotic agent produced by *Penicillium griseofulvum*, and luteoskyrin is an anti-bacterial agent produced by *Penicillium islandicum*.[10]

If there is substantial surface vegetation, bone is susceptible to plant root damage, although this will be strongly influenced by seasonal effects. Physical damage by plant roots can mark, warp, and even break bones but the exact mechanism of biochemical plant root damage is obscure.[83] It is probable that plant roots manufacture mucilaginous substances that promote the growth of microorganisms when secreted. Certain microorganisms, including fungi, will discharge enzymes into the soil which catalyses the reaction that dissolves hydroxyapatite in bone and facilitates its absorption into the plant root system. A low pH will promote these chemical changes. Plants and their root systems constitute complex physical and chemical processes that efficiently breakdown the external and internal structure of human bone.[84] While it is appreciated that plant activity in the tropics is at a greater level than in the UK, the principle of vegetation acting as a decomposition vector of human skeletal remains is valid.

Environmental Controls that Promote and Inhibit Putrefactive Decay

There are a large number of inter-related factors that will affect the rate and nature of cadaveric decay. These principally include the condition of the body at the time of burial and the nature and circumstances of the burial environment.[85] A comprehensive survey of the issues has been reviewed by Mant,[85–87] which is a synthesis of results from over 150 exhumations carried out in Germany after the Second World War. These burials were made under a range of different circumstances and burial conditions: for instance, burial was often immediately after death rather than allowing for the normal postmortem interval of several days. In most cases, the dates of death and interment were known. It was not possible to carry out laboratory analyses of the tissues recovered, and the results are based on gross changes. From this data it is possible to examine the influence of a variety of factors on the decomposition of buried human remains. Some generalization can be made, although attention must be made to individual circumstances.[14] Thin bodies will skeletalize more rapidly than more fleshy ones in the same conditions. Antemortem or postmortem wounding makes cadavers more susceptible to invasion by extra-corporeal organisms than bodies that are buried with the skin intact, and will have a more rapid rate of skeletalization.[85]

The rate of decomposition of a body on the ground surface is more rapid than that of a buried body. This is due to the soil limiting the access by extra-corporeal microorganisms and larger animals as well as reducing the rate of gaseous diffusion. An oxygenated environment will increase the rate of human decomposition. Exposure above ground, even for a short period, will allow insects and carnivorous larvae to colonize the body and rapidly attack the soft tissue, a process which will continue after burial. Ambient temperatures above the ground are higher, there is more oxygen and less carbon dioxide, and access to the body is easy for scavenging mammals.

During initial cadaver decomposition, when the soft tissues lose their morphological structure, aspects of the burial environment that affect soil biology such as oxygen availability predominate and localized soil chemistry may be modified and dominated by the biochemistry of soft tissue decomposition. When the bulk of soft tissue decay has ended, then generalized soil chemistry may have a greater direct effect, for instance, on the corrosion of associated metals or in bone diagenesis. The long-term factors relate to later phases of decay in which soil chemistry has a greater effect than either soil biology or the gaseous composition of the burial atmosphere. These factors have been studied both archaeologically[5,47,86] and forensically.[5,85,87]

It has been suggested by Mant[86] and Mann et al.[30] that, in the short term, up to 2 years, the soil type is not a particularly important factor governing cadaveric decay.[85] However, experimental work conducted using contrasting burial sites[76] has indicated that in addition to factors relating to microclimate and seasonality, depositional conditions including soil do have a marked effect on decomposition rates.[47] Decomposition is accelerated in porous, permeable, and light soils, which allow a relatively free exchange of oxygen and water from the atmosphere, and reductive gases such as carbon dioxide, hydrogen sulphide, ammonia, and methane from the body.

In general, the deeper the burial, the better the preservation of the body.[47] This is a result of a stable, low temperature; poor gas diffusion; and inaccessibility to floral and faunal agents of decay. However, the action of soil pressure in the burial context can warp bones and this has implications for osteometric analysis in both palaeopathology and forensic osteoarchaeology. Quantifying the extent of this phenomenon is, however, virtually impossible.

Mant[85] observed that a corpse buried and surrounded by certain vegetable matter – straw, pine branches – showed more rapid decomposition than others buried without this material. The straw and pine needles introduced additional bacteria that aided decomposition and surrounded the body with a layer of air. It is also thought that the vegetable matter acts as an insulator, retaining the heat produced by decomposition and generating heat through its own breakdown.[85]

Temperature

Ambient temperature has a profound effect on cadaver decomposition, and in tropical climates rigor may be complete in 2 h while cold will cause it to persist. Bodies sunk in cold water will retain rigidity for a long time, as cold water tends to retard putrefaction. Temperature is a major factor because the microbial processes that occur both internally and externally in a corpse will be affected by this.[30] When temperatures are warm, human decomposition has been documented to occur within 4 min.[31] Contrary to this, at cold temperatures these processes usually begin after 4–7 days.[85] At temperatures below −5°C, decomposition is prevented, as both enzymatic and microbial action will be halted. In the event of death being caused by viral or bacterial infection, not only will the body temperature be higher but bacteria may be widespread throughout the cadaver and hasten postmortem decomposition.

The effect of temperature varies with latitude, season, and depth of burial. In climates where the ground freezes in winter, the burial environment during that period is one of preservation rather than decomposition. Data on putrefaction rates in a temperate climate for a cadaver of average physique have been supplied by Mant.[47,85,87] The onset of putrefaction does not appear for some 36 h in an unrefrigerated body, while in cold but not freezing temperatures the first signs of putrefaction do not appear for 5–7 days. In summer weather putrefactive changes may be pronounced after 24 h.[85]

Moisture

Natural mummification due to rapid drying of the tissues is well attested in both the archaeological[42] and forensic literature.[8] In temperate climates it usually occurs when there is a good air flow and does not usually occur in bodies that have been buried. Desiccation of a substrate to below a critical threshold leads to inhibition of microbial activity but usually does occur when some autolytic and putrefactive change has already occurred – thus the tissue will have been subject to both chemical and mirostructural change prior to dessication. Rehydration of tissue and subsequent histology can reveal these changes.

Contrasting Depositional Environments (Soil Burial vs. Surface Exposure)

The impact of different environmental conditions (buried, surface-exposed, and water-deposited remains) on entomological activity has long been of interest.[88–90] While the depositional environment will affect the rate of decomposition, and in some cases lead to a stasis in breakdown, generally all bodies follow the same basic sequence of decay. Forensic taphonomists have produced a classification of decay sequences that can be applied to a broad range of environmental situations.[10,91]

Few depositional contexts allow for the domination and mutual exclusion of either putrefactive decay or the action of insects. This is particularly evident in the case of surface exposure and shallow burials. Even bodies in confined spaces (e.g., a car with closed doors/windows) will be accessible by a varied insect population. Bass[91] gives a detailed summary for the summer decay rates for a body exposed on the surface at the Anthropological Research Facility at Knoxville, Tennessee.[91]

First Day (Fresh)

In addition to the fly activity, early external signs of decompositional change are the colouration of major veins under the skin that turn dark green or blue, and the exudation of body fluids from the nose, mouth, and anus due to early putrefaction of contents of the intestinal tract.

First Week (Fresh to Bloated)

In addition to active maggot activity, including maggot masses under the skin in the regions of oviposition, the skin will show signs of slippage, and hair will begin to detach from the scalp. The discoloration of the veins become more prominent and an odour of decay becomes apparent. The by-products of decomposition include gas products that initially form in the intestines as a result of the rapid decomposition of their contents, and the gut cavity becomes distended. The distension phase is referred to as a "Bloat". Discoloured natural liquids and liquefying tissues are made frothy by the gas; some may exude from the natural orifices, forced out by the increasing pressure of gases. Molds begin to appear on the surface of the body. The average duration of the decay phases of human remains is known to vary according to season, with the bloat phase being most rapid during the summer months compared with spring or autumn.[10]

First Month (Bloated to Decay)

As the skin starts to breakdown the body cavities will rupture, and the subsequent deflation of the corpse following rupture and purging is known as "Post bloat" or decay stage. Insect activity is diminished. If the body is clothed or covered, the soft tissue will decay to expose the underlying bones. If the is not covered, the skin will get dry and leathery, with maggots protected by the dry outer tissues from direct effects of sunlight. If the body is lying supine, the chest cavity (ribs and sternum) will be held together by a combination of the dried skin and connective tissue. Outer surfaces will continue to be colonized by moulds.

The First Year (Dry)

The skeleton will continue to be exposed, and bone will start to bleach in the sunlight.

First Decade (Bone Breakdown)

It is important to point out at this stage that the wooded hillside on the banks of the Tennessee river in Knoxville that houses the Anthropological Research Facility with its continental US climate differs greatly to the maritime climate of the United Kingdom, which itself has many different geoclimatic conditions.[76] Much of the background work on soft tissue decay and other related factors of interest in forensic cases have been addressed to bodies on the ground surface. Buried bodies are contained in a much less predictable decay environment. Within the less complicated field of material biodeterioration, it is still difficult to produce systematically replicable results for the burial of materials in soil.[92]

The Microclimate Associated with Human Decomposition

The concept of the micro-environment (microcosm) of the grave has been explored by various researchers, with the human body seen as a major nutrient source for microorganisms.[76,93–95] In particular, the decomposition of the body is seen to affect the survival/decomposition of associated death-scene materials. The chemical and biological interactions of a body, with associated materials in a specific soil, are very difficult to model in a realistic manner. The result is that we can describe what we know in a specific set of circumstances; it may be possible to predict general trends within a specific soil type (provided factors of soil moisture and microbiology are largely similar) but it is unlikely that valid prediction can be made between widely different geographical regions or differing burial situations.

Soil conditions at different burial sites have a marked effect on the condition of the buried body, but even within a single site variation can occur; the process of soft tissue decomposition modifies the localized burial microenvironment in terms of microbiological load, pH, moisture, and changes in redox status.[76] The tissues become increasingly liquid, and in the case of a body buried directly in the soil, a mucus sheath will form around the corpse consisting of liquid body decomposition products and a fine silt fraction from the soil.[76,96]

The formation of a highly concentrated island of fertility, or cadaver decomposition island (CDI), is associated with increased soil microbial biomass, microbial activity (C mineralization), and nematode abundance. Each CDI is an ephemeral natural disturbance that, in addition to releasing energy and nutrients to the wider ecosystem, acts as a hub by receiving these materials in the form of dead insects, exuvia and puparia, faecal matter (from scavengers, grazers, and predators), and feathers (from avian scavengers and predators).[95]

Differential Decomposition

The biochemical and microbiology processes that occur on and within a human corpse are very complex. The shorter the timescale between interment and recovery, the more likely soft tissue is preserved. However, it should not be assumed that the presence of extensive soft tissue will indicate a recent death, as in specific burial environments soft tissue remains can be preserved for thousands of years. A skull recovered during commercial extraction of a peat bog in Cheshire during 1983 was examined by a Forensic Science Service pathologist, who noted intact hair and skin, an identifiable eye ball, and pultaceous matter inside the cranial vault. Police suspicions were roused by these well-preserved human remains since a long, unsolved crime was being investigated. However, archaeological dating techniques identified the skull as originating from around the third century A.D.[97] Similarly, the example of Lt. Col Shy killed and subsequently embalmed during the American Civil War is a further cited case.[42]

Before consideration of particular circumstances that have led to soft tissue preservation over long timescales, it is necessary to consider the nature of soft tissue that has been subject to partial decomposition. It was originally thought that natural mummification and the formation on hydrolysed but not oxidized fat (adipocere) were mutually exclusive processes. However, it has been demonstrated by Mant[14] that both tissue types can be encountered from cadavers in forensic cases.

Soil, with its varied oxygenation, water content, redox potential, ion exchange capacity, and pH variation, as well as the nature of the body, its biochemistry, fat content, cause of death, time interval between death and burial, whether it is clothed or unclothed, wrapped in a polythene sheet, buried shallow or deep, affect forensic analysis and interpretation of data obtained from human remains. In short, it is very unwise to draw direct predictive parallels between one specific case and another. Experimental work can indicate general trends for the specific parameters tested.[76]

Mant[86] observed significant retardation of decomposition in clothed bodies buried directly in the soil without a coffin. Clothing will partially negate the effects of the general soil environment and delay the process of decay. Textiles around the body also impede access of burrowing carrion scavengers. Even after 2 years in shallow graves, those parts of the body covered by clothing frequently showed good preservation. It was also observed that adipocere formation was uniform and putrefactive liquification rare and that muscle tissues and muscle attachments to bone were still well preserved in areas such as the thighs and buttocks where the thick layer of fat was only in the process of hydrolysis and hydrogenation.

It has been suggested that, in general, the time required for the decomposition of corpses takes between 3 and 12 years.[98,99] If conditions are less favourable, the time delay is much higher and can be hundreds or even thousands of years before skeletalization of a human corpse[100] Following putrefaction, the decomposition process continues through liquefaction and disintegration, leaving skeletonized remains. Skeletonization proceeds until eventually only the harder, resistant tissues of bone, teeth, and cartilage remain. Bacteria and fungi aid to skeletonize the corpse.[100]

Both forensic pathologists and archaeological scientists are familiar with depositional environments that can retard the decomposition of soft tissues over long timescales.[13] The desiccation of tissue below thresholds for microbial activity will lead to preservation. This natural mummification is well documented in the forensic sciences literature.[13,15] Mummified bodies usually exhibit a marked reduction in tissue bulk, often accompanied by darkened skin resembling dried leather. Since tissue water loss is from exposed surfaces, there is often a difference in water content between core and peripheral tissues. This was directly recorded by Janaway and Wilson (publication being written) in recent experimental burial of pig cadavers in the costal desert of Southern Peru. After 2 years of burial, directly in the sand, the exterior tissues had formed a hard, desiccated layer, while interior of the body core remained moist. This differential desiccation is also observed in archaeological mummified bodies from the same region. It should be noted that desiccated tissue rarely has not been subject to putrefactive change prior to the moisture threshold dropping to the point where microbial activity is significantly inhibited. In extreme cases, a skeleton may be articulated because of intact ligaments and covered by a dried out skin of once-liquefied tissue lacking any residual morphological structure. This has been observed in both archaeological bodies and is also well documented at the Anthropological Research Facility at Knoxville, Tennessee.[12,73,101] Owing to surface area/volume effects, different parts of a body placed in desiccating environment will lose water at different rates. For instance, it is not unusual to observe well-developed mummification of hands, feet, and limbs while the trunk is still subject to major putrefactive change. An example from recent casework is instructive. The body of a young woman, who had been killed by blunt force trauma to the head, had lain in a cool, dry cellar for a number of months. The body was partially clothed and there had been considerable blowfly activity. While adult flies were actively hatching from the pupae within the cellar, there was no longer significant larval activity in the body. The head had been covered, and thus excluded the blow flies, although there was considerable putrefactive change accelerated by the trauma. The relationship between trauma and soft tissue decay was documented by Mant over 50 years ago.[87] The body was naked from below the waist, and the exposed uterus and internal tissues had been destroyed because of extensive feeding by fly larvae. The exposed limbs and lower body hair was desiccated and well preserved in an advanced state of mummification. Thus at the time of autopsy this single body exhibited massive tissue loss from putrefactive change, massive tissue loss due to the feeding of a maggot mass, but relatively intact tissue due to partial desiccation.

Under damp conditions, hair is readily attacked by keratinolytic microorganisms. Under dry condition human hair it is often preserved over long timescales, while still liable to attack, but usually not total destruction by insects such as the Dermestid beetle (*Anthrenus* spp. or Clothes moth larvae (*Tineola bissiella*).[40]

In addition to desiccation, low temperature regimes will inhibit microbial activity and therefore reduce putrefactive change.[29] Bodies have been preserved by both freezing due to the natural environment as well as the use of domestic freezers. Care must be taken to distinguish between tissue that is largely hydrated but frozen, and tissue that has desiccated because of the cold, dry conditions that are, for instance, found in many mountainous and arctic regions. Freeze-dried human tissue has survived over hundreds of years as is the case of the Greenland mummies and frozen bodies, buried in the 1840s, that have been exhumed from the Canadian arctic. In this case, at a macroscopic level the bodies exhibited good levels of soft tissue preservation, but microscopically little histological structure remained.

Conclusion

Clearly the human microbiota has a role to play in decomposition of the host. In fact, the indigenous microorganisms ultimately lead to the demise of their host. The microorganisms that were once classified as the indigenous human flora then persist within the environment and become free to colonize another host. The "microorganism and human cycle" then begins again.

References

1. Crell FLF. Some experiments on putrefaction. Philos Trans R Soc 1771;61:332–344.
2. Pringle J. Further experiments on substances resisting putrefaction; with experiments upon the means of hastening and promoting it. Philos Trans R Soc 1749;46:550–558.
3. Efremov EA. Taphonomy: a new branch of paleontology. Pan Am Geologist 1940;74:81–93.

4. Boddington A, Garland AN, Janaway RC, eds. *Death, Decay and Reconstruction*. Manchester: Manchester University Press. 1987.
5. Garland AN, Janaway RC. The taphonomy of inhumation burials. In C Roberts, F Lee and J Bintliff eds. *Burial Archaeology: Current Research, Methods and Developments*, pp. 15–37. Oxford: British Archaeological Reports. 1989.
6. Lyman RL. *Vertebrate Taphonomy*. Cambridge: Cambridge University Press. 1994.
7. O'Connor T. *Taphonomy: From Life to Death and Beyond: The Archaeology of Animal Bones*. Stroud: Sutton Publishing, pp. 19–27. 2000.
8. Haglund WD, Sorg MH, eds. *Forensic Taphonomy: The Postmortem Fate of Human Remains*. Boca Raton: CRC Press. 1997.
9. Haglund WD, Sorg MH. *Advances in Forensic Taphonomy: Method, Theory and Archaeological Perspectives*. Boca Raton: CRC Press. 2002.
10. Micozzi MS. *Postmortem Changes in Human and Animal Remains: A Systematic Approach*. Springfield, IL: Charles C. Thomas. 1991.
11. Tibbett M, Carter DO, eds. *Soil Analysis in Forensic Taphonomy: Chemical and Biological Effects of Buried Human Remains*. Boca Raton: CRC Press, Taylor & Francis. 2008.
12. Rodriguez WC, Bass WM. Decomposition of buried bodies and methods that may aid in their location. J Forensic Sci 1985;30:836–852.
13. Knight B, Simpson K, eds. *Simpson's Forensic Medicine*. London: Arnold. 1997.
14. Mant AK, ed. *Taylor's Principles and Practice of Medical Jurisprudence*. London. Churchill Livingstone. 1984.
15. Dix J, Graham M. *Time of Death, Decomposition and Identification an Atlas*. Boca Raton: CRC Press. 2000.
16. Child AM. Microbiological and Chemical Alteration of Archaeological Mineralised Collagen. Ph.D., University of Wales, Cardiff. 1993.
17. Huffine E, Crews J, Kennedy B, Bomberger K, Zinbo A. Mass identification of persons missing from the break-up of the former Yugoslavia: Structure, function, and role of the International Commission on Missing Persons. Croat Med J 2001;42:271–275.
18. Alonso A, Martin P, Albarran C, Garcia P, de Simon LF, Iturralde MJ, Fernandez-Rodriguez A, Atienza I, Capilla J, Garcia-Hirschfeld J, Martinez P, Vallejo G, Garcia O, Garcia E, Real P, Alvarez D, Leon A, Sancho M. Challenges of DNA profiling in mass disaster investigations. Croat Med J 2005;46:540–548.
19. Gilbert MTP, Bandelt HJ, Hofreiter M, Barnes I. Assessing ancient DNA studies. Trends Ecol Evol 2005;20:541–544.
20. Poinar HN, Stankiewicz BA. Protein preservation and DNA retrieval from ancient tissues. Proc Natl Acad Sci USA 1999;69:8426–8431.
21. Vass AA, Smith RR, Thompson CV, Burnett MN, Wolf DA, Synstelien JA, Dulgerian N, Eckenrode BA. Decompositional odor analysis database. J Forensic Sci 2004;49:760–769.
22. Carter DO, Tibbett M. Taphonomic mycota: Fungi with forensic potential. J Forensic Sci 2003;48:168–171.
23. Gill-King H. Chemical and ultrastructural aspects of decomposition. In WD Haglund and MH Sorg eds. *Forensic Taphonomy: The Postmortem Fate of Human Remains*. Boca Raton: CRC Press, pp. 93–108. 1997.
24. Janssen W. *Forensic Histopathology*. Berlin: Springer. 1984.
25. Forbes SL. Decomposition chemistry in a burial environment. In M Tibbett and DO Carter eds. *Soil Analysis in Forensic Taphonomy*. New York: CRC Press, Taylor & Francis, pp. 203–223. 2008.
26. Evans WED. *The Chemistry of Death*. Springfield, IL: Charles C. Thomas. 1963.
27. Polson CJ, Gee DJ, Knight B. *The Essentials of Forensic Medicine*. Oxford: Pergamon Press. 1985.
28. Payen G, Rimoux L, Gueux M, Lery N. Body putrefaction in "air tight" burials. IV. Microbiologic findings and environment. Acta Med Leg Soc (Liege) 1988;38:153–163.
29. Janaway RC. The decay of buried human remains and their associated materials. In J Hunter, C Roberts and A Martin eds. *Studies in Crime: An Introduction to Forensic Archaeology*. London: Batsford, pp. 58–85. 1996.

30. Mann RW, Bass WM, Meadows L. Time since death and decomposition of the human body: variables and case and experimental field studies. J Forensic Sci 1990;35:103–111.
31. Vass AA. Beyond the grave – understanding human decomposition. Microbiol Today 2001;28:190–192.
32. Janaway RC. The preservation of organic materials in association with metal artefacts deposited in inhumation graves. In A Boddington, ANGarland and RCJanaway eds. *Death, Decay and Reconstruction: Approaches to Archaeology and Forensic Science*. Manchester: Manchester University Press, pp. 127–148. 1987.
33. van Haaren FWJ. Churchyards as sources for water pollution. Moorman s Periodieke Pers 1951;35:167–172.
34. Reynold AE, Cahill GF. *Handbook of Physiology: Adipose Tissue*. Washington, DC: American Physiological Society. 1965.
35. Gresham GA. *A Colour Atlas of Forensic Pathology*. London: Wolfe Publishing. 1973.
36. Ambrose SH, Krigbaum J. Bone chemistry and bioarchaeology. J Anthropol Archaeol 2003;22:193–199.
37. Collins MJ, Nielsen-Marsh CM, Hiller J, Smith CI, Roberts JP, Prigodich RV, Weiss TJ, Csapo J, Millard AR, Turner-Walker G. The survival of organic matter in bone: a review. Archaeometry 2002;44:383–394.
38. Sealy J. Body tissue chemistry and palaeodiet. In DR Brothwell and AM Pollard eds. *A Handbook of Archaeological Sciences*. Chichester: Wiley, pp. 269–279. 2001.
39. Kushwaha RKS, Guarro J, eds. *Biology of Dermatophytes and other Keratinophilic Fungi*. Bilbao: Revista Iberoamericana de Micologia. 2000.
40. Wilson AS. The decomposition of hair in the buried body environment. In M Tibbett and DO Carter eds. *Soil Analysis in Forensic Taphonomy: Chemical and Biological Effects of Buried Human Remains*. Boca Raton: CRC Press, 2008. pp. 123–151.
41. Wilson AS, Dodson HI, Janaway RC, Pollard AM, Tobin DJ. Selective biodegradation in hair shafts derived from archaeological, forensic and experimental contexts. Br J Dermatol 2007;157:450–457.
42. Aufderheide AC. *The Scientific Study of Mummies*. Cambridge: Cambridge University Press. 2003.
43. Santoro T, Stotzky G. Sorption between microorganisms and clay minerals as determined by the electrical sensing zone particle analyzer. Can J Microbiol 1968;14:299–307.
44. Tomita K. On the production of hydroxy fatty acids and fatty acid oligomers in the course of adipocere formation. Nippon Hoigaku Zasshi – Jpn J Leg Med 1984;38:257–272.
45. Nanikawa R. Über die Bestandteile von natürlichen und experimentell hergestellten Leichenwachsen. Z Rechtsmed 72:194–202. 1973.
46. Takatori T, Ishiguro N, Tarao H, Matsumiya H. Microbial production of hydroxy and oxo fatty acids by several microorganisms as a model of adipocere formation. Forensic Sci Int 1986;32:5–11.
47. Henderson J. Factors determining the state of preservation of human remains. In A Boddington, AN Garland and RC Janaway eds. *Death, Decay and Reconstruction: Approaches to Archaeology and Forensic Science*. Manchester: Manchester University Press, pp. 43–54. 1987.
48. Mellen PF, Lowry MA, Micozzi MS. Experimental observations on adipocere formation. J Forensic Sci 1993;38:91–93.
49. O'Brien TG, Kuehner AC. Waxing grave about adipocere: soft tissue change in an aquatic context. J Forensic Sci 2007;52:294–301.
50. Pfeiffer S, Milne S, Stevenson RM. The natural decomposition of adipocere. J Forensic Sci 1998;43:368–370.
51. Fiedler S, Graw M. Decomposition of buried corpses, with special reference to the formation of adipocere. Naturwissenschaften 2003;90:291–300.
52. Forbes SL, Stuart BH, Dent BB. The effect of the method of burial on adipocere formation. Forensic Sci Int 2005;154:44–52.

53. Vane CH, Trick JK. Evidence of adipocere in a burial pit from the foot and mouth epidemic of 1967 using gas chromatography-mass spectrometry. Forensic Sci Int 2005;154:19–23.

54. Martins MT, Pellizari VH, Pacheco A, Myaki DM, Adams C, Bossolan NR, Mendes JM, Hassuda S. Bacteriological quality of groundwaters in cemeteries. Rev Saude Publica 1991;25:47–52.

55. Rothschild MA, Schmidt V, Schneider V. Adipocere – problems in estimating the length of time since death. Med Law 1996;15:329–335.

56. Craig OE, Love GD, Isaksson S, Taylor G, Snape CE. Stable carbon isotopic characterisation of free and bound lipid constituents of archaeological ceramic vessels released by solvent extraction, alkaline hydrolysis and catalytic hydropyrolysis. J Anal Appl Pyrol 2004;71:613–634.

57. Heron C, Evershed RP, Goad LJ. Effects of migration of soil lipids on organic residues associated with buried potsherds. J Archaeol Sci 1997;18:641–659.

58. Waksman SA, Starkey RL. *The Soil and the Microbe*. New York: Wiley. 1931.

59. Hare PE. Organic geochemistry of bone and its relation to the survival of bone in the natural environment. In AK Behrensmeyer and AP Hill eds. *Fossils in the Making: Vertebrate Taphonomy and Paleoecology*. Chicago: University of Chicago Press, pp. 208–219. 1976.

60. Hedges REM. Potential information from archaeological bone, its recovery and preservation. In K Starling and D Watkinson eds. *Archaeological Bone, Antler and Ivory*. London: UKIC, pp. 22–23. 1987.

61. O'Connor TP. On the structure, chemistry and decay of bone, antler and ivory. In K Starling and D Watkinson eds. *Archaeological Bone, Ivory and Antler*. London: UKIC, pp. 6–8. 1987.

62. Von Endt DW, Ortner DJ. Experimental effects of bone size and temperature on bone diagenesis. J Archaeol Sci 1984;11:247–253.

63. Cronyn JM. *The Elements of Archaeological Conservation*. London: Routledge. 1990.

64. Child AM, Pollard AM. Microbial attack on collagen. In E Pernicka and GA Wagner eds. *Archaeometry'90*, Basel: Birkhauser Verlag, pp. 617–625. 1991.

65. Garlick JD. Buried bone: the experimental approach in the study of nitrogen content and blood group activity. In DR Brothwell and E Higgs eds. *Science in Archaeology*. London: Thames & Hudson, pp. 503–512. 1969.

66. Rottlander RCA. Variation in the chemical composition of bone as an indicator of climatic change. J Archaeol Sci 1976;3:83–88.

67. Beeley JG, Lunt DA. The nature of the biochemical changes in softened dentine from archaeological sites. J Archaeol Sci 1980;7:371–377.

68. Collins MJ, Waite ER, Van Duin ACT. Predicting protein decomposition: the case of aspartic-acid racemization kinetics. Philos Trans R Soc Lond B 1999;354:51–64.

69. Nielsen-Marsh C, Gernaey A, Turner-Walker G, Hedges R, Pike A, Collins M. The chemical degradation of bone. In M Cox and S Mays eds. *Human Osteology in Archaeology and Forensic Science*. London: Greenwich Medical Media, pp. 439–454. 2000.

70. Gennard DE. *Forensic Entomology: An Introduction*. Chichester: Wiley. 2007.

71. Rodriguez WC, Bass WM. Insect activity and its relationship to decay rates of human cadavers in East Tennessee. J Forensic Sci 1983;28:423–432.

72. Smith KGV. *A Manual of Forensic Entomology*. Ithaca: Cornell University Press. 1987.

73. Reeve J, Adams M, eds. *The Spitalfields Project: Across the Styx, Volume 1 – The Archaeology*. York: Council for British Archaeology. 1993.

74. Haglund WD. Dogs and coyotes: postmortem involvement with human remains. In WD Haglund and MH Sorg eds. *Forensic Taphonomy: The Postmortem Fate of Human Remains*. Boca Raton: CRC Press, pp. 367–381. 1997.

75. Haglund WD. Rodents and human remains. In WD Haglund and MH Sorg eds. *Forensic Taphonomy: The Postmortem Fate of Human Remains*. Boca Raton: CRC Press, pp. 405–414. 1997.

76. Wilson AS, Janaway RC, Holland AD, Dodson HI, Baran E, Pollard AM, Tobin DJ. Modelling the buried human body environment in upland climes using three contrasting field sites. Forensic Sci Int 2007;169:6–18.

77. Wells C. Pseudopathology. In DR Brothwell and A Sandison eds. *Diseases in Antiquity*. Springfield, IL: Charles C. Thomas, pp. 5–19. 1967.
78. Wedl C. Ueber einen Zahnbein und Knochen keinenden. Pilz Sber Akad Wiss Wein 1864;50:171–193.
79. Hackett CJ. Microscopical focal destruction (tunnels) in excavated human bone. Med Sci Law 1981;21:243–265.
80. Hillson S. *Teeth*. Cambridge: Cambridge University Press. 1986.
81. Jans MME, Nielsen-Marsh CM, Smith CI, Collins MJ, Kars H. Characterisation of microbial attack on archaeological bone. J Archaeol Sci 2004;31:87–95.
82. Sagara N, Yamanaka T, Tibbett M. Soil fungi associated with graves and latrines: toward a forensic mycology. In M Tibbett and DO Carter eds. *Soil Analysis in Forensic Taphonomy: Chemical and Biological Effects of Buried Human Remains*. Boca Raton: CRC Press, Taylor & Francis, pp. 67–107. 2008.
83. Morse D, Duncan J, Stoutamire J. *Handbook of Forensic Archaeology and Anthropology*. Tallahassee, FL: Bill's Book Store. 1983.
84. Warren CP. Plants as decomposition vectors of skeletal human remains. Proc Indiana Acad Sci 1976;85:65.
85. Mant AK. Knowledge acquired from post-war exhumations. In A Boddington, AN Garland and RC Janaway eds. *Death, Decay and Reconstruction: Approaches to Archaeology and Forensic Science*. Manchester: Manchester University Press, pp. 65–78. 1987.
86. Mant AK. *A Study in Exhumation – Data*. MD, University of London, London. 1950.
87. Mant AK. Recent work on post-mortem changes and timing death. In K Simpson ed. *Modern Trends in Forensic Medicine*. London: Butterworths, pp. 147–162. 1953.
88. Payne JA. A summer carrion study of the baby pig Sus scrofa Linnaeus. Ecology 1965;46:592–602.
89. Payne JA, King EW. Insect succession and decomposition of pig carcasses in water. J Georgia Entomol Soc 1972;7:153–162.
90. Payne JA, King EW, Beinhart G. Arthropod succession and decomposition of buried pigs. Nature 1968;219:1180–1181.
91. Bass WM. Outdoor decomposition rates in Tennessee. In WD Haglund and MH Sorg eds. *Forensic Taphonomy: The Postmortem Fate of Human Remains*. London: CRC Press, pp. 181–186. 1997.
92. Turner RL. Important factors in soil burial test applied to rotproofed textiles. In AJ Walters and H-v-d Plas eds. *The Biodeterioration of Materials*. Essex, A.H. Walters, H-vd Plas, H. Eleonora. Barking: Applied Science Publishers, pp. 218–226. 1972.
93. Hopkins DW, Wiltshire PEJ, Turner BD. Microbial characteristics of soils from graves: an investigation at the interface of soil microbiology and forensic science. Appl Soil Ecol 2000;14:283–288.
94. Schoenen D. Decomposition from the public health viewpoint with special reference to interference with natural biological disintegration processes in burial underground. Schriftenr Ver Wasser Boden Lufthyg 2003;65:1–74.
95. Carter DO, Yellowlees D, Tibbett M. Cadaver decomposition in terrestrial ecosystems. Naturwissenschaften 2007;94:12–24.
96. Turner B, Wiltshire P. Experimental validation of forensic evidence: a study of the decomposition of buried pigs in a heavy clay soil. Forensic Sci Int 1999;101:113–122.
97. Turner RC. Discovery and excavation of the Lindow bodies. In IM Stead, JB Bourke and DR Brothwell eds. *Lindow Man: The Body in the Bog*. London: British Museum Press, pp. 10–13. 1986.
98. Prokop O. *Forensische Medizin*. Berlin: Volk und Gesundheit. 1966.
99. Schoenen D. Wachsleichenbildung: ein mikrobielles Problem. Wasser Boden 2002;54:12–15.
100. Berg S, Mueller B, Schleyer F. Leichenveränderungen, Todeszeitbestimmung im frühpostmortalen Intervall: Leichenzersetzung und -zerstörung. In B Mueller ed. *Gerichtliche Medizin*. Berlin: Springer, pp. 45–106. 1975.
101. Vass AA, Barshick SA, Sega G, Caton J, Skeen JT, Love JC, Synstelien JA. Decomposition chemistry of human remains: a new methodology for determining the postmortem interval. J Forensic Sci 2002;47:542–553.

Index

A

A. actinomycetumcomitans, 132
Aciduric microorganisms, 136, 145
Acinetobacter spp., 316
Actinobacillus actinomycetemcomitans, 132
Actinomyces naeslundii, 133
Actinomyces spp., 132, 133
Activation-induced cytidine deaminase
    (AID), 206
Acute bacterial diarrhoeal infections, 281.
    See also Bacterial diarrhoea
Acute gastroenteritis, in children, 280–281
Adaptive intestinal immunity, 195
    antimicrobial actions of IgA, 195–197
    GALT
        and associated lymphoid tissue, 208–210
        effects of aging, 201
        intestinal B lymphocytes, 199–201
        intestinal epithelium, aging of, 201–207
        enterocytes, 201–202
        GALT B cells and GC, 204–207
        intraepithelial lymphocytes, 203–204
        toll-like receptor, 202–203
    intraepithelial lymphocytes, 197–199
ADD. *See* Attention deficit disorder
Adenosine triphosphate (ATP), 314
ADHD. *See* Attention deficit hyperactivity
    disorder
Adults and children, probiotics role in, 278.
    See also Probiotics
Ageing
    biology, 1
    disease and infection
        chronic conditions, 7
        death causes, 7–8

inflammation, 9
    sensitivity, 9
human development, 9–10
mechanistic theories
    damage-based theories, 3–4
    DNA-damage theory, 5–6
    energy consumption hypothesis, 4
    free radical theory, 4–5
    genetic principles, 2
    programmed theories, 2–3
microorganisms, 6
Age-related changes in human salivary flow
    rates, 137
Age-related comorbid conditions, 96
Age-related differences in salivary IgA
    subclasses, 143
Age-related effects on oral microflora, 140
Alveolar macrophage (AM), 102
Alveolar-to-arterial gradient for oxygen, 95
Alzheimer disease, 97
Amantadine, 117
Anaphylactic hypersensitivity, 117
Anthrenus spp., 330
Antibiotic-associated *C. difficile*
    colitis, 236
Antibiotic-associated *C. difficile*
    pseudomembranous colitis, 236
Antibiotic-associated CPEnt colitis, 249
Antibiotic-associated CPEnt diarrhoea, 249
Antibiotic-associated diarrhoea (AAD),
    224–225
    aetiology of infectious, 225–226
    Candida spp., 228
    cytotoxin-producing *Klebsiella oxytoca* in
        gut, 228

Fatty acid metabolism, in autism, 301–302.
    See also Autism, in children
FCA. *See* Freund's complete adjuvant
Ferulic acid, 72–73
Feverfew, 72, 73
Firmicutes, 156, 157
Flu hemagglutinin, 116
Flu vaccines, 118
Follicular dendritic cells, 100
Free radical theory, 4–5
Freund's complete adjuvant, 300
Fructooligosaccharides (FOS), 167
Fulminant *C. difficile* colitis, 236–237
Fusobacterium nucleatum, 133
Fusobacterium spp., 132

G

GABA. *See* Gamma-aminobutyric acid
β-Galactosidase, 278, 279
GALT. *See* Gut associated lymphoreticular
    tissue
GALT B cells, 204–207
Gamma-aminobutyric acid, 300
Gastric carcinogenesis, 264
Gastric malignancies, risk factor of, 279
Gastrointestinal disorders and *Helicobacter
    pylori,* 263
Gastrointestinal (GI), 275, 292
    immunity, 175
Gastrointestinal tract (GIT), changes in, 275.
    See also Autism, in children
    microbiological link, 296–297
    peptide component and autistic
        enterocolitis, 296
    sulphation deficit, 295
GBS. *See* Guillain–Barré syndrome
Genetic predisposition, in autism, 293.
    See also Autism, in children
Gingival crevicular fluid (GCF), 141
Gliadin protein, 295
Glucocorticoids, 98
Glucose adducts, 96
Glucose intolerance, 96
Glucosyltransferase (GTF), 143
Gluten protein, 295
Glycoprotein antigens, 114

Gram-negative bacteria
    children and adults, 17
    infant's gut, 24
    mouth, 21
    respiratory tract, 28
    skin, 18
    UTI (including vagina), 30
Gram-negative rods, 103, 106
Gram-positive bacteria
    mouth, 21
    skin, 18
    small intestine, 23
    UTI (including vagina), 29
Green tea, 73
Guillain–Barré syndrome, 298, 299
Gut-associated lymphoid tissue (GALT), 176
Gut associated lymphoreticular tissue, 296
    aging, 210–213
    effects of aging on, 201
Gut microbiota, activities of, 154
    immune system, 159–160
    metabolic activities, 157–159
    nutrition, 154–157
Gut physiology, 276–277

H

Haemophilus influenzae, 299, 301
Helicobacter pylori, 263–264, 277, 278, 296
    age and acquisition of, 268
    infection, 279–280
    medical significance of, 264–265
    pathogenicity of, 265–266
    prevalance of, 264
    transmission and epidemiology of,
        266–268
    transmission routes of, 263
Helicobacter pylori-related cancer,
    co-factors in, 264
Hemophilus influenzae, 103, 116, 180
Hepatic encephalopathy (HE), 301
Herpes virus, 298
Herpes zoster, 50
5-HIAA. *See* 5-Hydroxyindoleacetic acid
Highly unsaturated fatty acids, 301
H5N1 virus, 114
Homovanillic acid, 294